INTERNATIONAL SERIES IN
EXPERIMENTAL PSYCHOLOGY
General Editor: H. J. EYSENCK

VOLUME 26

Response Variability to Psychotropic Drugs

OTHER TITLES IN THE SERIES IN EXPERIMENTAL PSYCHOLOGY

NOTICE TO READERS

Dear Reader

If your library is not already a standing order customer or subscriber to this series, may we recommend that you place a standing or subscription order to receive immediately upon publication all new issues and volumes published in this valuable series. Should you find that these volumes no longer serve your needs your order can be cancelled at any time without notice.

The Editors and the Publisher will be glad to receive suggestions or outlines of suitable titles, reviews or symposia for consideration for rapid publication in this series.

ROBERT MAXWELL
Publisher at Pergamon Press

Response Variability to Psychotropic Drugs

Edited by

W. JANKE

University of Wurzburg, Federal Republic of Germany

PERGAMON PRESS

OXFORD · NEW YORK · TORONTO · SYDNEY · PARIS · FRANKFURT

U.K.	Pergamon Press Ltd., Headington Hill Hall, Oxford OX3 0BW, England
U.S.A.	Pergamon Press Inc., Maxwell House, Fairview Park, Elmsford, New York 10523, U.S.A.
CANADA	Pergamon Press Canada Ltd., Suite 104, 150 Consumers Road, Willowdale, Ontario M2J 1P9, Canada
AUSTRALIA	Pergamon Press (Aust.) Pty. Ltd., P.O. Box 544, Potts Point, N.S.W. 2011, Australia
FRANCE	Pergamon Press SARL, 24 rue des Ecoles, 75240 Paris, Cedex 05, France
FEDERAL REPUBLIC OF GERMANY	Pergamon Press GmbH, Hammerweg 6, D-6242 Kronberg-Taunus, Federal Republic of Germany

First edition 1983

Library of Congress Cataloging in Publication Data

Main entry under title:
Response variability to psychotropic drugs.
(International series in experimental psychology;
v. 26)
"Based on papers delivered at a symposium on response variability to psychotropic drugs at the 22nd World Congress of Psychology in Leipzig in 1980"—Pref.
1. Psychopharmacology—Congresses. 2. Chemotherapy—Psychological aspects—Congresses. I. Janke, W.
II. World Congresses of Psychology (22nd: 1980: Leipzig, Germany) III. Series. [DNLM: 1. Behaviour-Drug effects—Congresses. 2. Psychopharmacology—Congresses. 3. Psychotropic drugs—Pharmacodynamics—Congresses. W1 IN835JE v. 26 / QV 77 R434 1980]
RM315.R46   1983   615'.788   82-24644

British Library Cataloguing in Publication Data

Response variability to psychotropic drugs.—(International series in experimental psychology; v. 26)
1. Psychopharmacology—Congresses
I. Janke, W. II. Series
615'.78   RM315
ISBN 0-08-028907-X

In order to make this volume available as economically and as rapidly as possible the authors' typescripts have been reproduced in their original forms. This method unfortunately has its typographical limitations but it is hoped that they in no way distract the reader.

Printed in Great Britain by A. Wheaton & Co. Ltd., Exeter

PREFACE

This book is based on papers delivered at a symposium on response variability to psychotropic drugs at the 22nd World Congress of Psychology in Leipzig in 1980.

The description and explanation of drug response variability according to psychological factors is highly interesting and important for both *theoretical* and *practical* reasons.

The *theoretical* importance of drug response variability applies both to *pharmacology* and to *psychology*. Within the context of *pharmacology*, the theoretical importance relates mainly to the problem of finding out which sources are primarily responsible for behavioral drug response variability and how they interact. These sources refer to factors ranging from drug resorption and tissue distribution, to drug metabolism, elimination, and the specific drug effects at CNS receptor sites. At each step of the long path through the organism drug response differences can be observed and their contribution to the final observed behavioral response examined.

In *psychology*, drug response variability is particularly important for personality theory. Each drug response variability study contributes to our understanding of the biological foundations of individual differences.

The *practical* importance of the large intersubject and intrasubject behavioral drug response differences relates in particular to pharmacotherapy. The practical consequences of the huge drug response variability are highly dramatic considering that up to now, in spite of a tremendous number of research projects, it was not possible to isolate a set of parameters (e.g. plasma drug level, neurophysiological, or behavioral) by which individual responses to drug treatment might be predicted to any remarkable extent. Therefore, at the present time, any pharmacotherapy is more or less based on trial and error. This book shows that much work has to be done before we are able to devise predictor batteries which might be helpful in a practical sense.

The papers collected in this book give an overview of the research of a number of investigators who have been busy in research on differential psychopharmacology for many years. The emphasis is on research carried out on healthy subjects. Drug response variability in sick patients has been discussed only in one chapter by Wittenborn. This paper, however, shows some of the central problems of *differential pharmacotherapy*. Moreover, many of the basic problems involved in drug response variability are the same or at least similar in sick and healthy subjects.

I am grateful to those people who assisted me in editing this work: Firstly, I would like to thank Miss Bärbel Löll who organized the collection of the manu-scripts, who drew many of the figures, and who typed most of the papers. Many suggestions with regard to the organisation of the symposium and the book were made by Professor Gisela Erdmann (Berlin) and Professor Petra Netter (Giessen). Last but not least I would like to thank Professor K. J. Netter and Professor Petra Netter who accepted my invitation to write a chapter on pharmacokinetic factors, a topic which was not discussed extensively at the Leipzig symposium. This chapter is especially important, because drug response variability with respect to behavior can be understood only if one takes some fundamental pharmacological factors into consideration.

Würzburg   WILHELM JANKE

CONTENTS

Contents

LIST OF CONTRIBUTORS

Boucsein, W.
Department of Psychology, University of Duisburg
Federal Republic of Germany

Claridge, G.
Magdalen College, Oxford
Great Britain

Debus, G.
Department of Psychology, Technical University of Aachen
Federal Republic of Germany

Erdmann, G.
Department of Psychology, University of Düsseldorf
Federal Republic of Germany

Eysenck, H. J.
Institute of Psychiatry, Department of Psychology
University of London
Great Britain

Heinze, U.
Section to Psychology, Karl-Marx-University, Leipzig
German Democratic Republic

Janke, W.
Department of Psychology, University of Würzburg
Federal Republic of Germany

Krüger, H.-P.
Department of Psychology, University of Erlangen-Nurnberg
Federal Republic of Germany

Netter, K. J.
Department of Pharmacology, University of Marburg
Federal Republic of Germany

Netter, P.
Department of Psychology, University of Giessen
Federal Republic of Germany

Russell, R. W.
Department of Pharmacology and School of Medicine,
University of California, Los Angeles, USA

Strauß, E.-H.
Section to Psychology, Humboldt University, Berlin
German Democratic Republic

Warburton, D. M.
Department of Psychology, University of Reading
Great Britain

Wittenborn, J. R.
Interdisciplinary Research Center, Rutgers University,
New Brunswick, New Jersey, USA

Part I

**DRUG RESPONSE VARIABILITY:
PHARMACOLOGICAL FOUNDATIONS**

PHARMACOKINETIC FACTORS: SOME BASIC PRINCIPLES AND THEIR INFLUENCE ON PSYCHOTROPIC DRUG RESPONSE

K. J. Netter and Petra Netter

ABSTRACT

General principles of pharmacokinetics are outlined in order to illustrate the manner in which various somatic and behavioral factors can affect drug action. The phenomena and mechanisms of absorption, distribution, metabolism, and elimination of psychotropic drugs are described. In addition to differences in drug absorption due to sex, age, and body weight, interindividual differences in rates of absorption are reported for subjects scoring high and low on neuroticism, respectively. Furthermore, sex and age are discussed as resulting in differences in plasma levels, metabolism, and plasma half lives of drugs, as can be seen from studies applying multiple correlation or analysis of variance. Population and twin studies reveal genetic factors to be important for drug metabolism and elimination. In addition, behavioral variables like smoking, intake of alcohol and other drugs can be shown to enhance metabolism of drugs causing interindividual differences in response. A few examples of studies on the relationships between plasma levels of drugs and behavior or clinical response illustrate the methodological problems in establishing predictability of response from kinetic parameters.

KEYWORDS

Absorption; age; differential drug response and somatic factors; drug metabolism; interindividual differences; pharmacogenetics; pharmacokinetic factors; plasma half lives; plasma levels; sex.

INTRODUCTION

Variability in drug response is not only determined by interindividual differences in the pharmacodynamic aspects of a drug, such as differences in tissue sensitivity and intrinsic activity of the drug at the receptor site, but also to a great extent by differences in various aspects of pharmacokinetics. In order to understand how certain psychological, somatic, and environmental factors can influence the availability and metabolism of drugs, some general principles of pharmacokinetics shall be described.

3

1. PRINCIPLES OF PHARMACOKINETICS

In order to achieve their biological effects, drugs have to be present at the site of their action. This implies that drugs must be distributed throughout the body and reach the respective sites of action in concentrations that are pharmacodynamically effective. After oral medication, therefore, a drug has to be absorbed in the intestinal tract to reach the circulation, and finally pass through biological membranes in order to exert effects that are mediated within the cell. It is obvious that these processes require a certain amount of time. Therefore, all considerations about the character and onset of pharmacodynamic actions have to take the time factor into account. This applies to the beginning of the desired action as well as to its end. In pharmacotherapy, in most cases, the termination of the pharmacological action is equally as important as its beginning. Presently, no drug is known whose action will persist longer than the drug itself is present in sufficient quantity at its site of biological action. Colloquially speaking, it is safe to say that there is no such thing as a "hit and run" drug, with the exception perhaps of reactive metabolites that affect genetic material.

This situation requires the conscientious pharmacotherapist to consider the time dependent changes in concentration of a given drug at its site of action. This requires the study of the movement of drugs throughout the different areas of the mammalian organism (pharmacokinetics). The only "organ" that lends itself to the quantitative analysis of drug concentrations is blood which can be obtained by venipuncture. Therefore, most pharmacokinetic experimentation and considerations center around drug concentrations in blood plasma. Although drug action itself very rarely occurs in the blood, the determination of plasma levels has nevertheless proven to be a valuable tool in assessing the pharmacokinetic properties of a given drug, since there is a sufficient correlation between plasma level and pharmacodynamic action.

The general principles of pharmacokinetics are extensively described in respective text books such as those of Gilman, Goodman and Gilman (1980), Forth, Henschler and Rummel (1980), Melmon and Morrelli (1978), Goldstein, Aronow and Kalman (1974), and Gibaldi and Perrier (1975) as well as Atkinson and Kushner (1979). The first account of the evolving new field was that of Dost (1968).

In this brief survey the main pharmacokinetic parameters shall be introduced. They will be: absorption, distribution, and metabolism. Excretion via the kidney and the bile, the fourth step, will not be discussed in detail.

1.1 Absorption of Drugs

The rate and intensity of the gastro-intestinal absorption determines the effective strength of a pharmacodynamic action of a given drug. Therefore, it is of importance to consider that many variables influence the penetration of drugs through the gastro-intestinal wall.

1.1.1 Membrane transport. Since drugs have to traverse either a cellular membrane or layers of cells, one must consider the structure

of the membrane as lipid bilayers, which in the mammal have a complicated structure. Besides a double layer of hydrophobic fatty acids
the membranes contain transport proteins which contain specific mechanisms for transport of nutrients such as glucose, electrolytes and
other special substrates. Since drugs normally do not fit to the receptors for specialized transport mechanisms, drugs cross membranes
by passive diffusion along a concentration gradient. This happens either by using aqueous channels in the membrane or by dissolving in
the membrane. Such transfer is directly proportional to the concentration gradient across the membrane.

Furthermore, the lipid solubility of the drug in question is of importance, since only the lipid soluble portion of a drug may traverse a
membrane. Since most drugs are either weak acids or weak bases, the
ambient pH determines the amount of undissociated drug which penetrates
the cell membrane. In the case of a weak acid a decrease in pH (acidifi-
cation) would increase the amount of undissociated acid and, therefore,
increase its membrane passage. The opposite is true with bases. Thus,
also the pH determines the gastro-intestinal absorption of a drug.

1.1.2 Water solubility and rate of dissolution. Furthermore, solubility of a substance in aqueous solutions determines the amount of drug
that can be brought into contact with the absorbing surface. Therefore,
water solubility is an important factor, which overrides quantitatively
the subtle physico-chemical interrelations that take place at the membrane.
The rate of dissolution is of importance for the assessment of absorp-
tive potency for drugs that are given as tablets. This implies that
the galenic preparation of tablets, which determines the rate of their
dissolution, is of importance. In combination with the passage time
through the gut the dissolution rate determines the bioavailability
of a given drug. This has become especially important in the absorption
of digoxin, which is not easily absorbed and requires the full length
of gastro-intestinal passage time. Absorption is furthermore decisive-
ly determined by the degree of micronisation of the substance within
the tablet.

1.1.3 Gastric emptying and bioavailability. Another example, which
illustrates the influence of physiological function on drug absorption
is the gastric emptying. If, for instance, the opioid pethidine is injected, it will greatly delay gastric emptying and thereby also delay
the absorption of, for instance, indomethacin that has been given
orally. On the other hand, it becomes understandable from the above
considerations about the influence of pH on membrane passage that a
weak base like morphine after passage of the gastric wall in the reversed direction from the blood stream into the acid interior of the
stomach cannot return into the circulation, because in the acid milieu
of the gastric juice it will be dissociated and thus unable to penetrate the gastric wall again.

The factors discussed so far determine the amount of drug available to
the organism and thus the therapeutic value of a given drug preparation. They are comprised in the term bioavailability. This term denotes
the amount of drug that is actually available for gastro-intestinal absorption and consequently reaches the organism. The bioavailability,
according to the above mentioned principles, may be subject to`varia-

tion with the galenic preparation of the respective drug. In order to obtain a semiquantitative assessment of the proportion of a drug actually reaching the body, its bioavailability is measured. This can be done by following the plasma level curve from oral application to total elimination of the drug from the blood and determining the area under the curve. This area under the curve (AUC) represents a measure of the amount of drug absorbed. It can be compared with the area under the curve after intravenous injection of the same drug.
Bioavailability becomes an important determinant of drug quality when generic drugs are marketed after galenic preparation by manufacturers other than the original holder of the properietary name. Even in the hands of one manufacturer bioavailability may vary between different lots.

1.2   Distribution of Drugs and Blood Levels

1.2.1   Mode of application as a determinant of blood levels of drugs.
Oral ingestion of drugs represents the most convenient and economical and also the safest way of applying drugs. However, it must be considered that absorption might be variable on account of the factors outlined above. It, furthermore, requires the cooperation of the patient to maintain a stable drug therapeutic regimen.

The other major route of applying drugs is the parenteral injection which eliminates the factors associated with gastro-intestinal absorption. Especially with intravenous injection the therapist achieves accuracy of dosage and also an immediate action. From a pharmacokinetic standpoint this type of application eliminates any lag phase associated with gastro-intestinal absorption. Therefore, the blood level of an intravenously applied drug will immediately be very high before it rapidly declines in the phase of redistribution of the drug in the various compartments of the body. This rapid decline is usually followed by a slower decline which is determined by the elimination of the drug. Thus, intravenous application is valuable for emergency use, allows for a "titration" of a drug according to its effects, but is also the most dangerous way. Subcutaneous and intramuscular application take an intermediate position between either oral or intravenous application.

1.2.2   Compartments of drug distribution.   After a drug has reached the circulation it can penetrate into different compartments of the body. This is depicted in Fig. 1.

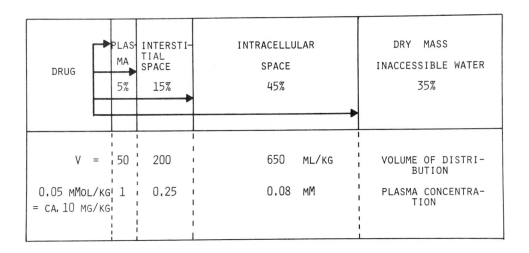

Fig. 1.   Volumes of distribution and plasma concentrations
          of a given drug (figured to be applied in a dose of
          0.05 mmol per kg) in different compartments of the
          body which cover the percentages of the total orga-
          nism given below their names. (Elimination processes
          are disregarded in this representation.)

The theoretical experiment serves to explain the two parameters:
volume of distribution and plasma concentration. In the upper half of
the figure the penetration of a drug into the various spaces is shown
along with the percentage volume these spaces occupy. It becomes clear
that when 0.05 mmol of a drug is given per kg, provided that it does
not leave the circulatory system, it distributes only over 5 % of the
body mass. Accordingly, its concentration will be rather high. The more
a drug also occupies other spaces the lower its concentration in the
plasma will become. Conversely, the volume of distribution provides
quantitative information on the space that a drug occupies per kg of
body mass. It is understood that the picture symbolizes the final
state of a distribution process disregarding simultaneous elimination.
After injection or oral ingestion the equilibrium will not be reached
immediately but rather after a period of redistribution into the various spaces.
The distribution of drugs into various compartments of the body is
depicted in Fig. 2.

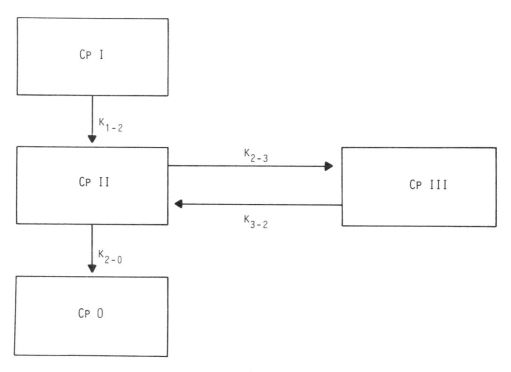

Fig. 2.   Basic pharmacokinetic model of the compartments
          influencing the distribution of a drug after intra-
          muscular injection (from Gladtke and v. Hattingberg,
          1973).
          Cp = compartment, explanation see text.

This is a graphical representation of the fact that drugs move through
various parts of the organism with varying velocity. The compartments
shown in the figure are not synonymous with any specific anatomical
entities. They represent spaces in which the drug or its metabolites
can be found at a certain concentration at a given time. The invasion
of a drug into compartment II (Cp II), for instance, is given by an
invasion constant (K_{1-2}) which determines the velocity of this transition. The main advantage of thinking in models of this kind is to
allow the mathematical expression of pharmacokinetic behavior of drugs.
In the end a drug or its metabolites will always reach the compartment
CpO which represents the elimination of the drug either by urine or
other means. The distribution of a drug can thus be described by the
various constants given in the figure. In this model by Gladtke and
v. Hattingberg (1973), Cp. I represents the entry compartment after
intramuscular injection, Cp. II the compartment of the vascular space,
Cp. III the extracircular space and as mentioned above, Cp. O the exit
compartment. The constant K_{2-0} is the elimination constant, while K_{2-3}
and K_{3-2} are the transition constants into other compartments. If K_{2-3}
and K_{3-2} are relatively large in comparison to K_{2-0}, then there is a
rapid equilibrium between Cp. II and Cp. III, and the pharmacokinetic
behavior of this drug is largely determined by K_{1-2} and K_{2-0}. If these
constants, however, are smaller than K_{2-0}, the pharmacokinetic behavior might be more complicated and especially characterized by the in-

volvement of so-called deep compartments. Such deep compartments exchange very slowly with the other compartments and, therefore, also
have the function of depot formation. Examples of such deep compartments are the bone matrix, which, for instance, accumulates lead, or
fatty tissues that accumulate highly lipid soluble compounds such as
DDT.

In a sense plasma and cellular proteins constitute another - silent -
compartment for drug distribution. They are able to bind drugs to a
very widely varying extent to non-specific binding sites and to reduce the amount of free drug in the respective body fluids. The only
pharmacodynamically active part of the drug is the free fraction which
in most cases covers merely about 5 - 20 % of the total drug. Since
there is rapid exchange between bound and unbound form the protein-
bound fraction is able to maintain a certain concentration of free
drug for a comparatively long time and thereby exerts a depot effect.
The non-specific binding occurs by either ionic or hydrophobic interaction. As a consequence of the fact that the amount of binding sites
is limited the relative proportion of bound drug decreases with increasing drug concentrations. In addition to plasma albumin, hemo-
globin and muscle proteins also bind drugs to a considerable extent,
whereby hydrophobic interaction is of predominant importance.

1.2.3   The Bateman-Curve.   Measurement of the time-dependent plasma
concentrations of a drug yields blood level curves of the type shown
in Fig. 3.

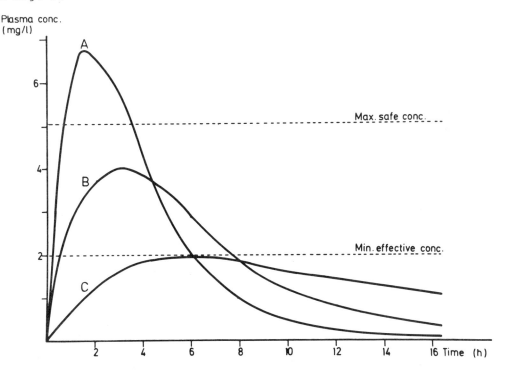

Fig. 3.   Time dependent change in plasma concentration
          (= Bateman-Curves) of three different drug-dosages.
          A = suprathreshold (potentially toxic) dosage;
          B = therapeutic dosage; C = subthreshold dosage
                                  (therapeutically ineffective)

This so-called Bateman-Equation results from the invasion and elimination reactions of a given drug. It thus represents a composite curve
which, however, is accessible to mathematical treatment. It is very
often used to describe the behavior of a drug provided that the analytical methodology is available that allows determination of concentrations in small volumes of plasma. Since the advent of the combination of gaschromatography and mass spectrometry (GC/MS) and other similarly sensitive and selective analytical methods, this is possible
for almost every chemical compound. Measurement of the Bateman-Curve
provides the possibility of predicting the pharmacodynamic effect of
a drug and of correlating it with the drug effect in a different compartment.

Figure 3 gives theoretical curves, the first of which represents
a suprathreshold dose which might even reach the toxic range of a
given compound, while curve B reaches and transgresses the therapeutic
limit of the plasma level in contrast to curve C which represents the
plasma level of a drug which never reaches therapeutic concentrations.

1.2.4 Elimination kinetics. The elimination half life of a drug is
of great importance in order to judge the time period of its clinical
efficacy. In principle, elimination mechanisms fall into two different
categories. In the first category the rate of elimination is independent of the concentration of the drug at the elimination site. The result is a zero order elimination kinetic in which equal amounts of
drugs are eliminated per time unit. Graphically this would be represented by a straight line with a downward slope in a concentration
versus time curve. An example for this type of elimination is the elimination of ethyl alcohol. This elimination behavior is the reason
for the relatively safe retrospective determination of the alcohol
blood level for forensic purposes.

The second category of elimination kinetics is described by the basic
fact that elimination is increased when the concentrations of the
drug or its metabolites are higher and decreased when they are lower.
This type of elimination is represented in Fig. 3, since the downward
slopes of the curves are not linear with time. The most common lineari-
sation procedure used is to apply a logarithmic ordinate scale. In
this so-called first order elimination kinetic a straight line would
result for the semi-logarithmic concentration versus time plot. First
order elimination kinetics are the common type of elimination for almost all drugs, because the concentrations at the eliminating sites
(enzymes, renal transport systems etc.) rarely reach the saturation
concentration so that with higher concentration at the elimination
site the elimination process will be more rapid.

1.2.5 Biological half life. To render these considerations more
practicable, the biological half life of a drug has become an important
constant that allows comparative clinical evaluation. For zero order
elimination, it is easily understandable that the blood level after
a certain time is reduced from 100 to 50%. Also for first order elimination, a half life can be determined from the semi-logarithmic plot
provided that the experimental values yield a straight line. Here at
any given time, the time period can be read from the graph during
which the blood level falls from a given value to half this value.

In practice, biological half lives of drugs in man can vary greatly. Thus, benzylpenicilline shows a half life at 30 min while diazepam requires about 10 hours and some of its metabolites even longer. Table 1 provides half lives of some psychotropic compounds.

TABLE 1   Half Lives of Some Psychoactive Compounds
          (extracted   from Kurz and others, 1980,p.56)

Substance	Hours
Propranolol	3.2
Imipramine	3.5
Reserpine	4.5
Diazepam	2 - 10
Oxazepam	6 - 25
Meprobamate	8
Chlordiazepoxide	18 - 24
Lithiumcarbonate	24 - 48
Phenobarbital	37 - 96
Protriptyline	54 -198

Figure 4 shows the situation for tritium labelled reserpine, where the semilogarithmic plot reveals that the total elimination depends on a rapid process with a half life of 4.5 hrs and a markedly slower process with a half life of 271 hrs. This demonstrates that obviously there are two processes involved in the elimination of reserpine. Conversely, transformation of the elimination curves into straight lines provides additional information on the existence of possibly more than one elimination process. Furthermore, this transformation, when applied after intravenous application, shows the extent and time required for redistribution of the drug into the various compartments. This is represented by a markedly steeper slope of the plasma concentration curve.

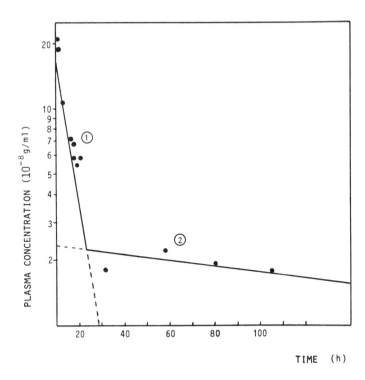

Fig. 4.   Evasion of tritium labelled reserpine in the human
          represented by a semi-logarithmic plot.
          1 = rapid elimination process ($t_{1/2}$ = 4.5 hrs)
          2 = slow elimination process ($t_{1/2}$ = 271 hrs)
          (from Maass and others, 1969)

1.2.6 The blood-brain-barrier. For the achievement of drug effects
in the central nervous system it is of utmost importance to know
whether or not a drug will permeate into the central nervous system
(CNS). With regard to this organ the situation is unique in that entry of drugs into the CNS is restricted. This restriction is similar
to that in the gastro-intestinal wall. The endothelial cells of the
brain capillaries are characterized by the absence of intracellular
pores and pinocytotic vesicles and a predomination of tight junctions.
Therefore, drugs have to traverse a greater barrier which is even enhanced by the structure of the surrounding glial cells that contributes to the slow diffusion of weak organic acids and bases into the
CNS. Strongly ionized substances such as quaternary amines or the various penicillines will normally not reach the CNS. This may represent a specific protective mechanism. Also, charged molecules like
those of neurotransmitters (e.g. dopamine) cannot overcome the blood-
brain-barrier. Therefore, in order to reach sufficient concentrations
of dopamine the precursor dopa (dihydroxyphenylalanine) is given in
rather large doses, since the blood-brain-barrier can be overcome by
the use of a specific amino acid transport system, which also trans-
ports dopa.

1.3 Metabolism of Drugs

A major way of elimination of foreign compounds is their metabolic
conversion. This reaction serves the purpose of rendering the parent
compound more easily excretable and at the same time less toxic. The
major metabolic pathways are given in Table 2 (see next page).

1.3.1 Oxidation.

Among these pathways the oxidative metabolism is
the most wide-spread and important. In this reaction oxygen from the
molecular oxygen of the air is incorporated into the drug molecule.
The complicated biochemical sequence of reactions is characterized by
the principle that one atom of the molecular oxygen is finally reduced
to water, thereby yielding the energy to activate the other oxygen
atom for incorporation into the foreign compound. Because the enzyme
catalysing this pathway performs a bifunctional catalysis it is termed
mixed function oxidase. The enzyme has been characterized as a hemoprotein occurring in greatest amounts in the parenchymal cells of the
liver. As a hemoprotein it readily combines with carbon monoxide and
exhibits a characteristic absorption band at 450 nm when reduced.
Hence, it has been named cytochrome P 450. Its intracellular location
is in the smooth endoplasmic reticulum. The necessary cofactors for
its action are obviously oxygen and a reducing factor, namely NADPH.
The resulting metabolites comprise a wide range of chemically altered
parent compounds such as those listed in the table. The mixed function
oxygenase or monooxygenase shows a biologically very important property in that it can be induced by a wide range of enzyme inducers. This
implies that cytochrome P 450 increases in quantity during treatment
of the animal with known enzyme inducers such as phenobarbital or a
number of carcinogens. This phenomenon will have the clinical implication that the duration of action of a drug which is eliminated by oxidative metabolism will be shortened. Conversely, alternative substrates
may exert an inhibitory effect, thus prolonging the pharmacodynamic
action of an oxidizable drug. The specificity of cytochrome P 450 for
various substrates is very low. This explains that it can function as
a detoxification enzyme towards many chemically different foreign compounds. Cytochrome P 450 not only occurs in the liver but (although in
much smaller quantities) in almost every organ, so that drug biotransformation may also occur outside the liver in other parts of the
organism.

1.3.2 Hydrolysis.

A second pathway of drug metabolism is the hydro-
lysis of esters and amines to the respective breakdown products. This
reaction is catalysed by tissue hydrolases that occur in wide distribution. Prominent substrates for this type of drug inactivation are
local anaesthetics such as procaine or the analgesic phenacetin.

1.3.3 Conjugation.

Conjugation reactions are among those that have
long been known and have been extensively described. The most prominent example is the conjugation with glucuronic acid to form glucuro-
nides of either the ester type or the ether type. The necessary biochemical requirement for this is an activated glucuronic acid that is
synthesized through various biochemical steps yielding in the end a
uridine diphospho compound (UDPGA). Similarly, conjugation with sulfate is a frequently occurring inactivation pathway especially for
phenolic compounds. Here also an energy requiring synthesis of the

14 K. J. Netter and P. Netter

TABLE 2 Pathways of Drug Metabolism in Man Illustrated by Selected Psychoactive Drugs

Pathways and required enzymes	paradigmatic psychoactive drugs								
	CPZ	imi	mia	am	bdz	prop	metq	mor	others
I. Oxydation: (mixed function oxygenases = cytochrome P 450)									
1. hydroxylation a) aromatic	x	x	x	x	d	x			phenytoin
N-dealkylation		x							
O-dealkylation									mescaline
b) aliphatic							x		
N-dealkylation	x	x			d				
O-dealkylation									codeine
2. epoxidation							x		
3. oxidation of heteroatoms									
N-oxidation			x				x		
S-oxidation	x								phenothiazines
4. oxidative deamination				x			x	x	
II. Hydrolysis (hydrolases)									
1. hydrolysis of esters									heroin, proca- ine, atropin
2. hydrolysis of amides									xylocaine
III. Conjugations (respective trans- ferases)									
1. glucuronidation	x				o l			x	valproic acid metabolite
2. sulfatation								x	steroids
3. acetylation									izoniazide phenelzine
4. methylation									epinephrine norepinephrine
5. conjugation with glutathione									(paracetamol)
IV. Reduction (cytochrome P 450, cytochrome c-reductase)					n				

CPZ = chlorpromazine, imi = imipramine, mia = mianserin, am = amphetamine,
bdz = benzodiazepines, prop = propranolol, metq = methaqualone, mor = morphine,
d = diazepam, o = oxazepam, l = lorazepam, n = nitrazepam

activated sulfate is neccessary. The resulting phospho-adenosyl-phospho-sulfate (PAPS) is able to provide the energy-rich sulfate moiety for the transferases. Acetic acid and methyl groups are also transferable according to a very similar scheme. In both cases, metabolic activation of the transferable moiety is necessary. In the first case this is acetyl-coenzyme A and in the latter S-adenosylmethionine (SAM). The last conjugative reaction listed here is a conjugation with glutathione (GSH) which recently has attracted great interest, since it was discovered that glutathione reservoirs in the liver can be exhausted by the application of large doses of drugs, such as paracetamol (acetaminophen), that are conjugated by GSH. Besides acetaminophen, many other compounds react with GSH with the aid of a respective transferase. This initial conjugation often is followed by further modifying reactions involving the glutathione molecule which in the end lead to mercapturic acids, that are finally excreted in the urine.

1.3.4 Reduction. A last pathway, and one of minor importance is that of the reduction of a few azo compounds and nitro groups. This reaction occurs to a small extent when oxygen is excluded and cytochrome P 450 or cytochrome c-reductase are present and active. Thus, nitrazepam may yield reduced metabolites. On the whole, however, this pathway, which also occurs in gut bacteria, plays a minor role compared to the other metabolic pathways mentioned above.

2.   FACTORS CAUSING INTERINDIVIDUAL DIFFERENCES IN
     PHARMACOKINETICS

Besides the physico-chemical factors described to be responsible for changes in drug absorption, distribution, metabolism, and elimination, several physiological and personality variables are associated with alterations of pharmacokinetic processes.
These factors may be due to specific genetic patterns, they may be unspecifically linked to age, sex, race or body build, they may be secondary physiological changes due to interindividually different behavior (such as nutrition, physical exercise, or smoking) or they may be due to acquired diseases and related medications. This chapter cannot provide a thorough review of these factors but will only briefly outline some examples of interindividual differences in pharmacokinetic parameters due to some of the factors described above.

Most studies, of course, derive their information on kinetics in humans from determinations of blood levels of drugs. These, however, represent the simultaneously occurring processes of absorption, distribution, metabolism, and elimination, as outlined in the first part of this paper, without providing clear evidence as to which of these processes the observed differences in plasma levels are due. Therefore, the distinction between the paragraphs might appear arbitrary but have been chosen in order to group results, if possible, with respect to the most predominant process or the one most likely to be responsible for the effect. Those papers referring to just "plasma concentration" have been grouped under a separate heading.

2.1 Factors Affecting Different Kinetic Processes Simultaneously

Some factors may be responsible for several pharmacokinetic processes

simultaneously. The most important of these is nutrition. Besides the
short acting influence fasting and different constituents of food
exert on absorption rates (Wallusch and others, 1978) or on drug metabolizing enzymes (Basu and Dickerson, 1974; Campbell and Hayes,
1974), long lasting states of malnutrition will affect kinetics of
drugs in a manyfold way. Although in our society starvation will rarely be found as a consequence of food deficiency, some pathological
states of behavior that require psychopharmacological treatment may
be associated with selective or general malnutrition. Thus, it seems
worthwhile to be aware of the bodily changes it may cause, changes
which alter the disposition, metabolism and also the pharmacodynamic
aspects of drugs in the body, as summarized in a graph by Krishnaswamy
(1978) (see Fig. 5).

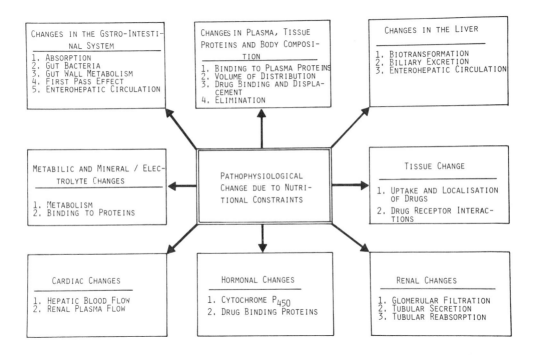

Fig. 5.   Changes in the pharmacokinetic and pharmacodynamic
          processes of drug action by malnutrition.
          (from Krishnaswamy, 1978)

2.2   Factors Affecting Absorption

2.2.1   Additional drug intake.   As outlined in section 1.1, pH and
gastric emptying determine the rate of absorption. Since antacids, as
for example a mixture of aluminium and magnesium hydroxides, could be
demonstrated to delay absorption of chlordiazepoxide in an experiment
by Greenblatt and others (1977a), subjects may vary in their response
to benzodiazepines according to whether they are treated for hyper-
acidity of the stomach. Since this is a fairly common complaint

especially in nervous and neurotic patients, subthreshold blood levels of tranquilizers may result from this type of treatment so that these subjects appear to be bad responders. Similarly, it has been reported that during attacks of migraine drug absorption may be delayed (Volans, 1978).

2.2.2 Personality traits. An example of differences in absorption according to personality is given in a paper by Nakano and others (1980) in which the absorption rate of diazepam was higher in neurotic than in non-neurotic subjects classified according to a questionnaire by Eysenck. The difference was no longer present after intraduodenal application of the drug suggesting higher rates of gastric emptying in neurotic subjects which was interpreted as a more sensitive response to the stress of the experimental situation.

Although there were only low and insignificant correlations between decrements in correct responses to a choice reaction time test and diazepam plasma levels in either group, the curves for the respective parameters showed an inverse relationship between 1.5 and 6 hrs after drug ingestion, as can be seen in Fig. 6.

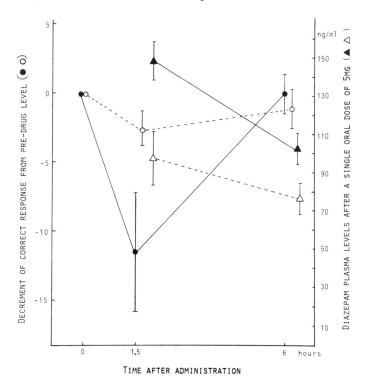

TIME AFTER ADMINISTRATION

Fig. 6. Change of correct responses in the Choice Reaction Time Test (left scale, circles) and diazepam plasma levels (right scale, triangles) 1.5 and 6 hors after oral ingestion of 5 mg of diazepam in 12 high (●▲) and 12 low neurotics (o △) subjects. Means ± SE. (mod. after Nakano and others, 1980)

Decrement in performance is greatest in the high neurotic group where
their diazepam level is at its maximum and becomes less with decreasing
plasma levels. The same is true for the low neurotic group, though less
pronounced.
A different absorption behavior was observed with respect to ethylal-
cohol in groups classified according to the same trait by Munkelt and
Lienert (1964). In this study subjects scoring high in neuroticism obtained lower blood levels of ethanol and reached their peaks evidently
also more slowly than non-neurotic subjects, as taken from differences
between two measurements at 30 and 90 minutes after ingestion of alcohol. This occurred in spite of dosing ethanol according to body weight
(850 mg/kg). In this experiment, performance deteriorated more in the
high neurotic subjects in spite of their lower blood levels. This was
taken as evidence that the unfavourable drink (brandy mixed into
grapefruit juice) may have caused pyloric contractions in the more
sensitive neurotics which may have resulted in a delayed absorption
of ethanol.

2.2.3 Somatic factors. Sex, age, and body weight may also be of importance for absorption. Thus, Greenblatt and others (1974) found much
greater variability in time to reach peak concentrations after oral
ingestion of 25 mg of chlordiazepoxide in females than in males and
suggested that this greater variability might be related to menstrual
cycle. In an elegant multiple regression analysis applied to three
different clinical groups receiving different oral dosages of chlordiazepoxide (CDX) (25 mg, 2 x 100 mg, 100 mg) for premedication purposes, the relative contributions of the factors age, sex, weight,
and time after medication as well as their mutual interactions were
computed with respect to CDX blood levels for each group separately
by Greenblatt and others (1977b). Low weight, older and - at least
in one group - male subjects achieved higher blood levels than heavier,
younger, and female ones. But simple correlations of the factors explained not more than maximally 15 % of the variance of CDX blood levels. In the largest group receiving the lowest dose of CDX, interaction effects age by weight, and in the two smaller, higher dosed groups
second order interactions age by sex by weight accounted for considerable proportions of variance of CDX blood levels. Further indirect
evidence for statistical interactions of factors can be taken from
the following observations: In group B, receiving 2 x 200 mg of the
substance, sex emerged as the factor contributing the most significant
part of variance to values of CDX blood levels (females obtaining much
higher levels than males), while in group A (25 mg) the sex effect
was reduced to zero. This may be taken as evidence that dose level
also interacts with sex of subjects, similarly as time after dose did
in group B. Part of this variation in blood levels, however, is due
to metabolic differences and will be discussed in section 2.4.

2.3 Factors Affecting Volumes of Distribution, Plasma Half Lives and
     Rates of Elimination

2.3.1 Age and sex. Several authors report prolonged half lives for
a variety of drugs in aged individuals. Thus, Kyriakopoulos (1976)
obtained a correlation of r = 0.62 between age and plasma half life
of lorazepam which very much resembles the value reported by Greenblatt and others (1978) from a study correlating age with chlordiazepoxide levels (r = 0.63) which could be confirmed by a study of their

own yielding also larger volumes of distribution and a reduced metabolic clearance in their group aged over 60 years as opposed to the
group below 30 years.

In a study by Greenblatt and others (1977) the volumes calculated for
the central compartment (V_1) and the total distribution space (V_d) of
50 mg of intravenously injected chlordiazepoxide - blood sampling being
performed for 72 hours - were found to be larger in females than in
males. But, as could be seen from the multiple regression analysis by
Greenblatt and others (1977b) reported in the section on absorption,
sex interacts with many other factors and evidently does not allow
generalization of observations from one drug to another.
Guidicelli and Tillement (1977),for instance, report higher plasma levels of phenobarbital and antiepileptics and lower excretion rates of
lithium in males, but steady state levels of antidepressants (nortriptyline and imipramine) to be higher in females. Much of the variance
due to sex differences may of course also be caused by differences in
body composition, hormone levels, and height. It is well established
for instance, that in groups of same sex subjects, shorter individuals
have shorter half lives of drugs (Evans, 1971).

2.3.2 Genetic factors. Half lives and clearance rates of phenylbutazone and antipyrine (Vesell, 1974), nortriptyline (Alexanderson and
others, 1969), alcohol (Kalow, 1975; Vesell and others, 1971), and
several other drugs have been observed to be very similar in identical
twins as compared to dizygotic twins yielding curves as depicted in
Fig. 7 by Vesell and others (1971).

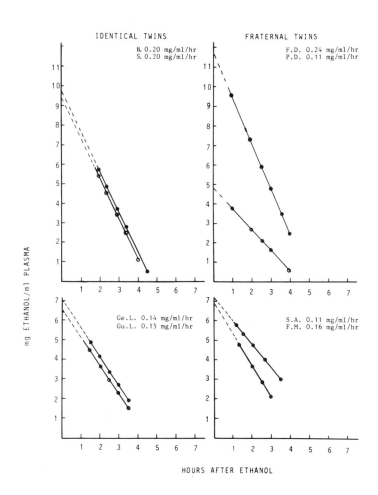

Fig. 7.   Ethanol disappearance from the blood plasma in two
          pairs of identical and fraternal twins. Each subject
          received 1 ml of 95 per cent ethanol per kg of body
          weight.(Mod. after Vesell and others, 1971)

Furthermore, there is great similarity in elimination rates of chemically dissimilar drugs, as documented by a correlation between rates
of clearance for antipyrine and phenylbutazone which ranged from
r = .29 after a single dose to r = .97 after chronic administration
(Davies and Thorgeirsson, 1971). The clearance rates of different
drugs correlate higher in identical twins than in dizygotic pairs
(Vesell and Page, 1968).
But as Alexanderson and others (1969) point out, the largest proportion
of the variance in half lives and elimination rates is due to differences in metabolic processes in the liver, as will be discussed in the
next section.

2.4 Factors Affecting Protein Binding and Metabolism of Drugs

2.4.1 Relevance of changes in protein binding. The ratio of the
bound to the free fraction of a compound is fairly high for most drugs
(for example 95%/5% for nortriptyline) and is a source of variance due
to the drug rather than to the individual. Increased binding will enhance hepatic clearance (Alvan, 1978).
But, although it is acknowledged that most of the variation in drug
plasma levels derives very little of its variance from subject related
differences in protein binding (Alexanderson and others, 1969; Evans
and Shand, 1973), it has to be kept in mind that the ratio of the bound
to the free fraction of the compound varies with time after application
(Curry and others, 1970a) so that factors interfering with this time
course will affect the amount of the free compound available for its
pharmacodynamic action.

Furthermore, protein binding of strongly bound drugs (like chlorpromazine and imipramine), will be affected by states of hypalbuminemia
which may be caused by inflammatory diseases or stress (Tillement and
others, 1978) and which occur more frequently in elderly subjects
(Tillement and others, 1978; Turner, 1978) and in neonates (Turner,
1978). Since elevation of free fatty acids in the blood may also displace a proportion of a protein bound drug from plasma albumin (Gugler
and others, 1974), substances causing elevations of free fatty acids
may increase the amount of free drug.

2.4.2 Sources of variance for metabolism by microsomal enzymes. Most
differences in plasma levels of drugs are due to individual differences
in the drug metabolizing enzyme systems of the endoplasmatic reticulum
of the liver. This can be demonstrated by the observation that there
are high negative correlations between in vitro rates of N-demethyla-
tion of ethylmorphine and cytochrome P 450 reductase activity of human
liver biopsy samples on one hand and respective plasma half lives of
antipyrine on the other (Davies and Thorgeirsson, 1971).
Differences in rates of drug metabolism can have various reasons:

(1) Research in pharmacogenetics has detected two ways of genetic con-
    trol of drug metabolism.
    (a) First there is a polygenetically controlled general influence
        on rate of drug metabolism. This can be detected by studies
        comparing plasma half lives or steady state plasma levels of
        certain drugs in identical and fraternal twins (Kalow, 1975;
        Vesell, 1974) as it was demonstrated for ethanol in Fig. 7.
        Furthermore, evidence for inheritance of rates of metabolism
        is derived from investigations establishing intraindividual
        stability of pharmacokinetic values upon repeated applications
        of the same drug to the same subjects (Wagner, 1973). This
        has been demonstrated among others for diazepam, ethanol, nor-
        triptyline and amobarbital. In studies using a sufficient num-
        ber of subjects, intraindividual variation is usually at least
        five times less than interindividual variation (Kalow, 1975).
        Similarly, high positive correlations between half lives of
        two different drugs metabolized by the same pathways point to
        genetic control of enzyme activities as was demonstrated, for
        example, for nortriptyline and desmethylimipramine (Åsberg
        and others, 1971) and for amobarbital and glutethimide (Kadar
        and others, 1973).

(b) A second mode of genetic influence is represented by mono-
    genic control of certain drug metabolizing enzymes. This may
    result in two genetically distinct subtypes of the same enzyme
    showing quantitative differences in activity. Whereas polyge-
    nic control is expressed in unimodal distributions of enzyme
    activities in a population, the second mode of influence is
    discovered by bimodal distributions of oxidation rates.
    In particular, two types of enzymes have been described that
    show the properties of b), namely liver alcohol dehydrogenase
    (Edwards and Evans, 1967) and N-acetyltransferase (Evans, 1971),
    which both are controlled by two allelic genes: About 10% of
    the Caucasian population possess a subtype of alcohol dehydro-
    genase characterized by a lower pH-optimum and a much higher
    rate of ethanol oxidation. This explains faster disappearance
    of ethanol from the plasma in subjects possessing the fast
    enzyme.
    Similarly fast and slow acetylators have been described (Evans,
    1971), the slow ones excreting isoniazide, phenelzine, sulfa-
    metazine and hydralazine more slowly than the rapid ones and
    developing more side effects when treated with equivalent doses
    of these substances. Lunde and others (1977) point out that
    this polymorphic acetylation which also affects drugs like
    nitrazepam (see Table 2) could explain the variations in hypno-
    tic effects observed in most samples of patients.

(2) The role of <u>age</u> in drug metabolism has been investigated and re-
    viewed by several authors with respect to the developing organism
    as well as to old age (Stevenson, 1973; Davies and Thorgeirsson,
    1971; Greenblatt and others, 1977b, 1978; Garattini and others,
    1973). It has been demonstrated that the newborn has not yet de-
    veloped the full activity of mixed function oxigenases for drug
    metabolism. Similarly, in old age these enzyme activities are
    gradually decreased again as could be shown from increased plasma
    half lives mentioned in sections 2.2 and 2.3 and from negative
    correlations between age and formation of chlordiazepoxide meta-
    bolites (Greenblatt and others, 1977b).

    The physician has to be aware of this when dosing psychotropic
    drugs, since increased levels of the drug may considerably enhance
    the effects and frequently lead to side effects which therefore
    are observed more frequently in older patients.

(3) As could be seen from the studies on excretion rates, <u>sex differ-
    ences</u> in drug disposition are more dependent on type of drug and
    intraindividual variation than the effects due to age. Thus,
    Guidicelli and Tillement (1977), for instance, observed that nor-
    triptyline was more rapidly metabolized in males and Duvoisin
    (1968) reports some results from different investigations in which
    Parkinson-like side effects after treatment with neuroleptics were
    observed more frequently in females than in males. Other drugs like
    antipyrine, however, are metabolized more slowly in males (O'Malley
    and others, 1971). Sex differences in metabolism of some drugs are
    reported to be dependent on the amount of circulating hormones,
    since testosterone and estrogens influence hepatic enzyme activi-
    ties via stimulation and inhibition respectively. This would be
    in line with the observation that estrogenic agents precipitate
    Parkinsonism in patients treated with phenothiazines (Duvoisin,
    1968). The proportion of variance contributed by sex in human drug

studies, however, is lower than the variance due to general genetic factors, as revealed by an analysis of variance on identical
and dizygotic twins performed by Alexanderson and others (1969).

(4) Environmental factors.
  The most important influence on variations in drug metabolizing
  enzymes, however, is derived from enzyme induction and inhibition
  by foreign compounds like other drugs, alcohol, nicotine, delta-
  9-tetrahydrocannabinol and steroid hormones, resulting in an increase or decrease of therapeutic efficiency of drugs by respective
  alterations of their metabolisms.With respect to metabolism of
  psychoactive drugs in the human increased enzyme synthesis
  by enzyme inducers is of greater clinical relevance than enzyme
  inhibition.

  The best known and most potent stimulators are phenobarbitone and
  other barbiturates, which have been shown to increase, among others,
  the metabolism of chlorpromazine, diphenylhydantoin, and desmethylimipramine in man (Conney and Burns, 1972).Further inducers are
  glutethimide, meprobamate, diphenylhydantoin, phenylbutazone, anti-
  pyrene, and tolbutamide, some of which not only stimulate metabolism of other therapeutically applied drugs but also their own metabolic degradation (Conney and Burns, 1972; Stevenson, 1973).

  Psychologically important is the fact that nicotine may enhance
  metabolism of psychoactive drugs, which has been demonstrated by
  higher plasma levels of imipramine in non-smokers than in smokers
  (Perel and others, 1976). Also, in subjects having smoked marihuana
  for at least one year, intravenously administered delta-9-tetra-
  hydrocannabinol showed a decreased plasma half life of 27 hours
  as compared to 56 hours in subjects who had never tried the drug
  (Lemberger and Rubin, 1975).

  The well known tolerance to ethanol which develops with chronic
  administration can also partly be explained by enhanced metabolism
  induced by ethanol itself. This enzyme induction is also responsible
  for the increase in metabolism of, for instance, benzodiazepines
  observed in heavy drinkers and for the accelerated disappearance
  of meprobamate from the blood of subjects receiving 46 % of their
  daily calorie intake from ethanol for one month in an experiment
  reported by Sellers and Holloway (1978). Therefore, behavioral
  habits like drinking, smoking, intake of sleeping pills etc. linked
  to other personality variables like anxiety or extraversion may
  cause correlations between psychological factors and drug response.

2.5 Blood Levels of Drugs and Clinical Response

The aim of investigation of interindividual differences in absorption,
metabolism and elimination of a drug is to explain part of the variance
in peaks and time course of blood concentrations of the drug, the assumption being that by obtaining a prediction for blood levels part
of the variance of clinical response can also be explained.

But as will be shown, the variance of clinical response can only partly be explained by differences in the kinetic parameters, since there
is a great deal of controversy as to whether blood levels do correspond
to clinical effects or not.

With respect to this question many papers have been published which try to related blood levels of diazepam or chlordiazepoxide and its metabolites to antiaggressive (Gottschalk and Kaplan, 1972; Gottschalk and others, 1973a) or to antianxiety effects (Curry, 1974; Dasberg and others, 1974; Gottschalk and Kaplan, 1972; Gottschalk and others, 1973a; Lin and Friedel, 1979; Smith and others, 1976),to decrements in performance (Curry, 1974; Hillestad and others, 1974) and to biochemical changes such as those of glucose, free fatty acids (FFA), hormones, and liver enzymes (Gottschalk and others, 1973a) or 3-methoxy-4-hydroxy-phenylglycol (MHPG) excretion in urine (Smith and others, 1976). Similarly, efforts have been reported to establish relationship between chlorpromazine (Clark and Kaul, 1976; Cooper, 1978; Curry, 1969, 1974; Curry and others, 1970a, 1970b; Gottschalk and others, 1973b), butaperazine (Cooper, 1978), thioridazine (Cooper, 1978; Gottschalk and others, 1973b,1975) or nortriptyline levels (Alexanderson and others, 1973) and improvement of psychiatric symptomatology. Two reviews on correlations between blood concentrations of neuroleptics or antidepressants and clinical response by Modestin and Petrin (1976) and by Glassman and Perel (1978) yielded the following results (Table 3):

TABLE 3   Results of Correlation Analyses between Blood Levels of Neuroleptics and Antidepressants and Clinical Response or Side Effects (after Modestin and Petrin, 1976, and Glassman and Perel, 1978)

Type of Correlations observed	Neuroleptics		Antidepressants		
	Modestin and Petrin therapeutic effects	side effects	Modestin and Petrin therapeutic effects	side effects	Glassman and Perel therapeutic effects
Intraindividual Positive	3		1		-
Interindividual Positive	5	2	5	4	4
Negative	0		2		0
U-shaped	1		1		4
Zero	6		3		1
Total	15	2	14	4	9

The failure to establish significant correlations may, however, be due to the fact that overall blood levels do not represent the correct parameter reflecting concentrations at the site of drug action. Levy (1973), for example, demonstrated that the amount of intravenously injected lysergic acid diethylamide (LSD) present in a slowly accessible peripheral compartment identified in a three compartment system showed a linear and significant negative correlation with performance in a mathematical test, whereas general blood levels were only insignificantly related to test response. Similarly, dystonic side effects caused by butaperazine (Cooper, 1978) were shown to be predictable from drug concentrations in the red blood cells rather than from plasma levels, in a study attempting to establish plasma level-response relationships.

Furthermore, different behavioral responses seem to reach their peaks at different levels of concentrations varying again with type of compound chosen for investigation, as was demonstrated for different types of benzodiazepines and their effects on muscle relaxation and aggressivity in mice by Garattini and others (1973).

On the whole it seems that physiological reactions, such as pupil size, blood pressure, heart rate, sweat gland activity, EEG parameters and salivary activity show better correlations with blood concentrations of drugs than psychological test parameters as summarized for studies on chlorpromazine by Curry (1973). The failure to obtain substantial correlations between plasma levels and behavioral response may be due to disregard of one of the 11 rules which according to Sjöquist and Bertilsson (1973) have to be followed when studying drug kinetics - effect relationships. These rules concern:

a) the elimination of confounding factors or experimental error such as additional diseases or therapy, preexisting drug tolerance in members of the experimental group or other reasons for lack of group homogeneity;

b) the use of specific and sensitive techniques for the assessment of plasma concentrations and clinical response as well as careful timing of blood sampling;

c) precise knowledge about whether the parent compound or its metabolites are effective and whether the free and not the bound fraction of the compound reflects the concentration at the receptor site.

Therefore, prediction of clinical response from plasma levels, which is especially important in chronic treatment must take these sources of error into account and must be specified for subgroups formed according to the factors outlined in this chapter which are relevant for differences in pharmacokinetics.

REFERENCES

Alexanderson, B., D. A. P. Evans, and F. Sjöquist (1969). Steady-state plasma levels of nortriptyline in twins: influence of genetic factors and drug therapy. Br. Med. J., 4, 764-768.

Alexanderson, B., M. Åsberg, and D. Tuch (1973). Relationship between steady-state plasma concentration of nortriptyline and some of its pharmacological effects. In D. S. Davies, and B. N. C. Prichard (Eds.), Biological Effects of Drugs in Relation to their Plasma Concentrations. University Park Press, Baltimore. pp. 191-199.

Åsberg, M., D. A. P. Evans, and F. Sjöquist (1971). Genetic control of nortriptyline kinetics in man (a study of relatives of propositi, with high plasma concentrations. J. Med. Genet., 8, 129-135.

Alvan, G. (1978). Individual differences in the disposition of drugs metabolised in the body. Clin. Pharmacokinetics, 3, 135-175.

Atkinson, A. J.,Jr., and W. Kushner (1979). Clinical pharmacokinetics. Ann. Rev. Pharmacol. Toxicol., 19, 105-128.

Basu, T. K., and J. W. T. Dickerson (1974). Inter-relationships of nutrition and the metabolism of drugs. Chem. Biol. Interact., 8, 193-206.

Campbell, T. C., and J. R. Hayes (1974). Role of nutrition in the drug metabolizing enzyme system. Pharmacol. Rev., 26, 171-198.

Clark, M. L., and P. N. Kaul (1976). A preliminary report of clinical
    response and blood levels of chlorpromazine and its sulfoxide during
    CPZ therapy in chronic schizophrenic patients. In L. A. Gottschalk
    and S. Merlis (Eds.), Pharmacokinetics of Psychoactive Drugs: Blood
    Levels and Clinical Response. Spectrum Publ., New York. pp. 191-197.
Conney, A. H., and J. J. Burns (1972). Metabolic interactions among
    environmental chemicals and drugs. Science, 178, 576-586.
Cooper, T. B. (1978). Plasma level monitoring of antipsychotic drugs.
    Clin. Pharmacokinetics, 3, 14-38.
Curry, S. H. (1969). Interpatient variation in physiological availabi-
    lity of CPZ as a complicating factor in correlation studies of drug
    metabolism and clinical effect. In
    The Present Status of Psychotropic Drugs. Excerpta Medica Foundation,
    Amsterdam. pp. 72-76.
Curry, S. H. (1973). Action and metabolism of chlorpromazine. In D.S.
    Davies and B. N. C. Prichard (Eds.), Biological Effects of Drugs in
    Relation to their Plasma Concentrations. University Park Press,
    Baltimore. pp. 202-210.
Curry, S. H. (1974). Concentration-effect relationships with major and
    minor tranquilizers. Clin. Pharmacol. Ther., 16, 192-197.
Curry, S. H., J. M. Davis, D. S. Janowsky, and J. H. D. Marshall (1970a)
    Factors affecting chlorpromazine plasma levels in psychiatric pa-
    tients. Arch. Gen. Psychiat., 22, 209-215.
Curry, S. H., J. H. D. Marshall, J. M. Davis, and D. S. Janowsky (1970b)
    Chlorpromazine plasma levels and effects. Arch. Gen. Psychiat. , 22,
    289-296.
Dasberg, H. H., E. von der Kleijn, P. J. R. Guelen, and H. M. v. Praag
    (1974). Plasma concentrations of diazepam and its metabolite N-des-
    methyldiazepam in relation to anxiolytic effect. Clin. Pharmacol.
    Ther., 15, 473-483.
Davies, D. S., and S. S. Thorgeirsson (1971). Mechanism of hepatic drug
    oxidation and its relationship to individual differences in man.
    Ann. N.Y. Acad. Sci., 179, 411-420.
Dost, F. H. (1968). Grundlagen der Pharmakokinetik. Thieme, Stuttgart.
Duvoisin, R. C. (1968). Neurological reactions to psychotropic drugs.
    In D. H. Efron (Ed.), Psychopharmacology - A Review of Progress
    1957 - 1967. US Department of Health Education and Welfare, Washing-
    ton. pp. 561-573.
Edwards, J. A., and D. A. P. Evans (1967). Ethanol metabolism in sub-
    jects possessing typical and atypical liver alcoholdehydrogenase.
    Clin. Pharmacol. Ther., 8, 824-829.
Evans, D. A. P. (1971). Inter-individual differences in metabolism of
    drugs: The role of genetic factors. Acta Pharmacol. Toxicol., 29,
    56-163.
Evans, D. A. P., and D. G. Shand (1973). Disposition of propranolol.
    Independent variation in steady-state circulation, drug concentra-
    tions, and half life as a result of plasma drug binding in man.
    Clin. Pharmacol. Ther., 14, 494-500.
Forth, W., D. Henschler, and W. Rummel (1980). Allgemeine und spezielle
    Pharmakologie und Toxikologie, 3rd ed. Wissenschaftsverlag, Bibl.
    Inst. Mannheim.
Garattini, S., F. Marcucci, P. L. Morselli and E. Mussini (1973). The
    significance of measuring blood levels of benzodiazepines. In D.S.
    Davies, and B. N. C. Prichard (Eds.), Biological Effects of Drugs
    in Relation to their Plasma Concentrations. University Park Press,
    Baltimore. pp. 211-225.
Gibaldi, M., and D. Perrier (1975). Pharmacokinetics. Marcel Dekker,
    New York.

Gilman, A. G., L. S. Goodman, and A. Gilman (Eds.) (1980). The Pharmacological Basis of Therapeutics, 6th ed. Macmillan, New York.

Gladtke, E., and H. M. v. Hattingberg (1973). Pharmakokinetik. Springer, Berlin.

Glassman, A. H., and J. M. Perel (1978). Tricyclic blood levels and clinical outcome: A review of the art. In M. A. Lipton, A. DiMascio, and K. F. Killam (Eds.), Psychopharmacology: A Generation of Progress. Raven Press, New York. pp. 917-922.

Goldstein, A., L. Aronow, and S. M. Kalman (1974). Principles of Drug Action: The Basis of Pharmacology. Wiley, New York.

Gottschalk, L. A., and S. A. Kaplan (1972). Chlordiazepoxide plasma levels and clinical response. Compr. Psychiatry, 13, 519-527.

Gottschalk, L. A., E. P. Noble, G. E. Stolzoff, D. E. Bates, C. G. Cable, R. L. Uliana, H. Birch, and E. W. Fleming (1973a). Relationships of chlordiazepoxide blood levels to psychological and biochemical responses. In S. Garattini, E. Mussini, and L. O. Randall (Eds.), The Benzodiazepines. Raven Press, New York. pp. 257-280.

Gottschalk, L. A., E. P. Noble, and H. Elliot (1973b). Preliminary studies of relationships between psychoactive drug blood levels and clinical response: CPZ, meperidine and thioridazine. Psychopharm. Bull., 9, 40-43.

Gottschalk, L. A., R. Biener, E. P. Noble, H. Birch, P. E. Wilbert, and J. F. Her (1975). Thioridazine plasma levels and clinical response. Compr. Psychiatry, 16, 323-337.

Greenblatt, D. J., R. Shader, and J. Koch-Weser (1974). Pharmacokinetic determinants of the response to single doses of chlordiazepoxide. Am. J. Psychiat., 131, 1395-1397.

Greenblatt, D. J., R. I. Shader, K. Franke, D. S. MacLaughlin, B. J. Ransil, and J. Koch-Weser (1977). Kinetics of intravenous chlordiazepoxide: sex differences in drug distribution. Clin. Pharm. Ther., 22, 893-903.

Greenblatt, D. J., R. I. Shader, J. S. Harmatz, K. Franke, and J. Koch-Weser (1977a). Absorption rate, blood concentrations and early response to oral chlordiazepoxide. Am. J. Psychiat., 134, 559-562.

Greenblatt, D. J., J. S. Harmatz, D. R. Stanski, R. I. Shader, K. Franke, and J. Koch-Weser (1977b). Factors influencing blood concentration of chlordiazepoxdie: A use of multiple regression analysis. Psychopharmacology, 54, 277-282.

Greenblatt, D. J., R. I. Shader, S. M. MacLeod, and E. M. Sellers (1978). Clinical pharmacokinetics of chlordiazepoxide. Clin. Pharmacokinetics, 3, 381-394.

Gugler, R., D. W. Shoeman, and D. L. Azarnoff (1974). Effect of in vivo elevation of free fatty acids on protein binding of drugs. Pharmacology, 12, 160-165.

Guidicelli, J. F., and J. P. Tillement (1977). Influence of sex on drug kinetics in man. Clin. Pharmacogenetics, 2, 157-166.

Hillestad, L., T. Hansen, H. Nelson, and A. Drivines (1974). Diazepam metabolism in normal man: serum concentration and clinical effects after intravenous, intramuscular and oral administration. Clin. Pharmacol. Ther., 16, 479-484.

Kadar, D., T. Inaba, and L. Endrenyi (1973). Comparative drug elimination capacity in man - glutethimide, amobarbital, antipyrine and sulfinpyrazone. Clin. Pharmacol. Ther., 14, 552-560.

Kalow, W. (1975). Genetics and psychoactive drugs. In E. M. Sellers (Ed.), Clinical Pharmacology of Psychoactive Drugs. Addict. Res. Found., Toronto. pp. 105-115.

Krishnaswamy, K. (1978). Drug metabolism and pharmacokinetics in malnutrition. Clin. Pharmacokinetics, 3, 216-240.

Kurz, H., H. G. Neumann, W. Forth, D. Henschler, and W. Rummel (1980). Allgemeine Pharmakologie. In W. Forth, D. Henschler, and W. Rummel (Eds.), Allgemeine und spezielle Pharmakologie und Toxikologie, 3rd ed. Bibl. Inst., Mannheim.

Kyriakopoulos, A. A. (1976). Bioavailability of lorazepam in humans. In L. A. Gottschalk and S. Merlis (Eds.), Pharmacokinetics of Psychoactive Drugs: Blood Level and Clinical Response. Spectrum Publ., New York. pp. 45-60.

Lemberger, L., and A. Rubin (1975). The physiologic disposition of marihuana in man. Life Sci., 17, 1637-1642.

Levy, G. (1973). Relationship between pharmacological effects and plasma or tissue concentration of drugs in man. In D. S. Davies, and B. N. C. Prichard (Eds.), Biological Effects of Drugs in Relation to their Plasma Concentrations. University Park Press, Baltimore. pp. 83-95.

Lin, K. M., and R. O. Friedel (1979). Relationship of plasma levels of chlordiazepoxide and metabolites to clinical response. Am. J. Psychiat., 131, 18-23.

Lunde, P. K. M., K. Frislid, and V. Hansteen (1977). Disease and acetylation polymorphism. Clin. Pharmacokinetics, 2, 182-197.

Maass, A. R., B. Jenkins, Y. Shen, and P. Tannenbaum (1969). Studies on absorption, excretion, and metabolism of ^{3}H-reserpine in man. Clin. Pharmacol. Ther., 10, 366-371.

Melmon, K. L., and H. F. Morrelli (Eds.) (1978). Clinical Pharmacology, 2nd ed. Macmillan, New York.

Modestin, J., and A. Petrin (1976). Beziehungen zwischen Pasmakonzentration und klinischer Wirkung von Neuroleptika und Antidepressiva. Int. J. Clin. Pharmacol., 13, 11-21.

Munkelt, P., and G. A. Lienert (1964). Blutalkoholspiegel und psychophysische Konstitution. Arzneimittelforschung (Drug Res.), 14, 573-575.

Nakano, S., N. Ogawa, and Y. Kawazu (1980). Influence of neuroticism on oral absorption of diazepam. Clin. Pharmacol. Ther., 27, 370-374.

O'Malley, K., J. Crooks, E. Duke, and I. H. Stevenson (1971). Effect of age and sex on human drug metabolism. Brit. Med. J., 3, 607-609.

Perel, J. M., M. Shostak, E. Gann, S. J. Kantor, and A. H. Glassman (1976). Pharmacodynamics of imipramine and clinical outcome in depressed patients. In L. A. Gottschalk, and S. Merlis (Eds.), Pharmacokinetics of Psychoactive Drugs: Blood Levels and Clinical Response. Spectrum Publ., New York.

Sellers, E. M., and M. R. Holloway (1978). Drug kinetics and alcohol ingestion. Clin. Pharmacokinetics, 3, 440-452.

Sjöquist, F., and L. Bertilsson (1973). Plasma concentrations of drugs and pharmacological response in man. In D. S. Davies, and B. N. C. Prichard (Eds.), Biological Effects of Drugs in Relation to their Plasma Concentrations. MacMillan, London.

Smith, R. C., H. Dekirmenjian, J. Davis, R. Casper, C. Gosenfeld, and C. Tsai (1976). Blood level, mood and MHPG responses to diazepam in man. In L. A. Gottschalk, and S. Merli (Eds.), Pharmacokinetics of Psychoactive Drugs. Spectrum Publ., New York.

Stevenson, I. H. (1973). The significance and determinants of drug metabolism in man. Digestion, 8, 80-86.

Tillement, J. P., F. Choste, and J. F. Guidicelli (1978). Diseases and drug protein binding. Clin. Pharmacokinetics, 3, 144-154.

Turner, P. (1978). Influence of age on drug metabolism in man. In J. Gorod (Ed.), Drug Metabolism in Man. Taylor & Francis, London. pp. 119-125.

Vesell, E. S. (1974). Application of pharmacokinetic principles to the elucidation of polygenically controlled differences in drug response. In T. Teorell, R. L. Dedrick, and P. G. Condliffe (Eds.), Pharmacology and Pharmacokinetics. Plenum Press, New York. pp. 261-280.

Vesell, E. S., and J. G. Page (1968). Genetic control of dicumarol levels in man. J. Clin. Invest., 47, 2657-2663.

Vesell, E. S., J. G. Page, and G. T. Passananti (1971). Genetic and environmental factors affecting ethanol metabolism in man. Clin. Pharmacol. Ther.,12, 192-201.

Volans, G. N. (1978). Research Review: Migraine and drug absorption. Clin. Pharmacokinetics, 3, 313-318.

Wagner, J. C. (1973). Intrasubject variation in elimination half lives of drugs which are appreciably metabolized. J. Pharmacokinetics and Biopharmaceutics, 1, 165-173.

Wallusch, W. W., H. Nowak, G. Leopold, and K. J. Netter (1978). Comparative bioavailability: Influence of various diets on the bioavailability of indomethacin. Int. J. Clin. Pharmacol., 16, 40-44.

Part II

DRUG RESPONSE VARIABILITY: OVERVIEW OF CONTRIBUTING FACTORS

RESPONSE VARIABILITY TO PSYCHOTROPIC DRUGS: OVERVIEW OF THE MAIN APPROACHES TO DIFFERENTIAL PHARMACO-PSYCHOLOGY

Wilhelm Janke[1]

ABSTRACT

The purpose of the introductory paper is to give an overview about some basic problems of differential pharmacopsychology which is that sub-discipline describing and systematizing inter- and intraindividual differences in response to psychotropic drugs.

In the first part of the paper, some basic drug issues are discussed which refer to the concept of sensitivity to drugs (as an enduring individual characteristic). The issues tapped are the reliability of the drug response, the generalizability of the drug response to different kinds of drugs and to different environmental and situational conditions, and to different dependent variables.

The paper takes the position that the relationship between drug response and personality traits has to be discussed while bearing in mind that a psychotropic drug alters behavior by changing momentary (actual) neurochemical and accompanying neurophysiological and psychological processes. The change in a system a drug will induce is dependent on the actual state of this system. From this, it follows that the optimal predictor variables for predicting the response to a drug are indicators of momentary somatic and behavioral state. They are regarded as <u>direct drug response modifiers</u>. The prediction of a response to drug by any indirect predictor variable can be successful only insofar as it involves some relationship to the actual somatic (neurochemical and neurophysiological) and behavioral state. The two most important classes of predictor variables which are to be regarded as <u>indirect drug modifiers</u> are long-lasting individual characteristics (somatic and behavioral traits) and environmental including situational conditions. A short survey of the personality and environmental factors which have been investigated in the past will be given. An accentuation in this survey is given to studies which relate drug response to emotional tension (and related concepts as neuroticism, anxiety, stress).

---

[1] I am very grateful to Dr. Gisela Erdmann, Prof. Nicholas Longo, and Dr. Douglas Rush for some suggestions made reading this paper. Moreover, I have to thank Prof. G. Debus with whom I discussed most of the problems which are sketched in this paper.

KEYWORDS

Drug response consistency; drug response variability; environmental
factors; personality; situational factors; susceptibility to drugs.

I. INTRODUCTION

The topic of this book is concerned with a theme central to all disciplines engaged in assessing the effects of drugs: variability to
psychotropic drugs.

The variation in behavioral drug response between and within subjects
is so enormous that all disciplines (pharmacology, psychiatry and
psychology) engaged in behavioral drug research face the problem
that it is usually impossible to predict the intensity and quality
of a drug response only from the knowledge of the drug parameters,
e.g. kind of drug and dose level.

Additional information which is needed relates to a number of factors.
It is usually stressed that at least information about characteristics
of the subjects and about the environmental and situational conditions
under which the drug is given is needed to make a prediction about
drug actions possible.

The number of factors which may modify drug response is very large
and is increasing at a rapid rate as new factors are studied. Moreover, more and more significant interactions between the drug response
modifying factors are reported as factorial analysis of variance or
other multivariate techniques have come into increasing use.

The whole field (called differential psychopharmacology) is concerned
with the description, prediction and explanation of inter- and intra-
individual drug response differences as affected by these numerous
factors. The orientation is to a considerable degree empirical rather
than theoretical. There are only a few exceptions as seen in the work
of Eysenck (this volume) and those researchers closely allied to his
approach. Consequently, the present state of our knowledge about the
effects of most of these drugs is rather confusing.

The empirical work in differential psychopharmacology is directed to
two main goals:
(1) Drug response differences which occur in the same subject when a
specific drug is given at several times (intra-individual drug response variability).
(2) Drug response differences which occur in different individuals
when a specific drug is given at the same time (inter-individual drug
response variability).

The main task of this paper is to evaluate the contribution of psychological variables in the variability of the response to psychotropic
drugs. The discussion will concentrate particularly on inter-individual drug response differences; that is, to differences between subjects tested at the same time under the same environmental and situational conditions.

Less emphasis will be given to within-subject response differences;
that is, to drug response differences which occur in the same subject

when a specific drug is given at several times (intra-individual drug response variability).

First, some basic problems will be sketched which must be solved before psychological factors can be considered at all.

II. DRUG RESPONSE VARIABILITY AS A RESULT OF ENVIRONMENTAL AND SITUATIONAL FACTORS

One of the most embarrassing problems in psychopharmacology results from the fact that psychotropic drugs have varying effects according to the environmental conditions and situations in which they are given. Thus, response variability to psychotropic drugs is necessarily concerned with both inter-individual and intra-individual differences. Intra-individual drug response variability seems to be dependent to a large extent on environmental and situational factors. The influence of these factors on drug response is probably of higher importance than spontaneous variations due to errors of measurement. As may be concluded from the significant results of many studies, environment and situation related intra-individual variance can exceed inter-subject variance.

Inter-individual or inter-subject variance is also considerably influenced by environmental and situational factors: In every experimental or therapeutic drug study, it is impossible to arrange for all subjects or patients absolutely the same environmental and situational conditions. Even if we would succeed in reaching equality in the physical sense, the environment and situation would differ for each subject because of different perceptions and evaluations. Since it is safe to assume that the drug response will change with different environmental and situational conditions it is safe to say that one of the sources of inter-individual drug response variability in a drug trial is environmental and situational factors.

In Table 1a a listing of environmental and situational factors which have been shown to influence drug response is given. Table 1b completes the list for pharmacotherapeutic trials. The range of these factors is very large. They range from rather unspecific physical environmental factors which are unrelated to the specific set-up of the drug study - such as geographical or climatic conditions - to very specific cognitive factors of the experiment (e.g. characteristics of the tests used, mainly complexity, attractivity, subjective difficulty; information given to the subjects about the aim of the study). For chronic drug administration in patients, additional factors have to be taken into consideration as may be seen from Table 1b. Several reviews or extensive discussions have been published in the past (Evans, 1970; Janke and Debus, 1968; Janke and others, 1979; Yehuda, 1976). Reviews which refer mainly or exclusively to pharmacotherapy have been published by Debus and Janke (1978) and May and Goldberg (1978). A very important paper on methodological problems of differential pharmacotherapy was written by S. Fisher (1970).

TABLE 1 Environmental and Situational Factors Determining Drug Response

1a   Factors Efficient in Acute Drug Studies

Class	Examples of important factors
General environmental conditions	1 Geographical conditions 2 Climatic and physical conditions 3 Environmental chemicals 4 Time of year, time of day
General situational conditions (general trial conditions)	Social variables: 1 Groups vs. individual trial 2 Interpersonal communication between S and E 3 Sex, age and general personality traits of E
Specific situational conditions	Situational factors determining the specific state of S: 1 Sensorial-perceptual changes inducing factors, e.g. sensory stimulation or deprivation 2 Cognitive processes inducing factors 3 Emotion inducing factors, e.g. presence or absence of stressors 4 Motivation inducing factors, e.g. food restriction, sleep restriction
Specific trial conditions	1a Information on the aim of the trial b Information on the meaning of specific arrangements of the trial c Information on the meaning of measurement devices (tests) 2 Activities required or permitted 3 Characteristics of the measurement devices, e.g. complexity, subjective difficulty, attractivity 4 Degree of introspection needed 5 Attitudes and expectations of E

1b   Factors Efficient in Chronic Drug Studies and Influencing the Success of Therapy

Characteristics of the physician	Characteristics of the treatment milieu	Characteristics outside the treatment milieu
Personality characteristics	Amount and kind of non-psychopharmaco-therapy	Occupational environment
Opinions on psycho-pharmacotherapy in relation to other therapies	Interpersonal contact opportunities during treatment	Family environment
Experience with psycho-pharmacotherapy		Unusual occurrences during therapy
Specific drug-effect expectations		
Opinions and feelings about the patient		

It would be easy enough to find for each of some twenty environmental and situational conditions several studies which show its possible contribution to drug response. In spite of this, however, it is difficult to generalize the findings because the number of studies is very small for most factors if one differentiates with regard to kind of drugs. It seems possible to draw conclusions for only a very small set of factors from the available literature. Such conclusions seem to be e.g. (1) Tranquilizer increase their tension reducing properties if applied in stress inducing conditions (for a review see Debus and Janke, 1980). (2) Stimulants seem to have stronger effects on performance and subjective activity if administered under fatigue producing conditions (e.g. Holliday and Devery, 1961; Janke and Amelang, 1965).

It is expected that differential psychopharmacology will elucidate the influence of environmental and situational factors more clearly. The main questions which should be investigated in further experiments are the following:
(1) By which mechanisms is the influence of environmental and situational factors mediated? This question, which will be discussed more thoroughly in Section IV 3, points to fact that the influence of these factors on drug response can be understood only as an indirect one. A first possibility is that by changing the organismic behavioral and somatic state on which the drug acts, a change of drug effects will result. A second possibility is that environmental and situational factors induce specific perceptions and evaluations of drug response. These perceptions and evaluations then lead to altered drug response.
(2) To what extent do environmental and situational factors modify the intensity and quality of drug response? This question of how much the drug response is influenced by environmental and situational factors has been in the past more theoretically discussed than experimentally investigated. The many significant drug-environment interactions which have been enumerated in the past do not justify the conclusion that the influence of environmental and situational factors is very large in quantitative terms.
(3) To what extent and in which way do environmental and situational factors differ in different individuals? As has been discussed and empirically demonstrated, the same environmental and situational factors have different meanings in different subjects. The meaning of these subject-environment interactions for psychopharmacology has to be elucidated in future empirical work. One step in this direction is the paper of Krüger (this volume).

III. DRUG RESPONSE VARIABILITY AS A RESULT OF INDIVIDUAL CHARACTERISTICS

1. Overview of Factors

There is no generally accepted taxonomy of individual characteristics (for discussion see Janke and others, 1979) which may be regarded as drug response modifiers.

TABLE 2   Individual Characteristics as Drug Response Modifiers Which Have Been Studied Several Times

	long-lasting (traits)		short-lasting (states)	
	broad	specific (narrow)	broad	specific (narrow)
behavioral	-neuroticism -extra-/introversion -action-orientation	-anxiousness -suggestibility -need for arousal -drug effect expectation -drug experience -attitudes towards drugs	-emotional tension stress -activation	-fear, anxiety -anger -need for reward -drug effect expectation -perception of side effects
somatic — anatomical	body type			
somatic — physiological {sex, race}	-ANS-lability -ANS/CNS-arousability	-tachycardia -EEG abnormalities	-momentary arousal of ANS and CNS	-momentary arousal of specific systems
somatic — biochemical		-specific inborn errors of metabolism		

Table 2 gives a listing of traits and states, both on the somatic and behavioral level, which have been investigated in several experiments. For a review of behavioral factors see Janke and others (1979); for a review of somatic factors see Netter (this volume). As Table 2 shows it is possible to differentiate long-term (traits) from short-term (states) characteristics and broad from specific or narrow characteristics. Moreover, behavioral characteristics are differentiated from somatic characteristics which include anatomical-morphological, physiological and biochemical aspects. Long-term characteristics refer to patterns which are enduring. Short-term characteristics are usually called states, which are patterns that change with time and situation. The differentiation of broad from narrow characteristics may be exemplified by neuroticism or extra-introversion as broad characteristics and anxiousness or suggestibility arousal as specific or narrow traits. In psychopathology diagnostic categories such as depression or schizophrenia refer to broad characteristics. Specific symptoms, however, are conceived as narrow characteristics. The differentiation of the individual characteristics according to the reference system in Table 2 is partly arbitrary. This is particularly the case for the differentiation of somatic from behavioral characteristics since some somatic characteristics listed in Table 2 have to be considered as biological bases of some behavioral characteristics. One example may be ANS lability and neuroticism. In spite of this difficulty the differentiation seems meaningful, in particular under the view that operationally defined predictors of drug response are useful.

2. The Interpretation of Drug Response Variability by Means of Individual Characteristics

One of the most neglected topics in differential psychopharmacology is the interpretation of drug response variability by means of individual characteristics mentioned in Section I.

Two of the main problems in the interpretation of the interaction between drug response and individual characteristics refer (1) to the possibility that drug response variability may be caused by spurious factors and (2) to the generalizability of drug response. These two problems will be discussed in the next sections.

2.1 Drug Response Variability Due to "Spurious" or "Peripheral" Factors

2.1.1 Drug availability differences caused by peripheral factors

The basic question which has to be asked at the beginning of all interpretations of drug response variability is the following one: Is it possible that the variance which we want to explain by behavioral or somatic variables may be caused by factors which are completely unrelated to any of the actions of the drug on the central nervous system?

It is evident that when we try to explain drug response differences by psychological factors they must be mediated by processes which are directly related to the CNS and/or behavior. It is safe to say, however, that the drug availability is highly different for the same drug level at all levels of observation (e.g. blood) in different subjects because of pharmacokinetic and pharmacodynamic factors (see Netter and Netter; Netter, this volume).

The usual assumption is that tnere is a substantial correlation between
dosage level, concentration of the drug in the blood in nervous tissue,
on the one hand, and behavioral changes on the other hand. Substantial
correlations have been found sometimes, but not very frequently. (For
more information see Netter and Netter, this volume.) What do these
findings mean? Evidently, they mean that the stimulus "drug", the responses to which we want to analyse, does not have the same intensity
for all subjects. This, however, means that at least a part of the
inter-subject response variance is due just to stimulus differences.
This could, for example, be compared to the situation in which we want
to analyse the inter-subject response variance to noise but apply different noise levels to each of the subjects.

What would be necessary to avoid the problem of "spurious" drug response
variance is the definition of "drug" not on the distal, e.g. physical
level, but on a more proximal, e.g. organismic level. This would probably be at the level of drug receptors in the CNS. This, however, induces many questions which cannot be satisfactorily answered. All that
is possible in the usual experiments is to determine whether some of
the inter-individual variance in drug variance in the blood is due to
peripheral factors and to control these factors (e.g. food consumption
or day of time) thus trying to eliminate peripherally caused variance
(see chapter of Netter and Netter, this volume).

2.1.2 Drug response due to side effects.
The second factor which may result in "spurious" drug differences,
refers to somatic side effects or, to state it more exactly, the response of subjects to side effects.

Many drugs produce autonomic symptoms, e.g. sweating or dryness of the
mouth. An important symptom occurring frequently at the beginning of
drug action period is the feeling of dizziness. The subject usually
responds to these effects negatively, for example, with anxiety and
fear. This response may be dependent on personality traits such as
neuroticisim. This would lead to a correlation between drug response
and neuroticism which has no specific pharmacological basis.

The influence of side effects is particularly evident in experiments
with neuroleptics which induce many autonomic effects, and with stimulants and lithium. With lithium, for example, it was shown for normal
subjects that behavioral effects were not correlated with plasma levels of lithium but with nausea (Karniol and others, 1978).

2.1.3 Drug response variability due to unspecific psychological factors
Expectations of drug effects, attitudes and evaluation of possible
drug effects constitute yet another set of variables which influences
drug response variability and which may have nothing to do with the
specific pharmacological actions. These variables have been discussed
frequently under the heading "unspecific factors" in pharmacotherapy
(e.g. Rickels, 1968).

In the case of strong expectancy factors, the result may be an increase
of drug response variability. Moreover, the reaction of the subjects
to the drug induced change has to be regarded as an important source
of drug response variability. Whatever the drug's actions may be, it
is reasonable that some people respond emotionally when they feel
suddenly altered. This is probably true if the effects occur very
fast and are pronounced.

The discussion of psychological parameters such as expectations, attitudes and evaluative processes under the heading "spurious" factors may be easily misunderstood. It should be realized that psychological parameters may function also as factors which interact with the specific actions of the drug. In this role, they are not "spurious".

2.2 Inter-Individual Drug Response Variability Due to Differential Susceptibilities to Drugs

2.2.1 Definition and problems of drug susceptibility.
Having evidence that the inter-individual drug response variability in an experiment is not completely or predominantly the result of "spurious" or "peripheral" factors some basic problems have to be discussed. Interpretations of inter-subject response variability in terms of psychological factors or CNS related somatic factors assume — more or less explicitly — that different subjects have different susceptibilities to drugs which are the basis of inter-individual behavioral response differences. Drug susceptibility may be defined as the tendency of an individual to respond to a drug with a certain intensity and quality.

Given this definition of drug susceptibility two basic questions arise:
(1) Stability: The definition above involves stability of response over time. Do we have enough evidence to conclude that there are susceptibilities to drugs as long-term characteristics?
(2) Generalizability: Are susceptibilities to drugs rather specific, e.g. are they bound to a specific drug or type of drug, and to a specific situation in which the drug is administered?

2.2.2 Stability of the response to drugs.
The question of stability of the drug response has been, interestingly enough, rather rarely investigated in those designs which are commonly used in psychopharmacological studies. Results are available only from a few studies in which the determination of thresholds (e.g. sedation or stimulation thresholds) or the reactivity of the autonomic nervous system (e.g. physostigmine, methacholine, histamine) were made. These results show that sedation thresholds have rather high stability over (short) time periods (Claridge, this volume). The stability of the response to above mentioned autonomic drugs seems to be in the medium level.

It is hoped that we shall obtain in the near future more empirical data on this question for the commonly used psychotropic drugs, since in our own findings we had the feeling that the stability of drug response is disappointingly low. The study from which the feeling is derived was carried out by Janke and Netter (1981): 32 subjects were tested with an interval of 7 days after receiving a stimulant drug (16 subjects received 25 mg fenetyllin, 16 subjects 25 mg mefenorex). The interval between drug administration and testing was 120 minutes. The results were as follows (see Table 3): Significant but moderate correlations were obtained between regression-corrected change scores (Delta scores) for three activity scales and a mood scale of an adjective check list (Eigenschaftswörterliste by Janke and Debus, 1978). The correlations were $r = .41$, $r = .33$, $.45$ and $.36$. For two emotionality scales, the stability coefficients were $r = .14$ and $r = -.14$. For most performance tests the stability coefficients were also very low.

TABLE 3   Stability of Drug Responses

Correlations of raw-scores and of the delta-corrected change scores
between the values obtained after first and second application of
stimulant drugs.
Interval between the two sessions: 7 days, N = 32 (male subjects).

Scales of adjective check list	Raw scores		Delta-corrected changes
	pre-drug	post-drug	(post-drug/pre-drug)
Performance oriented activity	.62	.80	.41
Desactivation	.29	.68	.33
Extraversion/ introversion	.24	.56	.45
General well-being	.63	.79	.36
Aggressiveness	.35	.65	-.14
Anxiousness	.02	.09	-.14

It is possible that for other drugs different results might have been
obtained. For chlordiazepoxide Shader and co-workers (1972) report
that the emotional responses were very consistent when measured twice,
one week apart.

2.2.3 Generalizability of drug response.
Any theory which seeks to explain drug response variability has to
take into consideration to what extent the drug response is limited
to the specific conditions or may be generalized to other conditions,
e.g. to other drugs, situations, and response measures.

The kind of range of generalizability will determine basic features
of the theory, in particular the breadth and the psychological or
physiological orientation.

Generalizability of susceptibility to drugs can be differentiated with
respect to situations, response measures, and drugs. Table 4 illustrates the most important aspects.

The most simple questions with regard to the generalizability of susceptibility to drugs are directed to the consistency of response over
situations and dependent variables.

TABLE 4   Generalizability of Response to Psychotropic Drugs

Consistency with regard to:	Kind of consistency
1a Different drugs within a drug class (e.g. diazepam vs. oxazepam)	Intra-drug type consistency
1b Different drugs belonging to different drug classes	Inter-drug type consistency
- with same directions of effects	
- with different directions of effects	
- with qualitatively different effects	
2 Different situations	Situational consistency
- same classes (e.g. noise of low and high intensity)	
- different classes (e.g. stimulating vs. monotonous)	
3 Different response measures	Drug response measure consistency
- relating to the same constructs (e.g. emotional tension measured by objective or subjective devices)	
- relating to different constructs (e.g. activity, emotional stability)	

Generalizability of drug response over different situations. The first question cannot be answered at the present time since no empirical data are available. Thus, it remains to be seen if drug effects have any situational consistency. From the few analyses of variance with two situations (stress and non-stress) available, there appears to be significant interaction between situations and subjects and thus only low situational consistency.

Generalizability of drug response over different response measures. The second question - concerning the generalizability of response measures to drugs - can be partly answered: Correlational analysis of change measures usually reveals that there are several factors involved. All these data involve the difficulty of the low reliabilities of difference scores (drug minus placebo). Thus, any conclusions about the drug response generalizability must be preliminary.

With respect to the consistency of response measures relating to different constructs it appears necessary to differentiate susceptibilities regarding the activation and the hedonic (pleasure) dimensions. Regarding the generalizability of drug effects using different methods assessing the same construct (e.g. emotional tension) strong dissociations have been reported several times. The dissociations which have been found most frequently refer to objective versus subjective measures.

Consistency of drug response over different drugs. The next series of questions concerning the generalizability of drug response is more crucial than that put forward above. What are the findings regarding the generalizability of drug response if we consider different drugs, whether they belong to the same or different drug class?

Dependent on the size of the correlations between the different kind of drugs, the question of a trait susceptibility to drugs has to be answered.

The data available to answer this question leave much to be desired. Only a few studies seem to have investigated these fundamentally important questions.

Kornetsky and his group reported low to moderate consistency for global performance decrements and subjective symptoms of activation and desactivation for several drug conditions. The consistency was obtained for different dose levels of one drug, for drugs within a given drug class (depressants: secobarbital, chlorpromazine), and for drugs belonging to different classes (dextroamphetamine vs. chlorpromazine) (Kornetsky, Humphries and Evarts, 1957; Kornetsky and Humphries, 1957; Kornetsky and Mirsky, cited after Kornetsky, 1960). Kornetsky concluded that his findings relating to different drugs of the same class support the hypothesis that a responder to one drug is also a responder to others. Comparing the change scores for stimulants and depressants, he stated: "Although the correlation is not high it was in the predicted direction, suggesting that the intrinsic variable or variables that account for responsivity to drugs is the same for both depressants and stimulants." (Kornetsky, 1960, p. 311).

Since Kornetsky's statements are based only on findings with 8 to 12 subjects, we tried to replicate them with more subjects. The drugs used in our studies were from four classes: Stimulants, neuroleptics, tranquilizers and hypnotics. For each class, one typical drug was selected and given at two dose levels with the exception of the tranquilizers. The drugs were given in counterbalanced order to 32 unselected subjects in two experiments. The bases of the correlations were standardized difference scores, drug minus placebo (z-scores).

Table 5 shows the results for the different types of consistencies, e.g. referring to different levels of one drug, to different drugs all belonging to the group of psycholeptics, to drugs having stimulating or depressing properties.

The directions of almost all correlations are as expected: The highest correlations were found between the dose levels of the same drug and between tranquilizers and neuroleptics in low doses. Negative or zero correlations were obtained between stimulants and depressants. This suggests that subjects who responded strongly to stimulants responded strongly to depressants, but in the opposite direction. In sum, the data only partially support Kornetsky's statement of a general responde

TABLE 5 Generalizability of Drug Response under Various Conditions (Data: Janke, 1974)
N = 32; r.05 = .34; r.01 = .44

	Inter-dose level			Intra-drug class				Inter-drug class				
	Stimulant low/high dose	Depressant low/high dose	Neuroleptic low/high dose	Neuroleptic/Depressant low dose	Neuroleptic/Depressant high dose	Neuroleptic/Tranquilizer low dose	Tranquilizer/Depressant low dose	Stimulant/Depressant low dose	Stimulant/Depressant high dose	Stimulant/Neuroleptic low dose	Stimulant/Neuroleptic high dose	Stimulant/Tranquilizer low dose
Exp. I												
subjective performance	.23	.15	.62	.26	.11	.26	.57	-.37	.13	-.29	-.28	-.19
objective performance	.36	.34	.49	.22	.33	.37	.16	-.16	-.33	.14	-.39	.03
Exp. II												
subjective performance	.44	.24	.52	.11	.40	.56	.07	-.22	-.32	-.40	-.41	-.18
hand steadiness	.48	.52	.43	.45	.44	.53	.47	-.31	-.10	-.35	-.41	-.43
motor coordination	.35	.64	.32	.05	.16	.62	.07	-.25	-.08	-.60	-.08	-.45
Mean r	.37	.38	.48	.22	.29	.47	.27	-.26	-.14	-.30	-.31	-.24

Stimulant low dose respectively high dose : Methylphenidate 20 mg respectively 40 mg
Tranquilizer low dose : Meprobamate 400 mg
Neuroleptic low dose respectively high dose : Promazine 50 mg respectively 75 mg
Depressant low dose respectively high dose : Heptabarbital 200 mg respectively 400 mg

2.2.4 <u>The causes of differential susceptibilities to drugs.</u>
Differential psychopharmacology has shown that the causes for individual susceptibility to psychotropic drugs may be found in quite different factors. Only one group of these factors involves behavioral
or somatic <u>traits</u>.

In summary, empirical data show that <u>individual susceptibilities</u> to
drugs may be caused by one or more of the following factors:
(1) Congenital biochemical individuality factors
(2) Acquired somatic factors such as drug tolerance and drug dependence
(3) Developmental and age-related factors
(4) Behavioral factors

<u>Congenital biochemical individuality factors</u> which may lead to strong,
weak or paradoxical drug responses can be inferred from several sources
of empirical data. One example is <u>extreme responses</u>. Such extreme responses are exemplified by adverse reactions to barbiturates, anti-
convulsants or MAO-inhibitors. For each class of drugs the reasons for
these extreme reactions are deficits of specific enzymatic processes
(see the chapter by Netter, this volume): (1) MAO inhibitors like
phenelzine and isoniazid produce adverse reactions in those individuals which have reduced activity of an inactivating enzyme (N-acetyl-
transferase). (2) The anticonvulsant diphenylhydantoine is metabolized
insufficiently in some persons. This leads to continuous accumulation
of the unmetabolized drug and toxic symptoms (Omenn and Motulsky, 1975).

It should be noted that the metabolic factors which are responsible
for extreme responses are usually very specific. This means that they
might have no relationship to larger behaviorally relevant systems or
to other drugs.

A second example for biochemical individuality comes from <u>genetic</u>
studies. Evidently, drug susceptibility may be genetically determined
(for details see Netter; Russell, this volume).

The empirical data on the influence of genetic factors are almost exclusively limited to animal and clinical data. Only a few papers deal
with experimental studies in normal subjects (Omenn and Motulsky,
1975). These papers show that genetic factors pay an important role
at least in the determination of plasma levels of antidepressant drugs
(e.g. Alexanderson and others, 1969; Omenn and Motulsky, 1975).

Also the sedation threshold of normal subjects was reported to be
heavily dependent on heredity. Claridge and Ross (1973) compared 11
monozygotic and 10 dizygotic twins. It was found for amobarbital that
9 monozygotic twins had very similar thresholds (difference 1 mg/kg)
and only 2 pairs had a larger difference. In the group of dizygotic
twins, 8 pairs, however, had larger differences and only 2 pairs had
threshold differences of 1 mg/kg body weight.

Very important are those findings which show that certain enzymes
which might be regarded as indicators of sympathetic reactivity are
genetically determined. One of these enzymes is responsible for the
last step in noradrenaline synthesis (dopamine-beta-hydroxylase)
(Omenn and Motulsky, 1975, p. 200).

<u>Acquired biochemical individualities</u> maybe involved in individual sus-
ceptibilities to drugs in different areas. The most important example

of biochemical individuality can be seen after chronic drug administration as in the case of drug tolerance and drug dependence. Such
biochemical individuality may develop during all life periods, mainly
during prenatal life and early childhood (see Russell, this volume).

Developmental and age-related factors: A huge set of empirical data
which shows that drug susceptibility may be biologically determined
comes from studies of developmental biochemistry. During infancy and
aging many deviations from middle-age people have been described which
result in drug response differences (e.g. reduced binding of plasma
 proteins in children, reduced inactivation of barbiturates)(see
Netter; Russell, this volume).

Behavioral factors which are usually the result of an environmental
genetic interaction are listed in the last position not because they
are of minor importance or because they contribute to a lesser degree
to the explanation of drug response variability.The reason for the
listing position is the high degree of complexity of their influences
on drug response.

Whatever the "origin" of individual susceptibilities may be, two questions arise which seem to be important: (1) The specifity of the somatic basis of individual susceptiblities,and (2) the range of the
susceptibilities which are due to neuro-physiological and neurochemical
factors.

The first point refers to the question whether observed susceptibility
to specific drugs is the result of very specific neurochemical processes or whether they arise from more general physiological processes
mainly in the CNS and ANS.

While it is safe to state that there are huge individual differences
in the biochemical and physiological reactivity, it is just as true
that we do not know which differences in which physiological and biochemical subsystems are responsible for inter-individual drug differences. Thus, we have to admit that we do not know if and to what
extent somatically based differences are due to peripheral or central
or to specific or general factors. A thorough discussion of some important problems can be found in Netter's chapter (this volume).

The second critical question relates to the range of the susceptibilities for which somatic factors can be made responsible. Most biochemical, genetic and developmental discussions refer to extreme drug
responses. It remains unclear, however, if the whole range of responses
can be related to individual reactivities of neurochemical and neurophysiological systems.

IV. INTER-INDIVIDUAL DRUG RESPONSE TO BEHAVIOR TRAITS
     AND STATES

1. General Remarks

It has always been assumed that at least a part of the intersubject
variance in drug response is the result of psychological, neuro-physiological or neurochemical characteristics of the individual. The
importance of neurochemical and neuro-physiological variables as me-
diators is said to follow from the mechanisms of the drug actions.

48 W. Janke

The importance of psychological factors is derived from (1) their correlation with somatic processes, and (2) the influence of evaluation and coping strategies on the final drug responses.

The two main approaches to behavioral processes on drug response modifiers refer to traits on the one hand and to states on the other. In Table 2 (see Section III) a listing of traits and states, both on the somatic and behavioral level which have been investigated by several experiments, was given. Bearing the just discussed low stabilities and consistencies in mind, it may be immediately evident that the probability to discover a strong relationship between traits and drug response is low. Until now, however, the trait approach has been dominant in psychopharmacological research.

In the next sections some basic findings on the interactions between drug response and behavioral traits and states will be discussed. Somatic traits and states are omitted in the discussion because Netter (this volume) has reviewed this topic.

2. Behavior Traits as Predictors of Drug Response

2.1 Broad Traits as Predictors of Drug Response
More than 20 years ago Hans-Jürgen Eysenck (1957) proposed his drug postulate which stated a relationship between extraversion/introversion and response to drugs. This drug postulate has attracted many researches who have investigated the relationship between drug response and personality because it was based on a physiological theory of personality. Many confusing results of drug studies seemed to be explainable by the drug postulate. Since H. J. Eysenck describes his approach in a chapter of this volume the details will be omitted. The most important parts of Eysenck's theory (1957, 1963, 1967) are:
(1) There are antagonistic processes within the CNS, excitation and inhibition.
(2) Excitation and inhibition are inferred from behavioral processes observed at different levels, e.g. experimental phenomena such as after-image duration, behavioral traits, and attitudes.
(3) Extraversion/introversion is the expression of the excitation/inhibition balance. Eysenck assumes that high degrees of extraversion are found in people in whom inhibitory processes occur quickly, strongly and persistently, while excitatory processes occur slowly, weakly, and non-persistently. High degrees of introversion are found in people in whom the reverse is true.
(4) Drugs belonging to the stimulant class increase excitation and therefore have introverting effects, while depressants increase inhibition and therefore have extraverting effects.

The "drug postulate" has been investigated by Eysenck and many others in a number of experiments. In most of these experiments barbiturates (mainly phenobarbital and amobarbital) were used as depressant drugs. As stimulants, most investigators administered amphetamines. A considerable number of experiments showed results which have been predicted from the drug postulate. In some cases the predictions could not be verified. Evidently, however, the predictions may be improved by taking the test situation into account (Eysenck 1973; this volume). When this is done some of the critical arguments proposed by Janke (1964) or Legewie (1968) may be of minor importance.

Quite independently from Eysenck's thinking three other psychopharmacology groups began to study the drug-personality interactions. All
three groups did not start from a universal personality theory but
more from some occasional observations in psychopharmacological or
clinical studies. Kornetsky at Harvard (1957) correlated the response
to secobarbital, meperidin, chlorpromazine and LSD with four scales
of the MMPI. The results seemed to show that high psychastenia and
depression was related to higher drug response scores (Kornetsky and
Humphries, 1957).

The second group is the Boston group. As early as 1958 DiMascio and
his group in Boston published a paper on the dependency of the response to a tranquilizer (phenyltoloxamine) on a typological dichotomy
which relates to the orientation towards activity or passivity (DiMascio
and others, 1958). The typological dichotomy used is based on the belief that people react with coping processes when they perceive the
drug-induced changes. In the case where a drug has deactivating properties, it has a different meaning for the action-oriented and non-
action-oriented subjects. It is assumed that action-oriented people
may react with paradoxical excitement because they feel threatened
by the deactivation which may involve a breakdown of major defenses.

An important feature of DiMascio's model is that it takes into account
coping processes according to specific motivational structures. This
approach has been chosen by several investigators (Janke, 1964; Sarwer-
Foner, 1959, 1970; Lindemann and Felsinger, 1961; Bellak and others,
1968). A second important feature is the emphasis of the concept action-
orientation itself. The importance follows from the fact that on the
one hand, the most prevailing and unequivocal behavioral effects of
all drugs are variations on the activation dimensions. On the other
hand, these variations are evidently related to important motivational
constructs. The importance of activity variations is at least apparent
in normal subjects.

As large as the heuristic value of the model of DiMascio and co-workers
(1958) may be, there are severe difficulties: (1) The definition of
the personality types is very unclear. There is no clear set of tests
for measuring these types as they have been defined. The action-oriented
people seem to be extraverted non-neurotics whereas the non-action-
oriented people may be regarded as introverted neurotics. (2) The number of studies is small. Positive findings are exclusively from DiMascio
and his group. Other research groups have reported negative findings
several times (e.g. McDonald, 1967). The weakness of the approach used
has evidently been recognized by DiMascio himself because in the middle
60's he switched to the concept of emotional lability or anxiety as
defined by Taylor's manifest anxiety scale (DiMascio and Barrett,
1965).

Emotional lability, therefore, is the third concept which has been
studied beginning in the second half of the 1950's. In 1957, I began
to investigate the effects of neuroticism on all important types of
drugs. The first preliminary results were published in 1959 and in
a monograph in 1964. The experiments by Janke (1964) showed that neuroticism excerted a strong influence on drug response.

Generally speaking, the most important findings seem to be (for a more
extensive review see Janke and Debus, 1968; Janke and others, 1979):

(1) Higher magnitude of drug response was obtained in subjects with high neuroticism scores (emotionally labile subjects). This is particularly true for the magnitude of <u>performance</u> impairment by larger doses of sedating drugs or stimulants. But also with regard to <u>activation</u> dimension as measured by self-reports, interactions between neuroticism and drug response magnitude were observed: Emotionally labile subjects demonstrated more activation with stimulants and more de-activation with higher doses of sedative drugs.

(2) Drug effects on emotional responses - defined by scaling of subjective responses and semi-projective techniques - were different in emotionally labile and stable subjects for most drug conditions. The differences between the two personality groups were quantitative (intensity of response) as well as qualitative (direction of response) depending on the type of drug and situation.

(3) The most impressing results of all our experiments were that the quantity and quality of the relationship between neuroticism and drug response were not fixed (consistent). There was a change according to the drug type, to the dose level, to the situation in which the drug was administered and to the kind of dependent variable.

The three constructs - extraversion/introversion, action-orientation, neuroticism have been investigated in a number of experiments during the last 20 years. The most important findings have been extensively reviewed by Janke, Debus and Longo (1979).

The main features by which the research on the meaning of these constructs may be described are:

(1) There is a sufficient number of experiments which demonstrate the importance of extraversion/introversion and neuroticism, but only a very small number for action-orientation.

(2) The dependent variables in the extraversion/introversion experiments were almost exclusively performance measures. The drugs preferred are <u>stimulants</u> and <u>sedatives</u>. This use, which follows from Eysenck's theory and his preference for objective tests, seems to be important because these variables may not be sensitive for demonstrating the effects of some other drug types (tranquilizers). In investigating the effects of <u>neuroticism</u>, most experiments have used <u>tranquilizers</u>. Moreover, the batteries were used with specific stress on the measurement of emotional tension or anxiety-frequently subjective reports.

(3) Summarizing the whole set of findings on the role of the three <u>broad traits</u> under consideration, we conclude that the results are altogether disappointing because very often no or very complex relationship have been found. All three constructs have only moderate predictive power, evidently.

The lack of sufficient predictive power should give us cause to think of other possibilities for explaining variability of responses to drugs Such possibilities are (1) to take narrow and specific response traits or (2) to take a multivariate approach by combining traits with multiple regression methods or by taking a pattern approach, and (3) to abandon the trait approach and use states as predictors of drug respons All these alternative possibilities will be discussed in the next section.

2.2 Specific (Narrow) Traits as Predictors of Drug Response

It might be suspected from theoretical reasons that specific (narrow) traits such as anxiety, attitudes towards drugs, or expectation of specific effects, would lead to better predictions of drug response than broad traits.

Those specific traits which have been investigated so far refer to (1) anxiety and stress reactivity, (2) suggestibility, (3) experience with specific drugs (drug experience), and (4) attitudes towards drugs.

Altogether the number of studies with specific traits is too small to draw any conclusions about their predictive value (for a review see Janke and others, 1979). For this reason, Boucsein and Janke (1974) carried out a study with a great number of specific and broad predictors. The data of this experiment which are relevant in this context are discussed in the chapter by Boucsein (this volume).

From the multivariate statistical treatment which was carried out by Boucsein the conclusion can be drawn that specific predictors may have much higher predictive value for specific criterion measures than broad traits. The drug applied was 25 mg promethazine, a highly sedating antihistaminic drug. The drug was administered to 22 normal subjects under noise condition and to another group of 22 subjects under non-noise condition. The drug-placebo differences were correlated with a set of predictor variables, including scales for measuring neuroticism, extraversion, and more specific traits (e.g. mental activity, anxiety, phobic tendencies). In a stepwise multiple correlation procedure, the best set of predictors was found out for each situation for measures of performance and subjective activity.

Interestingly, several of the best predictors referred to rather specific or narrow traits. For the subjective reaction to the drug, neuroticism and extraversion were not the best predictors. Thus, it might be concluded that further studies have to be carried out with broad and narrow traits in order to confirm or disprove the preliminary findings on this question.

2.3 Combination of Traits by Multivariate Techniques

Many studies have been carried out in pharmacotherapy for predicting therapeutic change by multivariate techniques, usually by multiple regression techniques. Most research has been concerned with antidepressants and tranquilizers, and to a lesser degree, with neuroleptics. The best known are the contributions by Rickels and Wittenborn (for reviews and monographs see May and Wittenborn (1969), May and Goldberg (1978), Rickels (1968, 1978), Wittenborn and May (1966)). This approach is neatly illustrated by Wittenborn (this volume).

With normal subjects, the multiple regression approach has been used to a lesser extent. As an example, the study discussed by Boucsein (this volume) mentioned before may be used in order to illustrate some possibilities and limitations of the approach. The multiple approach seems to be promising. Multiple prediction was markedly better than prediction of criterion variance by any single predictor. However, it is to be expected that the findings are not replicable. This was evident in many clinical studies. Moreover, the findings, of Boucsein showed that it is necessary to find different predictor systems for different criteria and situations. Boucsein's findings demonstrated that the contribution of a predictor changes with the criterion

to be predicted and with the situation in which the drug is applied.
For each criterion and each situation the set of optimal predictors
was different. This is not the result of the multiple regression techniques. It can be seen immediately by inspecting the single-order correlations.

We can conclude from the multiple predictions approach that the inclusion of more than one trait may improve the prediction but in turn
hinders the generalizability of predictor systems.

Quite another approach, which may be more promising is to take patterns
of traits into consideration. One of the most promising pattern is
Eysenck's (neuroticism and extraversion/introversion). The importance
of taking both into consideration (extraversion and neuroticism) is
emphasized in particular by Claridge (1967) for the sedation threshold
(see also the chapter by Claridge, this volume). Also, response to
other drugs could be predicted better by the extraversion-neuroticism
pattern than by single traits, e.g. for nitrous oxyde (Rodnight and
Gooch, 1963) or for methyl pentinol (Bartholomew and Marley, 1957).
However, Rodnight and Gooch's study has only 23 subjects which makes
statistical treatment impossible.

2.4 Problems in Explaining Drug Response Variability by Long-Term Personality Characteristics (Traits)

The results which have been collected over the past 20 years on the
importance of the concepts investigated have been altogether disappointing. We can conclude the following with respect to the predictive power of traits: Whether we use a univariate or multivariate
approach, there is practically no possibility to explain drug response
variability by using personality characteristics. In the section to
follow, I will try to sketch the arguments against traits as efficient
predictors of drug response.

2.4.1 The problem of traits as independent variables.

Traits are concepts which can be varied only by selection and not by
experimental manipulation. Many - if not all - studies which try to
assert that a certain trait is a predictor are not matched with regard to other personality traits. Moreover, when selecting groups with
specific personality traits, allowance has to be made for the possibility that factors which are only peripheral but which correlate with
personality traits, are the critical variables which are responsible
for the covariation. Examples of this might be differences in eating
behavior between neurotics and non-neurotics which lead to higher
drug levels in the CNS. It must always be considered that many behav-
iorly correlated peripheral factors might explain drug response differences to a considerable degree.

2.4.2 Level of trait description.

Most experiments have been directed towards broad traits on the type
level in the sense of Eysenck. It is not clear if this is a bad or
a good strategy. On the one hand, broad traits are related to physiological constructs more than most specific traits. On the other hand,
some findings show that very specific traits are good predictors, e.g.
attitudes (see Boucsein, this volume). As Revelle (Revelle and others,
1980) has shown, extraversion/introversion may have different predictive
validities for the two components impulsivity and sociability. On the
other hand, some studies found that the predictability of drug respons

did not improve when very specific predictors were used (e.g. Debus and Janke, 1980; Pillard and Fisher, 1975).

2.4.3 Missing neurochemical foundations of traits.
Most, if not all, behavior traits cannot yet be expressed within an empirically based neurophysiological or neurochemical system. The system proposed by Eysenck, though physiologically oriented, cannot be put easily into neurophysiological or neurochemical terms which can be measured. The system is more a conceptual than a physiological one. This holds true for the systems which have been proposed by other authors.

From the reported low and non-replicable correlations on behavioral traits, and all kinds of physiological or biochemical data it might be concluded that at the present time we are not yet able to relate traits in a satisfactory manner to physiological and biochemical processes. The postulate of such a relationship, however, seems necessary for drug-personality interactions if we want to explain them by biological models and not psychodynamical (e.g. coping) models.

2.4.4 Traits are not invariant predictors of drug response.
As was indicated by findings mentioned earlier, trait predictors have no fixed role. The predictive value of them changes according to many factors. Three of them shall be sketched.
(1) The dependence on the situation in which the drug is administered.
(2) The dependence on the predictive value from the dose level of the drug.
(3) The dependence on the kind of response measure.

2.4.4.1 The predictive value of traits and the situation. Since the revival of the concept that the variation of behavior should be explained to a great extent by the interaction between subjects and situations, many psychopharmacological findings seem quite obvious and understandable. Apparently, the relationship between traits and drug response is not independent of the situation in which the drug is given. The empirical data which show these second order interactions, however, are not very convincing.

Both for the trait "neuroticism" and "extraversion/introversion" some findings are available. The first study to be mentioned with regard to neuroticism shows that the kind of tasks which have to be performed during the drug action may influence the relationship between neuroticism and emotional effects of tranquilizers (Janke, 1964). The study was the following one: Sixteen emotionally labile and 16 stable subjects were tested under low work load conditions 1 - 2 hours after taking the neuroleptic promazine (50 mg). Low work load conditions were defined by tasks which demanded only low mental exertion. In a second experiment carried out with the same number of subjects the same drug was given under high work load conditions. The following figure illustrates that emotionally labile subjects reported reduced "excitation" in an excitation scale under conditions of low work load. Stable subjects show the reverse findings.

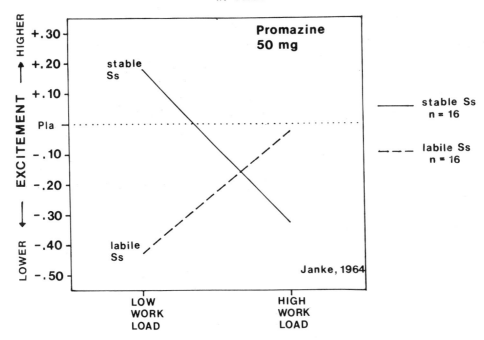

Fig. 1.   Effects of 50 mg promazine in two different con-
          ditions on self-reported excitement of 16 emotionally
          stable and 16 emotionally labile subjects (Janke, 1964).

The next finding is based on several experiments carried out by
Revelle (Revelle and others, 1980).
Figure 2 shows the effects of caffeine in the morning and the evening
on cognitive performance in high impulsive and low impulsive subjects.

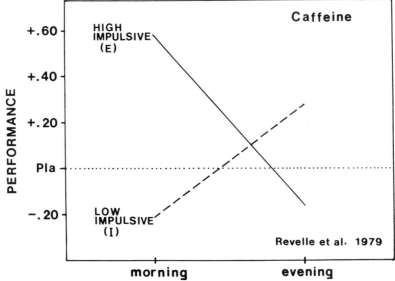

Fig. 2.   Changes of cognitive performance under caffeine
          in high and low impulsives (Revelle and others, 1980).

A clear interaction can be seen in Fig. 2. Positive effects in impulsives in comparison to negative effects in non-impulsives can be seen only in the morning. When caffeine is administered in the evening, the reverse is true.

The findings of both studies do not allow definitive conclusions. Paradoxically, a review of all the literature available does not reveal investigations which have definitely proved that the relationship between personality traits and drug response changes with the situation. Thus, the empirical evidence for the statement that drugs and personality traits have no fixed relationship is small and based mostly on the fact that many measures were not able to replicate the reported covariation. It is possible that the reason for this is that long-lasting characteristics of the traits show no or little relationship to drug response.

In this context, Eysenck's consideration of the dependence of the hedonic tone of mood from extraversion/introversion and level of stimulation are of interest in the relationship to the effects of nicotine (Eysenck, 1973; Eysenck, this volume).

2.4.4.2 The predictive value of traits and dose levels. The relationship between drug response and personality traits is essentially dependent on the dose level. With increasing dose levels of a barbiturate, differences between labile and stable subjects became, however, lower in studies by Janke (1964). Ideström and Schalling (1970), however, reported much more severe performance impairments of labile subjects in comparison to stable subjects with 300 mg amobarbital. With 150 mg amobarbital only few drug personality interactions occurred.

From some findings with extreme doses, it seems possible to conclude that there is curvilinear relationship between dose level and interindividual drug response variability, caused by personality traits. With very high doses some people react extremely insensitively and other highly sensitively.

2.4.4.3 The predictive value of traits and kind of response measures. One of the most embarrassing aspects with drug modifying factors results from the fact that any interactions between drug response and person or situation parameters are not the same with different dependent variables. In all multivariate studies which reported interactions, this was not indicated by all variables to a similar degree. Evidence for this type of higher order interaction (personality x situation x variable) was found for both personality traits and situational factors.
Usually the most pronounced interactions can be found in those variables which have a high sensitivity to drugs. For tranquilizing and sedating drugs these are self-reported mood variables and psychomotor tests (see McNair, 1973). For other drug types, it is unclear.

One example may illustrate the dependency of the relationship between drug response and neuroticism on the variables measured: Neuroticism interacted with drug response in 3 experiments in which a stimulant (methylphenidate, 400 mg), one tranquilizing (meprobamate), one neuroleptic drug (promazine, 50 and 70 mg), and one hypnotic drug (heptabarbital, 200 and 400 mg) were applied to the following percentages of variables: Motor performance (40%), subjective variables in high work load conditions (45%), subjective variables in low work load conditions (40%) and non-motor performance (27%).

The influence of the dimension <u>extraversion-introversion</u> on the response in different variables is unclear because performance variables
have been used, exclusively.

For the dimension <u>action-orientation</u>, the same conclusion as for neuroticism is possible: The prevailing influence of this trait is on
subjective variables.
It should not be concluded from the data on neuroticism and activation
that only subjective and motor variables reveal large drug response
variability depending on personality traits.

Surprisingly, several experiments in which attitudes and expectations
of the subjects were manipulated showed that performance and physiological variables were very sensitive in showing drug response differences. These experiments were carried out mainly with alcohol (for a
review see Marlatt and Rohsenow, 1980; Marlatt, 1976).

3. States as Predictors of Drug Response

3.1 General Remarks
The changing predictive validity and the shift of drug effects when
situational characteristics change, leads to the idea that psychological states would be better predictors than traits. But not only empirical findings support this idea. One of the most reasonable assumptions
is that the amount of change which might be induced by a drug is direct
ly dependent on the initial level and quality of the neurophysiological
and neurochemical systems upon which the drug acts. This assumption is
usually explicit or implicit in all drug-personality studies.

Figure 3 shows a model of drug response which illustrates that the
direct mediator of drug response is according to our view the present
behavioral and somatic state (Janke and others, 1979).

<u>Long-term</u> individual characteristics are principally only indirectly
related to drug response by the way they influence the state. This
behavioral, neurophysiological, and neurochemical state. This means
that only in the case where there is a direct relationship between a
personality trait (e.g. anxiousness) and state (e.g. anxiety) can we
find a substantial correlation between drug response and traits.
This, however, has to be expected only at some times and in certain
situations, which follows from the definition of a state.
According to Fig. 3, the present state determines a primary drug response. This response, however, is not the observed one. The reason
for this are "coping mechanisms" by which the drug response may be
changed in intensity or direction.
After coping mechanisms have done their job, the final drug response
may be measured. The kind of coping processes is probably influenced
by personality traits. However, it is not very likely that the coping
processes are influenced to a large degree by traits. It is more
probable that momentary situational characteristics and individual
states exert influence on coping processes. Examples of this influence
of the coping processes are found in experiments in which the momentary cognitive set is manipulated by instruction or experimental variations.

As it can also be seen from Fig. 3, <u>situational</u> and <u>environmental</u>
factors exert their influences on drug responses <u>indirectly</u> by in-

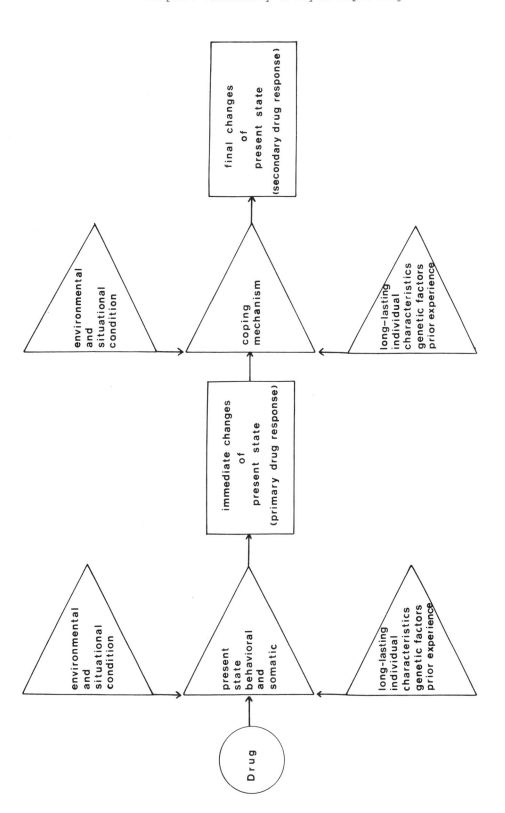

Fig. 3.   Model of drug response variation by individual characteristics and environmental factors.

fluencing the present state. Their roles as drug modifiers can be
understood best in terms of the psychophysiological changes induced
by them. This means that the essential modifiers of drug response
are the states and not the environmental and situational factors themselves. Compared to traits, environmental and situational factors as
predictors of drug response have the advantage that they refer to the
present state. The problem, however, is that they are defined on the
distal level and not on the organismic level.

A characterization of environmental and situational factors in purely
semantical or physical terms thus involves the problem that we do not
know whether they have really those effects on the individual which
we expect they have.
It seems likely that many studies reporting interactions between drug
response and environmental and situational factors could not be replicated because they defined their independent variables only on the
distal level - that is in physical or semantical terms.
An additional definition on the proximal, that is organismic level,
would have explained differences between studies with differing results for the same set of environmental and situational factors. The
problem of the experimentation with environmental and situational
conditions in psychopharmacology is thoroughly discussed by Krüger
(1981, this volume).

3.2 Relationship between States and Drug Response
Table 6 (see next page) lists states which have been discussed or investigated in the past and methods to induce them.
The characteristics which have been studied most frequently in the
past are the broad qualities emotional tension, general activation
and fatigue and a few specific emotional and motivational qualities
such as pain, anxiety and fear, anger, euphoria and depression,
dysphoria, need for arousal, hunger, frustration and conflict. Moreover, specific cognitive attributes have been induced, e.g. drug expectation, perception of side effects, etc.

The results of many studies show that most of these state variations
led to changes in drug response (for a summary see Janke and others,
1979; Debus and Janke, 1980).
This has been shown predominantly for stress and anxiety. A number
of experiments carried out within the Düsseldorf psychopharmacology
team (Janke, Debus, Boucsein, Lehmann, Erdmann, Stoll) have shown
that subjects in high arousal state(by high intensity intermittent
or continuous white noise) responded to depressant drugs with an increase of self-reported emotional stability. Subjects not stressed
did not respond at all or even with a decrease of stability.

TABLE 6 Frequently Used Behavioral States for Predicting Drug Response

	Induced State	Inducing Method
Emotional	Stress, emotional tension	High intensity noise, especially discontinuous noise
	Anxiety and fear	Threat of pain inducing stimuli, medical manipulation, physical danger (e.g. disasters), or anxiety provoking stimuli (e.g. animals, ferris wheel); anticipation of ego-threatening situations (e.g. examination, public speaking)
	Pain	Electric, thermal or chemical stimulation, postoperative states
	Frustration	Interruption of tasks
	Conflict	Confrontation with tasks or goals which are incompatible
	Anger	Offending or insulting the subject because of specific actions
	Elation, euphoria	Telling jokes, inducing funny situations (e.g. by stooges)
	Depression	Repeated presentation of unsolvable tasks
	Dysphoria	
Motivational	General activation	Any arousal inducing set of stimuli
	Fatigue	Presenting tasks with high work load
	Need for arousal	Presenting highly monotonous tasks or situations
	Hunger	Food deprivation
Cognitive	Expectation of strong drug effect	Giving information about the intensity of expected drug effects
	Stimulant, depressant or tranquilizer drug expectation	Giving information about the expected direction of drug effects (stimulant, depressant, tranquilizer)
	Expectation or perception of side effects	Giving information or cues for expected side effects

TABLE 7   Effects of Tranquilizing and Sedating Drugs in
9 Experiments with Stressed or Unstressed Subjects
(All Studies from Janke's Research Group)

Drug	Dose	Results of self-report of emotional lability		Author
		stressed subjects	unstressed subjects	
Chlordiazepoxide	10 mg	0	0	Dietsch, 1967
Diazepam	5 mg	0		Boucsein, 1976
Ethchlorvynol	250 mg	-	0/+	Janke and Glathe, 1964
Homofenazine	3 mg	-	0	Stoll, 1968
Homofenazine	6 mg	-	0	Stoll, 1968
Meprobamate	400 mg	-		Dietsch, 1967
Oxazepam	10 mg	-/0	0/+	Janke and Stoll, 1965
Oxazepam	20 mg	-/0	0/+	Janke and Stoll, 1965
Promethazine	25 mg	0	0	Boucsein and Janke, 1974

0 : no significant effects
- : significant reduction of emotional tension
+ : significant increase of emotional tension

Table 7 shows the results of nine experiments. Stressed subjects responded in half of the experiments in the expected direction, unstressed subjects, however, did not reveal this tendency. Quite on the contrary, three experiments showed a paradoxical increase of emotional
lability after administration of tranquilizing agents.

As an example for more specific states as predictors of drug response,
we may take anxiety. In a number of experiments it could be demonstrate
that the drug response differed greatly for subjects who were in the
state of anxiety than non-anxiety. However, several experiments failed
to find the expected results (for a summary see Debus and Janke, 1980).

3.3 Predictive Power of States Compared to that of Traits
Now, the question arises: Are states, as suggested, really better
predictors than traits?
Direct comparisons between the predictive power of traits and states
are usually not possible because of the lack of equivalent measurement techniques. An exception is perhaps state and trait emotional
tension. Some findings with respect to emotional tension shall be reported.

TABLE 8   Effects of Depressant Drugs on Emotional Tension
          in Subjects Differing with Regard to Their
          Emotional Tension

| | | | Drug effect | | |
			Relaxation	No Change	Tension
Emotional lability of subjects	High	Trait	8 (0.5)	7 (0.4)	1 (0.1)
		State	9 (0.6)	6 (0.4)	1 (0.1)
	Low	Trait	0 (0.0)	9 (0.6)	7 (0.4)
		State	3 (0.2)	8 (0.5)	5 (0.3)

The table shows the number of studies (in parenthesis for the percentage) which yielded the effects mentioned at the top of the
table.

In order to be able to make more or less direct comparisons between
the power of traits and states for predicting drug response, we counted the results of 16 studies which used trait measures of emotional
lability or similar constructs (mainly anxiety) and of 16 studies
which involved emotional tension as state. Table 8 shows that about
half of the studies revealed the expected reduction of emotional
tension with high emotional tension subjects whether conceived as
trait or as state. In contrast to these findings, subjects with low
emotional tension do not show any reduction or relaxation and in a
third to almost half of the studies, there is even an increase in
tension.

The conclusion to be drawn from this literature review is that traits
are not necessarily worse predictors than states. However, the state
was defined in some experiments only by the experimental conditions
and not by a real assessment of state before the experiment. In particular, with the state of anxiety many methodological and basic
problems in its assessment are involved (e.g., response sets).

It is likely that with other concepts, such as activity, the predicted
superiority of states would emerge. The reasons for this assumption
stems from many experiments which showed that the response to drugs
differed according to the present state of activity.

V. CONCLUSION

The overview of findings and problems in explaining drug response
variability by psychological factors was intended to illustrate that
at the present time we have to face more problems which are unsolved
than solved.
The many psychopharmacological studies which yielded significant interactions between drug response and behavioral and somatic variables
reveal that the interpretation of response variability to psychotropic
drugs is highly complex and that a simple prediction of the individual
reaction to a drug is impossible. It is our hope that in the future
new empirical data and theoretical analysis will be available which
will enable solutions for at least some of the problems which have
been sketched in this paper.

REFERENCES

Alexanderson, B., D. A. P. Evans, and F. Sjöquist (1969). Steady-state
    plasma levels of nortriptyline in twins: influence of genetic fac-
    tors and drug therapy. Br. Med. J.,4, 764-768.
Bartholomew, A. A., and E. Marley (1959). Susceptibility to methylpen-
    tinol: personality and other variables. J. Ment. Sci., 105, 955-970.
Bellak, L., M. Hurvich, M. Silvan, and D. Jacobs (1968). Toward an ego
    psychological appraisal of drug effects. Am. J. Psychiatry, 125,
    593-604.
Boucsein, W. (1976). Experimentalpsychologische Untersuchung zur Wir-
    kung von Tranquilizern (Diazepam und einer Prüfsubstanz) unter Be-
    rücksichtigung von Persönlichkeitsmerkmalen. Arzneim.-Forsch. (Drug
    Res.), 26, 28-31.
Boucsein, W. (1981). Multiple prediction of reactions to a psychotro-
    pic drug (promethazine) by personality traits. In W. Janke (Ed.),
    Response Variability to Psychotropic Drugs. Pergamon Press, Oxford.
Boucsein, W., and W. Janke (1974). Experimentalpsychologische Untersu-
    chungen zur Wirkung von Propiramfumarat und Promethazin unter Nor-
    mal- und Stressbedingungen. Arzneim.-Forsch. (Drug Res.), 24, 675-
    693.
Claridge, G. (1967). Personality and Arousal. Pergamon Press, Oxford.
Claridge, G. (1981). Sedation threshold and personality differences.
    In W. Janke (Ed.), Response Variability to Psychotropic Drugs.
    Pergamon Press, Oxford.
Claridge, G., and E. Ross (1973). Sedative tolerance in twins. In
    G. Claridge, S. Canter, and W. I. Hume (Eds.), Personality Differ-
    ences and Biological Variations. Pergamon Press, Oxford. pp. 115-
    131.
Debus, G., and W. Janke (1978). Psychologische Aspekte der Psychophar-
    makotherapie. In L. J. Pongratz (Ed.), Handbuch der Psychologie,
    Vol. 8/2. Hogrefe, Göttingen. pp. 2161-2227.
Debus, G., and W. Janke (1980). Methods and methodological considera-
    tions in measuring antianxiety effects of tranquilizing drugs.
    Progr. Neuro-Psychopharmacol., 4, 391-404.
Dietsch, P. (1967). Der Einfluss verschiedener Situationen auf die
    Wirkung von Psychopharmaka. Unpubl. Diss., Gießen.
DiMascio, A., and J. Barrett (1965). Comparison effects of oxazepam
    in "high" and "low" anxious student volunteers. Psychosomatics, 6,
    298-302.
DiMascio, A., G. L. Klerman, M. Rinkel, M. Greenblatt, and J. Brown
    (1958). Psychophysiologic evaluation of phenyltoloxamine, a new

phrenotropic agent. Am. J. Psychiatry, 115, 301-317.

Evans, W. O. (1970). Interaction of factors in the external environment upon the actions of psychotropic drugs in humans. Fed. Proc., 29, 1994-1999.

Eysenck, H. J. (1957). Drugs and personality: I. Theory and methodology. J. Ment. Sci., 103, 119-131.

Eysenck, H. J. (1963). Personality and drug effects. In H. J. Eysenck (Ed.), Experiments with Drugs. Pergamon Press, Oxford. pp. 1-24.

Eysenck, H. J. (1967). Personality and drugs. In H. J. Eysenck (Ed.), The Biological Basis of Personality. Thomas, Springfield. pp. 263-318.

Eysenck, H. J. (1973). Personality and the maintenance of the smoking habit. In W. Dunn (Ed.), Smoking Behavior. Winston, Washington. pp. 113-146.

Eysenck, H. J. (1981). Psychopharmacology and Personality. In W. Janke (Ed.), Response Variability to Psychotropic Drugs. Pergamon Press, Oxford.

Fisher, S. (1970). Nonspecific factors as determinants of behavioral response to drugs. In A. DiMascio, and R. I. Shader (Eds.), Clinical Handbook of Psychopharmacology. Science House, New York. pp. 17-39.

Holliday, A. R., and W. J. Devery (1961). Effects of drugs on the performance of a task by fatigued subjects. Clin. Pharmacol. Ther., 3, 5-15.

Ideström, C.-M., and D. Schalling (1970). Objective effects of dexamphetamine and amobarbital and their relations to psychasthenic personality traits. Psychopharmacologia, 17, 399-413.

Janke, W. (1964). Experimentelle Untersuchungen zur Abhängigkeit der Wirkung psychotroper Substanzen von Persönlichkeitsmerkmalen. Akad. Verlagsgesellschaft, Frankfurt.

Janke, W., and M. Amelang (1965). Untersuchungen zur psychischen Wirkung eines zentralen Stimulans nach verschiedenen Graden psychischer Beanspruchunge. Psychol. Forsch., 28, 562-586.

Janke, W., and G. Debus (1968). Experimental studies on antianxiety agents with normal subjects: Methodological considerations and review of the main effects. In O. Efron, J. Cole, J. R. Lewine, and J. R. Wittenborn (Eds.), Psychopharmacology. A Review of Progress 1957-1967. U.S. Government Printing Office, Washington. pp. 205-230.

Janke, W., and G. Debus (1978). Die Eigenschaftswörterliste (EWL). Hogrefe, Göttingen.

Janke, W., and H. Glathe (1964). Experimentelle Untersuchungen zur psychischen Wirkung von Sedativa unter Normal- und Belastungsbedingungen. Psychol. Forsch., 27, 377-402.

Janke, W., and P. Netter (1981). Zur Wirkung von Psychopharmaka nach einmaliger und mehrmaliger Verabreichung: Ein Beitrag zur Problematik pharmakopsychologischer Akutversuche. In L. Tent (Ed.), Erkennen, Wollen, Handeln. Hogrefe, Göttingen. pp. 404-423.

Janke, W., and K.D. Stoll (1965). Untersuchungen zur Wirkung eines Tranquilizers auf emotional labile Personen unter verschiedenen Versuchsbedingungen. Arzneim.-Forsch., 15, 366-374.

Janke, W., G. Debus, and N. Longo (1979). Differential psychopharmacology of tranquilizing and sedating drugs. In Modern Problems of Pharmacopsychiatry, Vol. 14. Basel, Karger. pp. 13-98.

Karniol, I. G., J. Dalton, M. H. Lader (1978). Acute and chronic effects of lithium chloride on physiological and psychological measures in normals. Psychopharmacology, 57, 289-294.

Kornetsky, C. (1960). Alterations in psychomotor functions and individual differences in responses produced by psychoactive drugs. In L. Uhr., and J. G. Miller (Eds.), Drugs and Behavior. Wiley, New York. pp. 297-312.

Kornetsky, C., and O. Humphries (1957). Relationship between effects
    of a number of centrally acting drugs and personality. Arch. Neurol.
    Psychiat., 77, 325-327.
Kornetsky, C., O. Humphries, and E. V. Evarts (1957). Comparison of
    psychological effects of certain centrally acting drugs in man.
    Arch. Neurol. Psychiat., 77, 318-324.
Krüger, H.P. (1981). Differentielle Pharmakopsychologie ohne differen-
    tielle Psychologie? In W. Janke (Ed.), Beiträge zur Methodik in der
    differentiellen, diagnostischen und klinischen Psychologie. Hain,
    Meisenheim.
Krüger, H.P. (1981). What differentiates a differential psychology?
    In W. Janke (Ed.), Response Variability to Psychotropic Drugs.
    Pergamon Press, Oxford.
Legewie, H. (1968). Persönlichkeitstheorie und Psychopharmaka. Hain,
    Meisenheim.
Lindemann, E., and J. M. v. Felsinger (1961). Drug effects and person-
    ality theory. Psychopharmacologia, 2, 69-92.
Marlatt, G. A. (1976). Alcohol, stress, and cognitive control. In I.G.
    Sarason, and C. D. Spielberger (Eds.), Stress and Anxiety, Vol. 3.
    Hemisphere Publ. Co., Washington. pp. 271-296.
Marlatt, G. A., and D. J. Rohsenow (1980). Cognitive processes in al-
    cohol use: Expectancy and the balanced placebo design. In N. K.
    Mello (Ed.), Advances in Substance Abuse. JAI Press, Greenwich.
May, P. R. A., and S. C. Goldberg (1978). Prediction of schizophrenic
    patients' response to pharmacotherapy. In M. A. Lipton, A. DiMascio,
    and K. F. Killam (Eds.), Psychopharmacology. Raven Press, New York.
    pp. 1139-1153.
May, P. R. A., and J. R. Wittenborn (Eds.) (1969). Psychotropic Drug
    Response. Thomas, Springfield.
McDonald, R. L. (1967). The effects of personality type on drug re-
    sponse. Arch. Gen. Psychiat., 17, 680-686.
McNair, D. M. (1973). Antianxiety drugs and human performance. Arch.
    Gen. Psychiat., 29, 611-615.
Netter, P. (1981). Somatic factors as predictors of psychotropic drug
    response. In W. Janke (Ed.), Response Variability to Psychotropic
    Drugs. Pergamon Press, Oxford.
Netter, K.J., and P. Netter (1981). Pharmacokinetic factors: Some basic
    principles and their influence on psychotropic drug response. In
    W. Janke (Ed.), Response Variability to Psychotropic Drugs. Pergamon
    Press, Oxford.
Omenn, G. S., and A. G. Motulsky (1975). Pharmacogenetics: Clinical
    and experimental studies in man. In B. E. Eleftheriou (Ed.), Psycho-
    pharmacogenetics. Plenum Press, New York. pp. 183-228.
Pillard, R. C., and S. Fisher (1975). Chlordiazepoxide and phenobarbi-
    tal in a model anxiety-inducing situation. Compr. Psychiatry, 16,
    97-101.
Revelle, W., M. S. Humphreys, L. Simon, K. Gilliland (1980). The inter-
    active effect of personality, time of day, and caffeine: A test of
    the arousal model. J. Exp. Psychol. (Gen.), 109, 1-32.
Rickels, K. (1968). Non-specific Factors in Drug Therapy. Thomas,
    Springfield.
Rickels, K. (1978). Use of antianxiety agents in anxious outpatients.
    Psychopharmacology, 58, 1-17.
Rodnight, E., and R. N. Gooch (1963). A new method for the determina-
    tion of individual differences in susceptibility. In H. J. Eysenck
    (Ed.), Experiments with Drugs. Pergamon Press, Oxford. pp. 169-193.
Russell, R. W. (1981). Genetic and early environmental factors in re-
    sponse variability to psychotropic drugs. In W. Janke (Ed.), Respon
    Variability to Psychotropic Drugs. Pergamon Press, Oxford.

Sarwer-Foner, G. (1959). Theoretical aspects of the mode of action of the tranquilizing drugs in schizophrenia. In N. Kline (Ed.), Psycho-pharmacology Frontiers. Little, Brown & Co., Boston.
Sarwer-Foner, G. (1970). Psychodynamics of psychotropic medication - An overview. In A. DiMascio, and R. I. Shader (Eds.), Clinical Hand-book of Psychopharmacology. Science House, New York. pp. 161-182.
Shader, R. I., A. DiMascio, and J. S. Harmatz (1972). Single versus repeated dosage of the minor tranquilizer chlordiazepoxide. Am. J. Psychiat., 128, 126-127.
Stoll, K. D. (1968). Tranquilantien-Reaktionen unter variierten Bean-spruchungs- und Belastungsbedingungen. Unpubl. Diss., Gießen.
Wittenborn, J. R., and P. R. A. May (Eds.) (1966). Prediction of Re-sponse to Pharmacotherapy. Thomas, Springfield.
Wittenborn, J. R. (1981). Relationships between personality and phar-macotherapeutic responses among depressed patients. In W. Janke (Ed.), Response Variability to Psychotropic Drugs. Pergamon Press, Oxford.
Yehuda, S. (1976). The influence of behavioral and environmental fac-tors on drug effects. In D. I. Mostofsky (Ed.), Behavior Control and Modification of Psychological Activity. Prentice-Hall, Englewood. pp. 297-313.

SOMATIC FACTORS AS PREDICTORS OF PSYCHOTROPIC DRUG RESPONSE

Petra Netter

ABSTRACT

The main somatic factors contributing to variation in psychotropic drug response are 1) genetic influences - partly linked to race, 2) age, 3) sex, 4) body build and related pre-drug physiological states, 5) influences of additional pharmacologically active compounds, pretreatment and disease. The contribution lists examples for each of these factors the emphasis being placed on studies investigating behavioral effects in healthy humans, but with an endeavour to relate results to underlying pharmacokinetic processes and to psychiatric observations and laboratory research.

A genetic influence on drug action could be demonstrated by examples from family and twin studies as well as from population and race studies yielding evidence for differences in behavioral effects caused by single genes or by polygenic control of kinetic parameters and receptor sensitivity. The studies were grouped according to the level of dependent variables from gross behavioral to metabolic parameters.

Age effects can be shown with respect to the greater sensitivity in the developing as well as in the aging organism, the former being largely due to incomplete development of the enzyme system, the latter resulting from a general principle of slowing processes that comprise all types of kinetic parameters, but higher as well as lower receptor sensitivities.

Sex differences are reported for various psychotropic drugs, females being frequently more affected than males due to slower metabolism which may be linked to the inhibiting influence of female sex hormones. On the other hand many drug studies show pronounced drug by sex interactions pointing to drug dependent different mechanisms of facilitation of sex effects.

Body build: Some studies also reveal influences of body build with respect to tolerance for alcohol or reaction to stimulants, eurymorphs being less impaired in performance and andromorphs feeling more stimulated by fenetylline.

<u>Drug interaction</u>: Intake of additional drugs as well as caffeine, nico-
tine and alcohol may change response to psychotropic drugs. A main
source of this effect is the induction of drug metabolism by some compounds but also competition at the receptor or interaction with enzymes
at the receptor site. These may result in an enhancement or reduction
of psychotropic drug response. Changes of response after chronic treatment can also partly be explained by enzyme induction or by a decrease
in receptor sensitivity. Renal and liver diseases are additional factors
accounting for increased response largely by slowing down metabolism
and excretion of drugs.

        KEYWORDS

Somatic factors; genetic factors; age; sex; race; physical constitution; drug interaction; pre-drug physiological state; disease.

    1. INTRODUCTION

The object of this contribution is to compile some of the results in
the psychopharmacological literature demonstrating the influence of
somatic factors of subjects on interindividual differences in drug
response.

In clinical studies the nature and severity of disease, of course, was
acknowledged to be one of the most important somatic factors responsible
for variation in drug response. Differences in reaction to psychotropic
drugs served as a tool to define subtypes of diseases as it was the
case with different types of depression (Pare and Mack, 1971; Raskin
and others, 1974). Furthermore, pre-therapeutic symptomatology was investigated with respect to its predictive value for therapeutic outcome (Cole and others, 1968; Galbrecht and Klett, 1968; Klett and
Moseley, 1965).

Since this contribution, however, is mainly concerned with observations
in healthy humans, studies performed on psychiatric patients and laboratory animals will not be referred to in detail and may only occasion-
ally be mentioned briefly for comparison, if required (for a discussion
of work carried out with animals see Russell, this volume).
Studies in non-psychiatric samples that take somatic factors into
account are comparatively rare. One reason for this may be that many
somatic factors are rarely accessible by therapeutic intervention, if
they turn out to produce unfavourable effects in the subject.

Another reason presumably originates from the difficulty to trace the
physiological or biochemical substrates of an observable difference in
response between groups of different sex, age, body build, or ethnic
origin. Furthermore, most of the somatic factors are highly confounded
with one another as well as with behavioral variables which can emerge
as causes or consequences of the somatic factors, and which can by
themselves lead to additional physiological conditions such as those
produced by dietary, smoking, and drinking habits (for the discussion
of behavioral variables see Janke, this volume).

If we try to list somatic factors that have been investigated with
respect to drug response in non-psychiatric samples, we may come to
the following network of interrelated sources of variance (Fig. 1),

from which - for reasons of simplification - the behavioral variables
involved have been excluded.

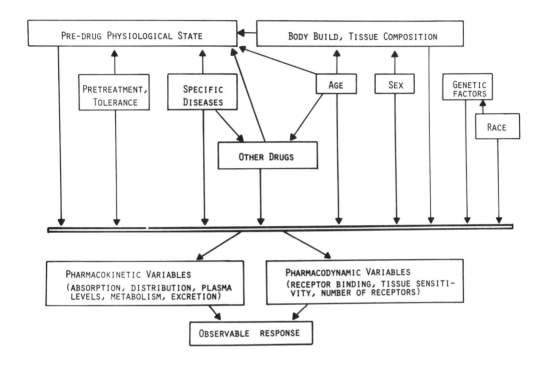

Fig. 1.   Somatic factors influencing drug response and their
           interrelations. The link between these factors and the
           observable response may be pharmacokinetic as well as
           pharmacodynamic in nature.

All of these factors may either interact with pharmacokinetic or with
pharmacodynamic steps of the route which a drug takes through the organism. Whereas in most cases pharmacokinetic changes can be identified by some direct or indirect measurement, changes of drug-receptor
interactions can hardly be detected in the human. Thus, in many studies
drug reactions which are found different as a consequence of one of
the factors listed above are not explained by underlying pharmacological mechanisms.

The differences to be discussed will be confined to observable symptoms
and behavior responses rather than to pharmacokinetic findings which
have been presented in a previous chapter and which, as could be demonstrated, do not always turn out as reliable predictors of behavioral drug response.

2. GENETIC FACTORS AND ETHNIC DIFFERENCES

2.1 Types of Gene Action and Approaches to the Study of Genetic Influence

Genetic factors may influence drug effects in three different ways:
by affecting drug disposition, pharmacodynamic drug action and liabi-
lity to self-medication (Kalow and Le Blanc, 1975).
While the last aspect can be studied separately (Eriksson, 1975), pharmacokinetic and pharmacodynamic effects of a drug may result in the
same changes of behavior or symptomatology which, therefore, can frequently not be traced back to their specific underlying mechanisms.
The possibility to identify the specific underlying mechanism of drug
response varies with type and specificity of gene action, number of
genes involved and type of response considered (which again depends
on choice of subjects or species). Figure 2 illustrates different levels of operation of genetic influence and the types of responses
yielding access to the study of genetic factors involved in drug action.

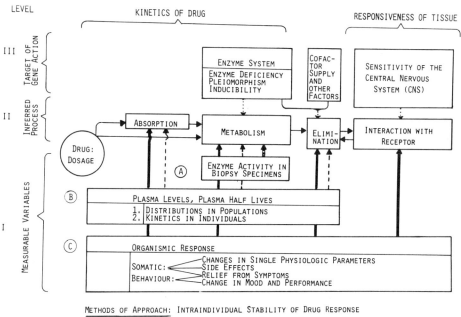

Fig. 2.   Levels of inference in research on genetic factors in
          psychopharmacology. The blocks A, B, C at the level of
          measurable variables (level I) cover that range of
          processes on level II and targets of gene action on
          level III which may be inferred from them.
          ➡ = inferences to be drawn from organismic response variables
          ---➤ = inferences to be drawn from kinetic parameters
          ➡ = inferences to be drawn from in vitro studies on metabolism
          ⟶ = chronological sequence
          ·····➤ = causal relationship

It becomes evident that gross organismic response, the reaction in
which psychologists are predominantly interested, can be due to many
different factors which bar inference to the underlying genetic origin.
On the other hand, the closer the level of observable variables to the
underlying physiological cause the less it seems related to psychology.
Genetic sources of both kinetic and somatic or behavioral response may
be studied by intraindividually repeated measurements, by selective
breeding or twin and kinship studies or by comparisons of different
groups of populations.

2.2 Approaches Using Organismic Response (Type C Variables in Fig. 2) for Pharmacogenetic Inference

Although genetic control of behavior has been widely studied in psychology, psychological differences in drug response have rarely been at-
tacked in the field of psychology.
It must be emphasized, however, that any experiment using type C variables as the only source of inference cannot decide whether observed
differences are due to genetic variation in metabolism or in physiological endowment of the target organ.

2.2.1 Intrafamily comparisons.
One well-known example of genetic inference from drug behavior similarity in humans is the result obtained by Glass (1954) when studying
the effect of caffeine on improvement in a target aiming task (throwing a needle into a series of small rings drawn on paper) in two identical twin boys. Consecutive performance scores of both boys obtained
after five cups of coffee and control conditions are depicted in
Fig. 3.

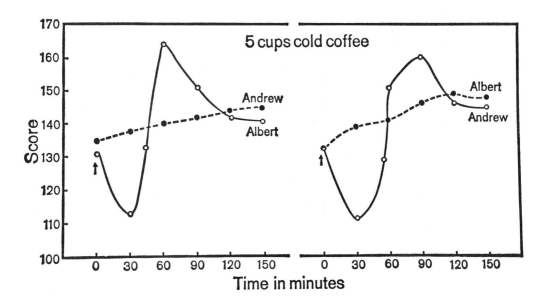

Fig. 3.   Effect of caffeine on the performance task of
          target-aiming in a pair of identical twins.
          o + solid lines = after 5 cups of coffee
          ● + dotted lines = under no-drug conditions

Of course, the results would need to be contrasted with those of a control group of non-related persons or fraternal twins in order to confirm that the characteristic sinus curve of performance obtained with caffeine is specific for these twins and not specific for caffeine in general. But also twin studies comparing the sedation threshold for amobarbital in mono- and dizygotic twins arrive at very much higher intrapair similarities for monozygotic than for dizygotic twins (Claridge and Ross, 1973).

An example of inference on genetic control of response to psychotropic drugs by studying kinship similarities is given by a study by Angst (1964) who observed that relatives of depressed patients suffering from the same disease as the patient himself tend to show response or nonresponse to the same drugs as the patient.

Corresponding results have been obtained in animal studies using selective breeding to demonstrate genetic control of tolerance to alcohol as measured by the impairment of motor activity (Worsham and others, 1977).

2.2.2   Intergroup comparisons.
Populations or groups differing in drug response may either be defined by empirically observed clusters of the drug response itself or by other "genetic markers" such as race. An example of the first approach is given in a study of Ahrens (1971), who recorded EEG patterns after alcohol consumption in healthy subjects and was able to classify three groups: a) bioelectrically indifferent subjects, b) those responding by increase in theta waves, and c) those with a generally very sensitive EEG response with respect to various parameters.

Ethnic and race differences in drug response have frequently been used for establishing evidence of genetic influence (Omenn and Motulsky, 1975; Propping and Kopun, 1973). Many studies, of course, are performed on patients and thus mostly evaluate differences in response to psychiatric treatment, such as improvement in schizophrenics after phenothiazines (Cole and others, 1968; Goldberg and others, 1966; Holden and others, 1971), in groups of black and white depressed patients after antidepressants (Raskin and Crook, 1975), or in neurotic outpatients after anxiolytics (Downing and Rickels, 1974). In some studies, however, differences in response were also evident upon placebo treatment (Cole and others, 1968; Goldberg and others, 1966) indicating racial differences in perception of symptom change or influence of expectations rather than of genetic reactivity to drugs.
Behavioral differences between black and white healthy subjects have been reported for reactions to amphetamine in an experiment by Hubin and Servais (1966). Negroes showed more improvement in performance tasks in which learning was possible, whereas performance of white subjects was not improved by amphetamine. The law of initial values, however, may have been operating in these results, since the black subjects had lower performance levels than the whites under control conditions.

Further evidence for genetic control of drug action is derived from observations of differences in tolerance to alcohol in different ethnic groups.
Thus Wolff (1972) compared samples of Caucasoid, Japanese, Taiwanese, and Korean adults and infants with respect to reactions of flushing

and increases in optical density of the ear lobe upon intake of comparable amounts of alcohol. The mongoloid groups all showed higher in-
tensities of the autonomic responses than the Caucasians. Similar results are reported by Ewing and others (1973) who included heart rate
and subjective scores of discomfort (dizziness, weakness, and sleepi-
ness) when comparing alcohol effects in Caucasian and oriental groups,
and obtained more severe effects both in the physiological and self
report responses in the oriental groups. This corresponds well with
observations reported by the police that North American Indians and
Eskimos usually require a longer time to sober up after an alcoholic
debauch (Fenna and others, 1971).

Strain differences in animals have also been shown to contribute considerably to variation in drug response (Bovet and others, 1966;
Petrinovich, 1967; Russell, this volume), and the type of gene action
has been elucidated by this approach. Thus for instance amphetamine
effects on learning have been identified to be controlled polygenically
whereas effects of scopolamine and chlorpromazine on activity have
been shown to be determined by single gene loci (Elias and Pentz, 1975).

Also in humans the mode of action of genes can be inferred from the
type of distribution in response. Since these studies, however, mostly use kinetic parameters, they shall be referred to in the next
section.

2.3   Approaches Using Pharmacokinetic Parameters (Type B Variables in Fig. 2) for Pharmacogenetic Inference

Efforts to establish evidence for genetic influence on drug kinetics
have been more successful than those trying to elucidate intraindividual response variability due to differences in the CNS (Propping and
Kopun, 1973). As previously mentioned in the chapter on pharmacokinetic factors in this volume, plasma levels and plasma half lives of a
number of drugs have been shown to be determined to a considerable
extent by genetic factors as demonstrated e.g. by twin studies
(Alexanderson and others, 1969; Curry and Marshall, 1968; Vesell,
1972; Vesell, 1974; Vesell and others, 1971) and by studies demonstrating intraindividual stability in the elimination rates of the same
drug upon repeated application (Sjöquist and others, 1971; Vesell,
1973). Most of these investigations, however, have not related organismic response(type C variables) to the kinetic parameters.

2.3.1   Studies relating kinetic parameters to organismic response.
As outlined in the chapter on factors responsible for kinetic variation, genetic differences may be due to single gene effects or may be
polygenically controlled (Kalow, 1975; Propping and Kopun, 1973).
Single gene effects may be discovered by a bimodal distribution of
response or plasma concentration in a given population (LaDu, 1974)
representing deficiency or polymorphism of a specific drug metabolis-
ing enzyme. The consequence frequently is that within a normal therapeutic dose adverse reactions will be observed such as acute or chronic
toxicity, side effects, ineffectiveness of the drug, or unexpected
metabolites causing unexpected clinical symptoms (LaDu, 1974).

Numerous examples of enzyme deficiencies or pleimorphisms as discovered by adverse reactions to drugs in various populations are listed in

reviews on pharmacogenetics (Fuller and Hansult, 1975; Goedde, 1974; Motulsky, 1957; Vogel and Motulsky, 1979, p. 259). The two best known examples of genetic polymorphism relevant for psychotropic drug meta- bolism are a) the slow and rapid type of N-acetyl-transferase (Evans and White, 1964) and b) the typical and atypical alcohol dehydrogenase (Edwards and Evans, 1967) the latter of which is distributed to about 5 - 20% in Caucasians, but to an extent of 85% in the Japanese popula- tion (Propping and Kopun, 1973).

The rapid and slow types of N-acetyl-transferase were discovered among others by higher incidences of severe side effects on phenelzine in a number of subjects in psychiatric populations, the enzyme subtypes were then identified by differences in plasma half lives of isoniazid, hydralazine, and phenelzine in experimental studies, and their genetic origin was confirmed by correlations between plasma half lives of phenylbutazone in parents and their off-spring in family studies (Evans, 1971).

Correspondance between acetylator phenotype and clinical response, however, is not very convincing. Application of the MAO inhibitor phenelzine to depressed patients in a study by Evans and others (1965) yielded more side effects in slow acetylators than in rapid ones and no difference in recovery rates, whereas the same drug applied to neu- rotic depressed patients by Johnstone and Marsh (1973) revealed no difference in side effects but higher response rates in slow acetyla- tors (acetylation rates being determined by plasma half lives).

The two types of alcohol dehydrogenase differ in pH-optimum (the a- typical enzyme showing a severalfold higher in vitro activity at pH 8.8 (Omenn and Motulsky, 1975)). Efforts to relate the two types of alcohol dehydrogenase to the ethnic differences in response to al- cohol mentioned above (Wolff, 1972; Ewing and others, 1973; Fenna and others, 1971) left some unsolved puzzles which emerged, when Fenna and co-workers (1971) studied rate of decline and rate of metabolism of intravenously injected alcohol in Eskimos, Indians and Whites. They found significantly lower rates of elimination and metabolism (as cal- culated from kinetic parameters) in both Eskimos and Indians as com- pared to Whites. This difference was also maintained, when influence of previous consumption of ethanol and type of diet were controlled as sources of bias. The results correspond well with the observed physiological responses of the subjects, but they cannot be reconciled with the presence of atypical dehydrogenase since this would rather imply more rapid elimination rates in Eskimos and Indians.

2.3.2 Studies relating kinetic parameters to in vitro studies.
It is of course rare that liver biopsy samples can be obtained in humans for studying metabolism in vivo in order to relate it to somatic or behavior response.
An effort to relate ethanol elimination rates to genotype of liver alcohol dehydrogenase was undertaken by Edwards and Evans (1967). They could not demonstrate correlations between type of dehydrogenase and elimination rates of ethanol in healthy subjects. The reason for this given by Kalow (1975) is that the rate of ethanol metabolism is governed by the cofactor supply and not by the enzyme.
The examples mentioned served the general purpose to demonstrate how in pharmacogenetics the drug serves as a diagnostic tool for detecting underlying genetic differences in physiological dispositions of the individual.

3. THE INFLUENCE OF AGE

Responses to drugs in adult individuals differ from those in young
ones as well as from those in geriatric populations.

3.1 Differences Between Young and Adult Individuals

Studies trying to relate change of response to drugs from neonatal to
adult life suffer from the difficulty that behavioral parameters can
hardly be compared in newborns, children and adults. Most information
on this subject matter therefore is derived from clinical observations,
studies in animals and biochemical and pharmacokinetic work on both
animals and humans.

Paradoxical effects of drugs are said to be more frequent in the developing as well as in the aging organism (Irwin, 1964). The most
striking evidence of difference in response between children and adults
is frequently claimed to be the decrease in activity by stimulant drugs
like methylphenidate observed in children suffering from minimal brain
dysfunction. But as Wender (1978) points out, the major action of stimulants, an increase in alertness and concentration, is essentially
the same in children as in adults. This was also confirmed in healthy
boys aged 6-12 (Rapoport and others, 1978): They showed significant
improvement in memory, reaction time and cognitive tests accompanied
by a reduced motor activity when treated with 0.5 mg/kg dextroamphetamine.
The emotional changes, however, may be perceived differently, since
the children's repertoire of experience is less differentiated than
it is in adults' life.
Although a few studies report changing psychopharmacological response
with growing age in childhood, as for instance hallucinations upon
LSD-25 in older children and amphetamine-like stimulation in younger
ones (Bender, 1962), on the whole, response and side effects in psychiatric treatment of children according to Engelhardt and Polizos (1978)
are grossly similar to those of adults.

The more rapid onset of response to psychoactive drugs in children as
compared to adults can be explained by higher rates of absorption,
lower protein binding and faster excretion rates which have been described in 7-10 year old children for imipramine (Winsberg and others,
1974) and for nortriptyline in 5-12 year olds (Morselli, 1977). Also
theophylline reached lower plasma concentrations in 2-12 year old
children as described by Grygiel and Birkett (1980).
There is, however, more dramatic change from the early postnatal period to childhood. This refers to delayed effects of drugs applied at
different postnatal periods as well as to immediate clinical response.
An example of the first principle is given by an increase in motor
activity observed in adult rats that had been treated with 6-hydroxy-
dopamine and desmethylimipramine between days 3 and 14 of life, an
effect which was not observed if treated on days 20 or 23 of age
(Erinoff and others, 1979).
Deviant immediate clinical drug responses particularly emerge as toxic
effects in newborns whose mothers have been treated with antidepressants or benzodiazepines (Morselli, 1977). This can be explained by
the reduced oxidative capacity of the liver enzymes in neonates (Hänninen, 1975) which at birth has been found to be only 1/3 of that in
the adult human (Klinger, 1977).

3.2 Differences Between Adult Life and Old Age

Table 1 presents a number of studies which yield evidence that behavioral and somatic responses to psychotropic drugs seem to be more pronounced in older subjects than in younger ones, no matter, whether the drugs applied were barbiturates, morphine or benzodiazepines and whether response was measured by sleeping time, self ratings on pain, mood, sleep quality, or symptoms of hangover or by psychomotor tasks. These results correspond well with clinical findings from psychiatric samples that older patients develop more side effects upon a variety of neuroleptic and antidepressant drugs (Bech and others, 1979; O'Malley and others, 1980; Stevenson, 1973). Further evidence comes from results of studies on animals which report for instance that older rats show lower body temperatures after chlorpromazine (Saunders and others, 1974) and perazine (Fähndrich and Hadass, 1969) and higher body temperatures (Rommelspacher and others, 1972) as well as higher activity levels (Saunders and others, 1974; Ziem and others, 1970) after amphetamine which also seemed to last longer than in young rats (Ziem and others, 1970) in spite of lower concentrations reaching the brain (Honecker and Coper, 1975). Furthermore, longer sleeping times were observed after barbiturates in old rats (Kuhlmann and others, 1970) as well as lower doses of hexobarbital required to obtain the silent second in EEG measurements (Saunders and others, 1974) and higher vocalisation thresholds according to electric current intensity after application of morphine (Saunders and others, 1974). When trying to relate these findings to underlying causes it must be kept in mind that responsiveness to drugs in old age can be due to a) changes in drug disposition, b) altered tissue responsiveness, c) reduced responsiveness of homeostatic principles, d) concurrent influences of disease states and e) changes in body composition (O'Malley and others, 1980).

The findings reported above can most readily be reconciled with experimental evidence of changes in pharmacokinetics in the elderly: While drug absorption seems to be little affected by age (O'Malley and others, 1980), there are many investigations reporting age related changes in volumes of distribution with resulting increases in plasma half lives, reduced protein binding due to reduced albumin plasma levels with increasing age, slower drug metabolism and a decrease in renal clearance in the elderly (reviewed by Conney and others, 1974; Hayes and others, 1975; O'Malley and others, 1980; Turner, 1978). Table 2 lists some of these pharmacokinetic results obtained with pethidine, some benzodiazepines, antipyrine and amylobarbitone in humans. It has to be kept in mind, however, that the drug hits an organism which is also physiologically changed by age itself. Thus, the second source of variance contributing to different response of the aging organism may be due to changes in neurotransmitter contents in different brain regions (Carlsson, 1980), such as decreases of dopamine, 3-methoxytyramine and noradrenaline and an increase in monoamineoxydase as measured in human autopsy samples of the brain.

Further changes on the tissue level, like decreased glucose utilization, decreased content of cerebral lipids and proteins as well as a decreased rate of incorporation of precursors and an increased rate of protein degradation (Domino and others, 1978) may also contribute to an age dependent change in response to drugs. Although these data seem to be hard to reconcile with an increased behavioral or somatic response (since they would rather suggest a reduced capacity of the

TABLE 1   Studies investigating the influence of age on behaviour and somatic response

Authors, Year	Groups of Subjects (n)	Age in Years	Drugs (Dose, Application, Duration)	Dependent Variables	Results	Statistical Evaluation
Oduah, 1969	preoperative patients (20 young, 30 old)	$\bar{x}$ = 29.6 $\bar{x}$ = 63.9	thiopental (4.5 mg/kg i.v. single dose)	1. duration of sleep 2. plasma levels	1. longer in old group 2. higher in old group 15-240 min. post inject.	descriptive
Kohnen and others, 1979	healthy volunteers (8 per group)	old, young	pentobarbital (100 mg) promazine (25 mg) combination (125 mg) placebo (all orally, crossover, 1 day each)	1. self reports on sleep quality, indicators of 2. hangover	1. old ss.: better sleep with separate and combined drugs young ss.: unaffected 2. old ss.: no hangover after separate drugs, feeling better after combined young ss.: no effect	Friedman rank analysis of var.
Belville and others, 1971	postoperative patients from 5 hospitals (712)	<30 up to >80	morphine (10 mg) pentazocine (20 mg) combin. (30 mg) (single trials)	differences in self ratings on pain intensity from first predrug pain level	Increased relief with increasing age between 40 and 80 years for both drugs; inverse relationship between 30 and 40 years	stepwise regression
Kalko, 1980	postoperative cancer patients (947)	18-29 30-49 50-69 70-89	morphine (8 mg} i.m. 16 mg} single trial)	1. pain relief 2. duration of relief	1. Increase with age 2. Increase with age	analysis of variance
Reidenberg and others, 1978	patients being prepared for cardioversion (23)	31-90	diazepam (i.v. titration single trial)	1. dose 2. plasma level } necessary for nonresponse to vocal stimuli with response to pain stimuli retained	1. negative correlation with age 2. negative correlation with age	correlation, regression
Salzmann and others, 1975	male volunteers (40)	60-68 >68	diazepam (12 mg, orally, 2 weeks)	1. self ratings: anxiety 2. self ratings: sedation 3. self ratings: fatigue 4. memory test	1. higher decrease in younger subjects 2. no effect 3. higher increase in older subjects 4. higher decrease in younger subjects	t-test correlation with age
Castleden and others, 1977	healthy subjects (15 each group)	<40 >69	nitrazepam (10 mg orally, 3 successive trials crossover with 3 placebo nights)	1. plasma half life 2. sleep quality, hangover 3. psychomotor test a) no. of mistakes b) total time	1. no difference 2. no difference 3. a) placebo - active drug difference greater in old ss. b) no difference	analysis of variance

TABLE 2 Studies Investigating the Influence of Age on Pharmacokinetic Parameters

Authors, Year	Groups of Subjects (n)	Age in years	Drugs (Dose, Application, Duration)	Dependent Variables	Results	Statistical Evaluation
Ilsalo and others, 1977	healthy volunteers (25) patients (12)	21-38 66-89	nitrazepam (5 mg orally, single dose)	1. peak concentration 2. volume of distribution 3. plasma half lives	1. lower in old group 2. higher in old group 3. longer in old group	t-test
Kangas and others, 1979	healthy volunteers (36) geriatric patients (22)	18-38 66-89	nitrazepam (5 mg orally, single dose and chronic (16 days))	1. peak concentration 2. volume of distribution 3. plasma half lives	1. lower in old group 2. higher in old group 3. longer in old group	t-test
Klotz and others, 1975	normal volunteers (33) patients with liver disease (21)	15-83	diazepam (0,1 mg/kg i.v. 10 mg orally, single dose)	1. plasma half lives 2. plasma clearance 3. plasma binding	1. increase with age 2. no effect 3. no effect	correlation
Chan and others, 1975	preoperative patients young (7) old (10)	< 40 > 70	pethidine (1,5 mg/kg u.m.)	1. urinary excretion 2. plasma and red cell concentration	1. higher excretion of parent compound in younger group 2. higher levels in older group	descriptive
Liddle and others, 1975	normal adults (26 per group)	20-40, geriatric	antipyrine (10 mg/kg orally, single dose)	1. plasma half lives 2. volumes of distribution	1. old: longer 2. only elderly females lower than the rest	t-test
O'Malley and others, 1971	geriatric patients (19) healthy controls (61)	> 70 20-50	antipyrine phenylbutazone (single trials each)	plasma half lives	old: longer half lives	t-test
Irvine and others, 1974	healthy males (8 per group)	< 40, > 65	amylobarbitone (200 mg, orally, single dose)	1. plasma levels 2. urine metabolites	1. older subj.: higher levels 2. older subj.: lower quantity	t-test

brain for neuronal information processing), theories of age related hypersensitivity of receptors are discussed concurrently with those of hyposensitivity of receptors (Storrie and Eisdorfer, 1978).

4. SEX DIFFERENCES

Findings of drug related sex difference are less uniform than the ones regarding age differences. This refers to behavioral or clinical response as well as to pharmacokinetic parameters and seems to be dependent on type of drug as well as on a number of nonspecific factors.

4.1 Evidence for Higher Drug Susceptibility in Females

4.1.1 Gross organismic response.
A larger group of results demonstrates higher reactivity in females as for instance those from clinical studies on schizophrenic patients reporting significantly better improvement with neuroleptics in females (Cole and others, 1968; Holden and others, 1971; Goldberg and others, 1966; Zubin and others, 1961) and greater frequencies of Parkinson-like side effects upon chronic treatment with phenothiazines (Ayd, 1961; Duvoisin, 1968).

Similarly, a number of studies on healthy volunteers yield evidence that females are more affected by psychotropic drugs than males. Slanska and others (1974) for instance report that upon a single oral dose of 100 mg pentobarbital female subjects reported more fatigue than males which also lasted much longer than in males and in some females was even observed 28 hours after drug application.
800 mg of meprobamate caused a significant decrease in performance in a tremometer task and in tapping speed as well as in mood in females, whereas males were not affected or rather improved by the drug (Munkelt, 1965). A similar tendency emerged in a study by Reisby (1972) where deterioration in eye coordination in the prism rod and Maddox Wing tasks was more pronounced after 800 mg of meprobamate in females than in males. The difference became significant only when meprobamate was applied in combination with alcohol.
Although Kelly and coworkers (1958) themselves cast doubt on their results with respect to sex differences obtained with 800 mg meprobamate their results may be taken as pointing to the same effect: Males were improved in reaction time in a driving test and felt more relaxed with the drug while females, as in the study by Munkelt (1965), felt emotionally upset or instable after the drug and were also deteriorated in psychomotor performance.
Similar results were obtained with alcohol by Myrsten and others (1972) and by Munkelt and others (1962). Females felt more irritated, tired and depressed and less happy, relaxed and alert (Myrsten and others, 1972) or more desactivated and emotionally imbalanced and could concentrate less well (Munkelt and others, 1962) 60 - 100 min after consumption of 720 or 800 mg/kg body weight of alcohol, respectively.
In the latter study the detrimental effect on performance became more pronounced in females, when 800 mg of meprobamate were given in combination with alcohol, whereas the alcohol induced impairment of performance in the males was partly compensated by meprobamate. It must be added, however, that there was a very pronounced interaction of drug and sex with the trait of emotional stability of the subjects

which we will not elaborate here, since personality factors are discussed elsewhere in this volume.

The observed results could be explained in several ways:
1. by slower metabolism and hence higher plasma concentrations of the
   drugs in females which can be due to
   a) genetic sex linked factors
   b) interactions of the drugs with female sex hormones
   c) greater drug-, alcohol- or nicotine-induced enzyme induction
      causing faster drug metabolism in males,
2. by higher receptor sensitivity in females,
3. by more sensitive cognitive perception of drug induced
   physical changes as aversive stimuli in females,
4. by higher reactivity in self descriptive emotional response
   in females.

4.1.2 Pharmacokinetic response.

Several pharmacokinetic studies have tried to shed light on the hypotheses listed under point 1. Examples of higher plasma levels in females can be taken from the following results: A study by Greenblatt
and others, 1977a) on a group of preoperative patients receiving an
oral dose of 2x200 mg of chlordiazepoxide revealed higher plasma levels in females.
In a clinical study on patients receiving chronic treatment with nortriptyline and imipramine (Giudicelli and Tillement, 1977) higher
steady state plasma levels were obtained in females. Unbound diazepam
after in vitro incubation with plasma of both sexes was also observed
to be higher in females than in males (Routledge and others, 1981),
and the blood alcohol levels obtained in the study by Myrsten and
others (1972) were also significantly higher in females.

Much of the endeavour in studying influence of sex on drug response
was of course directed to elucidation of the nature of these kinetic
sex differences.

A number of studies in animals report higher rates of drug metabolism
in male rats and mice for different compounds (Kato, 1974) which is
corroborated by the finding that application of androgens enhances
the activity of the mixed function oxidases (Kato and Gillette, 1965)
and that starvation, which causes an impairment of androgen activity,
decreases drug metabolism of those microsomal enzymes which are highly sex-dependent (Kato and Gillette, 1965). This observation, however,
is only valid in male rats while in females starvation increases metabolism of hexobarbital (Campbell and Hayes, 1974) which might be
explained by depression of enzyme inhibiting estrogens, since the
effect was reversed after refeeding the animals.

Also in humans drug metabolism of some compounds has been reported
to be higher in males as for example that of nortriptyline (Guidicelli
and Tillement, 1977). Since, furthermore, contraceptives and pregnancy
(Stevenson, 1973) have been demonstrated to inhibit drug metabolizing
enzyme activity the observation reported by Guidicelli and Tillement
(1977), that premenopausal women need higher doses and obtain lower
serum levels of antidepressants than young women, may be interpreted
as an increasing drug metabolism with decreasing estrogen activity.
Regular intake of contraceptives has also been shown to be related
to larger fractions of unbound diazepam in plasma as compared to the

plasma of females who do not use sex hormones (Routledge and others, 1981).

Finally, the greater variability in time to reach peak concentrations of chlordiazepoxide observed by Greenblatt (1974) in females may be taken as an indication of relations between drug metabolism and menstrual cycle.
But unfortunately other studies failed to prove a direct relationship between plasma levels of a drug (antipyrine) and menstrual cycle (Riester, 1980).
Other explanations for lower metabolic activity in females such as greater induction of enzymes caused by a longer and more abundant use of enzyme stimulating compounds in males (such as alcohol and nicotine) may be valid but have not been evaluated with respect to sex differences in behavioral response in humans.

4.1.3 Receptor sensitivity, perception of drug induced changes and emotional reactivity.

The other hypotheses for higher reactivity in females listed in paragraph 4.1.1 are less well investigated.
Greater sensitivity of mental structures to sedative drugs may be inferred from the fact that in the study by Reisby (1972) as well as in the study by Munkelt (1965) performance in some achievement functions was impaired more severely with ethanol in females in spite of the fact that their mean alcohol plasma levels were the same as for males.
Results referring to self reports on mood (Myrsten and others, 1972; Munkelt and others, 1962; Slanska and others, 1974) are of course more likely to be influenced by irritation about perception of drug induced bodily and mental changes. This seems very likely, since in the studies by Myrsten and others (1972) females responded by larger increases of adrenaline upon ingestion of alcohol which might indicate greater physiological deviation than in males. Furthermore, females are known to admit irritation, anxiety and unfavourable effects and feelings more readily than males in all scales referring to somatic complaints, a fact which might also contribute to the differences in self ratings.

4.2 Evidence for Higher Drug Susceptibility in Males

4.2.1 Gross organismic response.

There is less evidence that males show greater reactivity to drugs than females than for the reverse observation.
An animal study on tolerance for ethanol (Wallgren, 1959) revealed an opposite effect to the one reported for humans: female rats in 3 different experimental series were less impaired in their performance than males. The author reports similar results from other studies for morphine and chlorpromazine.

A review of Goldberg and others (1966) on clinical observations lists five studies in which schizophrenic males improved more upon neuroleptics than females, Zubin (1961) mentions another two. But Goldberg and others (1966) point out that in 9 out of 16 studies there was a marked sex by drug interaction revealing sex differences with respect to placebo responses as well. This points to the site of cognitive factors, the role of expectations and suggestibility in sex related drug response. Also in reviews on predictors of the placebo response

(Lasagna and others, 1958; Honigfeld, 1964; Shapiro, 1964) sex and
placebo proneness are not described to be linked in a predictable
manner, but rather seem to interact with processes of attribution,
coping and belief and other experimental and personality factors which
also operate in response to active compounds.

4.2.2 Pharmacokinetic response.

Examples of results suggesting slower drug metabolism in males than in
females are: higher plasma levels of phenobarbital and antiepileptics
reported by Guidicelli and Tillement (1977) lower volumes of distribution (which would imply higher plasma levels) for intravenously applied
chlordiazepoxide observed by Greenblatt and others (1977b), lower excretion rates of lithium described by Guidicelli and Tillement (1977)
and lower rates of antipyrine metabolism in males shown by O'Malley
and others (1971). These studies and the ones in which no differences
were found in plasma levels of phenazone (Liddle and others, 1975),
alcohol(Munkelt and Lienert, 1964; Wallgren, 1959) would be in line
with the results from animal studies by Kato and Gillette (1965) that
only certain drug metabolizing enzymes are influenced by sex hormones.
On the other hand there is evidence of hormonal influence on the pharmacodynamic action of some drugs. Thus Wallgren (1959) reports several
findings indicating that estrogens increase resistance of brain tissue
to narcotic effects of alcohol by increasing alcohol induced oxygen consumption of the brain which is decreased in the absence of estrogens.

Furthermore, sex differences in kinetic as well as in behavior parameters very often only become evident by interactions with other factors like race (Goldberg, 1966; Raskin and Crook, 1975), age (Raskin,
1974; Raskin and others, 1970), emotional stability (Munkelt, 1965),
motivation (Aletky and Carlin, 1975) or dosage and time of drug application (Greenblatt and others, 1977a).

5. PHYSIQUE AND PRE-DRUG PHYSIOLOGICAL STATES AS SOURCES OF VARIANCE IN DRUG RESPONSE

Frequently body build or physique chosen as variables for grouping individuals raise associations with constitutional types according to
Kretschmer (1921) or Sheldon and coworkers (1940) which imply predictability of behavior from morphology. Although very little credit
is given to this typological approach in modern psychology, also pharmacologists mention constitutional factors as important sources of
variance in drug response. Constitution in this sense refers to morphological aspects like body build, weight and height as well as to
"vigor or feebleness, susceptibility to environmental influences,
readiness or lack of self defense, completeness or insufficiency of
self repair" (Irwin, 1964). These dispositions, of course, can only
be inferred from drug response and may be linked to morphological or
tissue components as well as to psychological dimensions such as neuroticism and anxiety. We shall just pick some morphological and some
physiological examples in order to demonstrate how psychotropic drug
effect can be influenced by both aspects of bodily constitution.

5.1 Body Build and Weight

Since the classical constitutional types were said to differ in to-

lerance of alcohol, Grüner and Ludwig (1960) took the effort to test
whether eurymorphs and leptomorphs showed different impairment by alcohol at identical blood levels of alcohol. Careful statistical analysis performed on a sample of 5,745 persons arrested for driving under
the influence of alcohol and a laboratory experiment performed on 10
extremely eurymorph and leptomorph volunteers each revealed the following results: Fat subjects were less impaired as revealed by general
ratings of the physicians who took the blood samples in the large
group and with respect to reaction times tested in the sample of the
laboratory experiment. Leptomorph subjects, on the other hand, whose
pre-alcohol performance was better in quality and quantity than that
of the eurymorph ones in the Bourdon test were less impaired in this
task than eurymorphs which indicates better maintenance of attention
and psychomotor speed. The authors relate their findings to differences
in autonomic reactivity of the two groups, eurymorphs showing higher
sympathetic and leptomorphs higher parasympathetic activity which implies that the first group can counterbalance the parasympathetic action of ethanol better than the second. Another dimension of body build
is that of bone-muscle versus fat ratio derived from the typology of
the sexes (von Zerssen, 1964). In a study on phenetylline by Munkelt
and Othmer (1965) andromorph males (as measured by a combined score
from biceps and calf circumferences, bone diameters and thickness of
skinfolds) felt more stimulated according to self ratings than gyneco-
morph ones although at their placebo levels they already felt more
vigorous, alert, extraverted and active than the more delicate gyneco-
morphs. Figure 4 shows the shifts in self ratings produced by phenetylline.

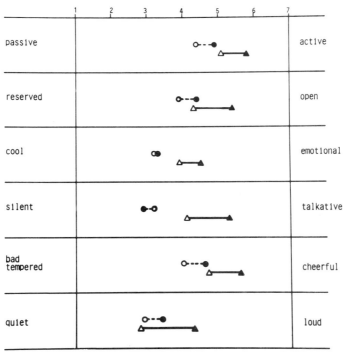

Fig. 4.   Self ratings on a semantic differential of andro-
          morph (△———▲) and gynecomorph (o------●) subjects
          after placebo (△ o) and 50 mg of phenetylline (▲ ●).

This is quite unique, since according to the law of initial values
drug induced increase should affect the lower level group more than
the one with higher initial values.
The andromorphs also obtained significantly greater increases in movement responses and form levels in the Holtzman Inkblot Test representing phantasy and accuracy of perception, respectively. These results
remind of the higher incidences of "coloured patterns phenomena" and
euphoria reported by the athletic type A personality subjects after
treatment with mescaline in an experiment by DiMascio and Rinkel (1963)
which, like the former, demonstrates the close relationship between
body build and personality factors.

As pointed out in the section on sex and age, body composition can
also turn out to be the relevant cause for sex and age differences
in drug response as pointed out by Turner (1978). Also in clinical
studies physique related differences in drug response have been observed. Thus, Bente and others (1968) report better recovery with
antidepressant drugs in depressed fat patients than in leptomorphs,
and Uhlenhuth and others (1968) in a multiple regression analysis
performed in order to identify non-specific predictors of antianxiety
effects of meprobamate, report that heavier male individuals (who in
addition were married and not well liked by their physicians) showed
the best clinical response. Similarly, in a longitudinal single case
observation on a depressed woman by Jobson and others (1978) efficacy
of tricyclic antidepressants was decreased in a period of starvation
of the subject and restored after her weight gain.

Some explanations may be given by kinetic considerations. Gillette
(1974) for instance, reports an example of a heavy person poisoned
with thiopental which even after complete dialytic removal of the drug
from the plasma kept redistributing back into the blood stream from the
deep compartments of fatty tissue.
The other end of the weight dimension - malnutrition and starvation -
and their role in reducing drug metabolism and changes in blood flow,
protein binding of drugs, drug receptor interactions and renal excretion (Basu and Dickerson, 1974; Campbell and Hayes, 1974) has been
discussed elsewhere in this volume (Netter and Netter, this volume).

5.2   Pre-Drug Physiological States

Numerous papers are concerned with predicting clinical response to
antidepressants and neuroleptics from pretherapeutic levels of symptomatology. Others are interested in antianxiety effects in subjects
differing in level of physiological arousal related to levels of trait
anxiety. Both aspects will be discussed elsewhere in this volume
(Janke, this volume). In most cases physiological states can be related to one of the more stable factors like age, sex, body build, or
to environmental influences like temperature, exercise, intake of additional drugs or food or the presence of stress factors. Sometimes,
however, experimental consideration of physiological factors not related to the dependent or independent variable reveal subtle interactions between drug effects and pre-drug physiological measures. Thus,
for instance, Koukko and Lehman (1979) could predict the degree of
euphoria and disturbances of body image produced by delta-9-tetra-
hydrocannabinol from certain patterns of the EEG. Similarly, Cooper
(1979) observed an antidepressant effect of levo-tryptophan only when
the 5-hydroxytryptamine levles were at their peaks.

6. THE INFLUENCE OF OTHER DRUGS, PRETREATMENT AND DISEASE

6.1 Drug Interactions

As outlined in a previous chapter on factors influencing pharmacokinetics, a number of environmental factors and drugs are known to change
drug response which may occur by alterations of tissue or receptor sensitivity, changes in absorption, distribution, plasma binding, metabolism or excretion and by blocking transport of another drug to the site
of action (Fann and Richman, 1975; Haraszti and Davis, 1978). All these
processes would be comprised in the term 'interaction' in its pharmacological meaning. The most widespread type of interaction occurs by
stimulating or inhibiting the oxygenases of the liver. Psychotropic
drugs can serve either as inducers of drug metabolism themselves or
may be affected by their own inducibility or by that of other compounds.
Among the substances known to inhance metabolism there are many psychotropic compounds such as barbiturates, meprobamate, delta-9-tetrahydro-
cannabinol, and in chronic or large doses also ethanol and caffeine,
respectively, and only a few are known to inhibt drug oxidation such
as oral contraceptives (see section 3) (Abernethy and Greenblatt,
1981; Conney and Burns, 1972) or chlorpromazine and other neuroleptics
(Haraszti and Davis, 1978).
Haraszti and Davis (1978) as well as Fraser and Dollery (1978) list
a number of studies, which were able to confirm some of these results
derived from laboratory research by clinical observations and by pharmacokinetic measurements. There seems to be agreement as to the inducing capacity of both benzpyrine and nicotine, the constituents of
cigarette smoke. It is reported that half lives of compounds which
are metabolized by oxidation can be increased by 25% (antipyrine) or
even by 75% (theophylline).

Fraser and Dollery (1978) report results according to which smokers
have been found to require higher doses of pentazocine and show less
unfavourable side effects, like drowsiness, after chlorpromazine, and
also plasma half lives of phenacetine were reduced in smokers.
Psychological experiments so far have not often taken smoking or use
of barbiturates or alcohol into account, if these variables were not
the aim of the study.
Caffeine has not been found to interact with other drugs (Patwardhan
and others, 1980) but clinical doses of caffeine have been claimed to
be below levels at which enzyme induction occurs (Fraser and Dollery,
1978).

While chronic alcohol consumption indeed seems to increase metabolism
of other drugs (Kalant and others, 1971; Sellers and Holloway, 1978),
the acute ingestion of ethanol rather seems to enhance or potentiate
the effect of other drugs predominantly of the sedative type. Well
known examples are enhancement of the effects of barbiturates
(Doenicke, 1962), benzodiazepines (Sellers and others, 1981), meprobamate (Reisby, 1972; Munkelt and others, 1962), amitriptyline
(Haraszti and Davis, 1978), and nomifensine (Taeuber and others, 1976).
This, however, is not only due to pharmacokinetic interactions, but
also to pharmacodynamic factors (Sellers and others, 1980).

Since equivalence of dosages between two structurally different but
similarly acting compounds is almost impossible to define, it is hard
to tell, whether the more pronounced effects described for a combina-

tion of drugs represent additive effects or potentiation. Thus, for
instance, promazine and barbital produced better sleep quality (Kohnen
and others, 1979) than the single compounds; diazepam and propranolol
had better anxiety reducing effects than each drug by itself (Oswald,
1979), and the activating antidepressant effect of imipramine was enhanced by thyroid hormone (Prange and others, 1969).

Another type of interaction is represented by competition at the receptor site. Thus, the anticholinergic effect of desimipramine anta-
gonizes the parasympathetic activity of propranolol (resulting in lack
of cardiac response to the betablocker), and blockade of the dopamine
receptor by phenothiazines counteracts the effectivity of L-dopa in
treatment of Parkinson's disease in patients treated for depression
simultaneously (Haraszti and Davis, 1978).

6.2 Pretreatment and Tolerance

Chronic pretreatment with psychotropic drugs may change their effects
by the development of either dispositional or functional tolerance
(Kalant and others, 1971). Whereas there is little evidence of dispositional change due to changes of absorption, distribution and excretion by psychopharmacological pretreatment, the mechanism of enzyme
induction described for interaction of different drugs in the previous
section is frequently also responsible for reduced response to the
same drug after chronic administration. Thus, plasma levels of delta-
9-tetrahydrocannabinol have been reported to be lower in subjects used
to cannabis for more than one year than in non-users (Lemberger and
Rubin, 1975), and also for barbiturates, benzodiazepines and meprobamate increase in metabolism may account for reduced effects after
chronic administration (Kalant and others, 1971). This phenomenon,
however, can serve as a better explanation for shortened duration of
action of these drugs than for the diminished immediate response,
since the latter is also observed, when plasma levels are kept high
by intravenous titration as demonstrated for alcohol (Kalant and
others, 1971).
No change in metabolism or accumulation in brain tissue was detected
after a chronic 20 day administration of amphetamine to rats (Ziem
and others, 1970), but probably most of the changes in response observed after chronic treatment are due to changes in receptor sensitivity (= functional tolerance according to Kalant and others, 1971),
as can be demonstrated by animal experiments on dexamphetamine and
apomorphine (Bailey and Jackson, 1978) and cocaine (Epstein and Altshuler, 1979).

Experiments on humans are, of course, mostly confined to psychiatric
patients on chronic drug treatment. Kornetsky (1960) reports on some
psychometric test results obtained under acute and chronic treatment
of schizophrenics with secobarbital and chlorpromazine. He was able
to demonstrate that secobarbital revealed a slightly greater decrease
in psychomotor performance (pursuit rotor, digit symbol, tapping speed
and tachistoscopic threshold) after chronic administration than with
the same dosages in the acute trial. Under chlorpromazine, however,
patients seemed to perform better after chronic treatment and to be
less sensitive to twofold increase of the dose than with a single
trial medication. This effect was most pronounced in perceptual speed.

An experiment comparing acute and chronic stimulant effects of methyl-

phenidate and fenetylline in healthy subjects by Janke and Netter
(1981) showed less pronounced drug-placebo differences in psychomotor
performance scores on day 8 as compared to day 1 of the treatment phase,
but partly more pronounced differences in perceptual speed, reaction
time and concentration, subjective scores of activation and in decrease
of psychosomatic complaints after one week of drug administration.

It must be taken into account, however, that development of functional
tolerance takes different times for different compounds and in addition
varies within the same drug for different measures of drug tolerance.
Some figures for development of tolerance to different psychotropic
drugs in man are mentioned by Kalant and others (1971). The criterion
used is not very clearly defined and mostly refers to onset of decrease
in sleeping time or of other typical physiological drug effects
(Table 3).

TABLE 3   Time for the Development of Tolerance to Various Psycho-
           tropic Drugs in Man (after Kalant and others, 1971)

Drug	Time for Development of Tolerance	Comment
Ethanol	2 - 3 weeks	
Short acting barbiturates (pentobarbital)	3 - 5 days	
Long acting barbitures (phenobarbital)	5 - 7 weeks	
Meprobamate	1 - 3 weeks	according to EEG signs
Amphetamine	less than 2 weeks	according to mood and loss of appetite
D-lysergic acid diethylamide (LSD)	3 - 13 days	

6.3 Disease

The influence of disease is often investigated with respect to possible
change of dosage required for patients suffering from liver cirrhosis,
heart or renal failure. These diseases, of course, have not been investigated with respect to their effect on change in psychometric
test response to psychotropic drugs, but more often with respect to
kinetic parameters.
There seems to be agreement that liver diseases may cause prolongation
of plasma half lives for diazepam (Greenblatt and others, 1978; Klotz
and others, 1975) as well as for phenylbutazone (Levi and others, 1968)
and lidocaine (Thomson and others, 1971), whereas impairment of renal
function does not seem to lead to immediate changes in drug disposition,
as shown by excretion of glucoronic acid (Kampf and others, 1980) and

may only be of importance in combination with heart failure (Thomson and others, 1971).

These diseases are not always discovered before psychotropic effects are tested and therefore have to be considered as sources of particularly wide variances in response.

As emphasized in Fig. 1, all these factors, especially disease, are confounded with some of the other factors discussed and sometimes cannot even be controlled, since they are invariably linked to age or certain pretreatment effects (liver cirrhosis for instance will occur in older subjects whose drug response will be highly affected by chronic alcohol ingestion).

REFERENCES

Abernethy, D. R., and D. J. Greenblatt (1981). Impairment of antipyrine metabolism by low-dose oral contraceptive steroids. Clin. Pharmacol. Ther., 29, 106-110.

Ahrens, R. (1971). On the forensic-psychiatric significance of alcohol loading tests under EEG control. Electroencephalogr. Clin. Neurophysiol., 30, 269-270.

Aletky, P. J., and A. S. Carlin (1975). Sex-differences and placebo effects: Motivation as an intervening variable. J. Consult. Clin. Psychol., 43, 278-282.

Alexanderson, B., P.D.A. Evans, and F. Sjöquist (1969). Steady state plasma levels of nortriptyline in twins: Influence of genetic factors and drug therapy. Br. Med. J., 4, 764-768.

Angst, J. (1964). Antidepressiver Effekt und genetische Faktoren. Arzneim.-Forsch. (Drug Res.), 14, 496-500.

Ayd, F. J. (1961). A survey of drug induced extrapyramidal reactions. J. Am. Med. Assoc., 175, 1054-1060.

Bailey, R. C., and D. M. Jackson (1978). A pharmacological study of changes in central nervous system receptor responsiveness after long-term dexamphetamine and apomorphine administration. Psychopharmacology, 56, 317-326.

Basu, T. K., and J. W. T. Dickerson (1974). Interrelationship of nutrition and the metabolism of drugs. Chem. Biol. Interact., 8, 193-206.

Bech, P., J. Thomsen, and S. Prytz (1979). The profile and severity of lithium-induced side effects in mentally healthy subjects. Neuropsychobiology, 5, 160-166.

Belville, J. W., W. H. Forrest, E. Miller, and B. W. Brown (1971). Influence of age on pain relief from analgesics. J. Am. Med. Assoc., 27, 1835-1841.

Bender, L. (1962). Children with schizophrenic response to LSD-25. Drug Trade News, 74, 1-15.

Bente, D., M. P. Engelmeier, K. Heinrich, H. Hippius, and W. Schmitt (1968). The role of non-specific factors in the drug therapy of depressive syndromes. In K. Rickels (Ed.), Non-Specific Factors in Drug Therapy. Thomas, Springfield. pp. 108-114.

Bovet, D., F. Bovet-Nitti, and A. Oliverio (1966). Effects of nicotine on avoidance conditioning of inbred strains of mice. Psychopharmacologia, 10, 1-5.

Campbell, T.C., and J. R. Hayes (1974). Role of nutrition in the drug metabolizing enzyme system. Pharmacol. Rev., 26, 171-198.

Carlsson, A. (1980). Altern und Neurotransmitter im Gehirn. 7. Rothenburger Gespräch vom 6./7. Nov. 1980.

Castleden, C. M., C. F. George, D. Marcer, and C. Hallett(1977). Increased sensitivity to nitrazepam in old age. Br. Med. J., 1, 10-12.

Chan, K., M. J. Kendall, M. Mitchard, and W. D. E. Wells (1975). The effect of aging on plasma pethidine concentration. Br. J. Clin. Pharmacol., 2, 297-302.

Claridge, G. (1970). Drugs and Human Behavior. Praeger Publ., New York.

Claridge, G., and E. Ross (1973). Sedative tolerance in twins. In G. S. Claridge, S. Canter, and W. I. Hume (Eds.), Personality Differences and Biological Variations. Pergamon Press, Oxford. pp. 115-131.

Cole, J. O., R. Bonato, and S. C. Goldberg (1968). Nonspecific factors in the drug therapy of schizophrenic patients. In K. Rickels (Ed.), Non-specific Factors in Drug Therapy. Thomas, Springfield. pp. 115-127.

Conney, A. H., and J. J. Burns (1972). Metabolic interactions among environmental chemicals and drugs. Science, 178, 576-586.

Conney, A. H., B. Craver, R. Kuntzman, and E. J. Pantuck (1974). Drug metabolism in normal and disease state. In T. Teorell, R. D. De-drick, and P. G. Condliffe (Eds.), Pharmacology and Pharmacokinetics. Plenum Press, New York. pp. 147-162.

Cooper, A. J. (1979). Tryptophan antidepressant physiological sedative: Fact or phancy? Psychopharmacology,61, 97-102.

Curry, S. H., and J. H. L. Marshall (1968). Plasma levels of chlorpro-mazine and some of its relatively non-polar metabolites in psychia-tric patients. Life Sci., 7, 9-18.

DiMascio, A., and M. Rinkel (1963). In M. Rinkel (Ed.), Specific and Nonspecific Factors in Psychopharmacology. Philosophical Library, New York. pp. 130-140.

Doenicke, A. (1962). Beeinträchtigung der Verkehrssicherheit durch Barbiturat-Medikation und durch die Kombination Barbiturat/Alkohol. Arzneim.-Forsch. (Drug Res.), 11, 1050-1054.

Domino, E. F., A. T. Dren, and W. J. Giardina (1978). Biochemical and neurotransmitter changes in the aging brain. In M. A. Lipton, A. DiMascio, and K. F. Killam (Eds.), Psychopharmacology: A Generation of Progress. Raven Press, New York. pp. 1507-1515.

Downing, R. W., and K. Rickels (1974). The role of race and socioeco-nomic class level. Psychopharmacol. Bull., 10, 64-65.

Duvoisin, R.C. (1968). Neurological reactions to psychotropic drugs. In D.H. Efron (Ed.), Psychopharmacology: A Review of Progress 1957-1967. US Government Printing Office, Washington. pp. 561-573.

Edwards, J. A., and D. A. P. Evans (1967). Ethanol metabolism in sub-jects possessing typical and atypical liver-alcohol dehydrogenase. Clin. Pharmacol. Ther., 8, 824-829.

Engelhardt, D. M., and P. Polizos (1978). Adverse effects of pharmaco-therapy in childhood psychosis. In M. A. Lipton, A. DiMascio, and K. F. Killam (Eds.), Psychopharmacology: A Generation of Progress. Raven Press, New York. pp. 1463-1469.

Elias, F. F., and C. A. Pentz (1975). The role of genotype in behavior-al responses to anesthetics. In B. E. Eleftheriou (Ed.), Psycho-pharmacogenetics. Plenum Press, New York. pp. 299-321.

Epstein, P. N., and H. L. Altshuler (1979). Changes in the effects of cocaine during chronic treatment. Res. Commun. Chem. Pathol. Pharmacol., 22, 93-105.

Eriksson, K. (1975). Alcohol inhibition and behavior: A comparative genetic approach. In B. E. Eleftheriou (Ed.), Psychopharmacogenetics. Plenum Press, New York. pp. 127-168.

Erinoff, L., R. C. Macphail, A. Heller, and L. S. Seiden (1979). Age-dependent effects of 6-hydroxydopamine on locomotor activity in the rat. Brain Res., 164, 195-205.

Evans, D. A. P. (1971). Inter-individual differences in metabolism of
    drugs: the role of genetic factors. Acta Pharmacol. Toxicol., 29,
    56- 163.
Evans, D. A. P., and T. A. White (1964). Human acetylation polymorphism.
    J. Lab. Clin. Stud., 63, 387-403.
Evans, D. A. P., K. Davison, and R. T. C. Pratt (1965). The influence
    of acetylator phenotype on the effects of treating depression with
    phenelzine. Clin. Pharmacol. Ther., 6, 430-435.
Ewing, J. A., B. A. Rouse, and E. D. Bellizzari (1973). Alcohol sen-
    sitivity and ethnic background. Paper presented at the 126th
    Annual Meeting of the American Psychiatric Association, May 1973,
    in Honolulu.
Fann, W. E., and B. W. Richman (1975). Some drug-drug interactions in-
    volving psychotropic agents. In B. E. Eleftheriou (Ed.), Psycho-
    pharmacogenetics. Plenum Press, New York. pp. 377-382.
Fähndrich, E., and H. Hadass (1969). Relationship between the perazine
    concentration in the liver, brain and blood and the pharmacologic
    effects under chronic perazine medication in rats of different age.
    Pharmakopsychiatr. Neuropsychopharmakol., 2, 110-119.
Fenna, D.,L. Mix, and O. Schaefer (1971). Ethanol metabolism in various
    racial groups. Can. Med. Assoc. J., 105, 472-475.
Fraser, H. S., and C. T. Dollery (1978). Influence of drugs and en-
    vironmental chemicals on drug metabolism in man. In J. W. Gorrod,
    and A. H. Beckett (Eds.), Drug Metabolism in Man. Taylor and
    Francis, London. pp. 107-117.
Fuller, J. L., and C. D. Hansult (1975). Genes and drugs as behaviour
    modifying agents. In B. E. Eleftheriou (Ed.), Psychopharmacogenetics.
    Plenum Press, New York. pp. 11-18.
Galbrecht, C. R., and C. J. Klett (1968). Predicting response of phe-
    nothiazines: The right drug for the right patient. J. Nerv. Ment.
    Dis., 147, 173-183.
Gillette, J. R. (1974). The importance of tissue distribution in phar-
    macokinetics. In T. Teorell, L. R. Dedrick, and P. G. Condliffe
    (Eds.), Pharmacology and Pharmacokinetics. Plenum Press, New York.
    pp. 209-231.
Glass, H. B. (1954). Genetic aspects of adaptability. In Association
    for Research in Nervous and Mental Disease (Ed.), Genetics and
    Inheritance of Integrated Neurological and Psychiatric Patterns.
    Res. Nerv. Ment. Dis., 33. Williams and Wilkins, Baltimore.
Goedde, H. W. (1974). Pharmakokinetik: Variabilität von Arzneimittel-
    wirkung und Stoffwechselreaktionen. Internist, 15, 27-39.
Goldberg, S. C., N. R. Schooler, E. M. Davidson, and M. M. Kayce (1966).
    Sex and race differences in response to drug treatment among schizo-
    phrenics. Psychopharmacologia, 9, 31-47.
Greenblatt, D. J., R. I. Shader, and J. Koch-Weser (1974). Pharmacokinet
    determinants of the response to single doses of chlordiazepoxide.
    Am. J. Psychiatry, 131, 1395-1397.
Greenblatt, D. J., J. S. Harmatz, D. R. Stanski, R. I. Shader, K.
    Franke, and J. Koch-Weser (1977a). Factors influencing blood con-
    centrations of chlordiazepoxide: A use of multiple regression ana-
    lysis. Psychopharmacology, 54, 277-282.
Greenblatt, D. J., R. I. Shader, J. S. Harmatz, K. Franke, and J. Koch-
    Weser (1977b). Absorption rate, blood concentrations and early
    response to oral chlordiazepoxide. Am. J. Psychiatry, 134, 559-562.
Greenblatt, D. J., J. S. Harmatz, and R. I. Shader (1978). Factors
    influencing diazepam pharmacokinetics: Age, sex, and liver disease.
    Int. J. Clin. Pharmacol. Biopharm., 16, 177-179.

Grüner, O., and O. Ludwig (1960). Konstitution und Alkoholwirkung. Ärztl. Forsch., 14, 303-311.

Grygiel, J. J., and D. J. Birkett (1980). Effect of age on patterns of theophylline metabolism. Clin. Pharmacol. Ther., 28, 456-462.

Guidicelli, J. F., and J. P. Tillement (1977). Influence of sex on drug kinetics in man. Clin. Pharmacogenetics, 2, 157-166.

Hänninen, O. (1975). Age and exposure factors in drug metabolism. Acta Pharmacol. Toxicol., 36 (Suppl. 2), 3-20.

Haraszti, J. S., and J. M. Davis (1978). Psychotropic drug interaction. In W. G. Clark,and J. del Giudice (Eds.), Principles of Psychopharmacology. Academic Press, New York. pp. 495-510.

Hayes, W. J., M. J. S. Langman, and A. H. Short (1975). Changes in drug metabolism with increasing age. I and II. Br. J. Clin. Pharmacol., 2, 69-78.

Holden, J. M. C., W. Hsu, T. M. Stil, and A. Keskiner (1971). Predictor patterns in the management of therapy resistent schizophrenics. Dis. Nerv. Syst., 32, 260-268.

Honecker, H., and H. Coper (1975). Kinetics and metabolism of amphetamine in the brain of rats of different ages. Naunyn Schmiedebergs Arch. Pharmacol., 291, 111-121.

Honigfeld, G. (1964). Non-specific factors in treatment: I. Review of placebo reactions and placebo reactors. Dis. Nerv. Syst. , 25, 145-156.

Hubin, P., and J. Servais (1966). Etude comparative des effets psycho-physiologiques de l'amphetamine chez sujets de race blanche et de race noire. Psychopharmacologia, 9, 118-136.

Ilsalo, E., L. Kangas, and I. Ruikka (1977). Pharmacokinetics of nitrazepam in young volunteers and aged patients. Proceedings of the BPS, 646-647.

Irvine, R. E., J. Grove, P. A. Toseland, and J. R. Trounce (1974). The effect of age on the hydroxylation of amylobarbitone sodium in man. Br. J. Clin. Pharmacol., 1, 41-43.

Irwin, S. (1964). Determinants of variability in drug response. Psychosomatics, 5, 174-178.

Janke, W., and P. Netter (1981). Zur Wirkung von Psychopharmaka nach einmaliger und mehrmaliger Verabreichung: Ein Beitrag zur Problematik psychopharmakologischer Akutversuche. In L. Tent (Ed.), Erkennen, Wollen, Handeln. Hogrefe, Göttingen. pp. 404-426.

Jobson, K., G. Burnett, and M. Linnoila (1978). Weight loss and a concomitant change in plasma tricyclic levels. Am. J. Psychiatry, 135, 237-238.

Johnstone, E., and W. Marsh (1973). Acetylator status and response to phenelzine in depressed patients. Lancet, I, 567-570.

Kaiko, R. (1980). Age and morphine analgesia in cancer patients with postoperative pain. Clin. Pharmacol. Ther., 28, 823-826.

Kalant, H., A. E. LeBlanc, and R. G. Gibbins (1971). Tolerance to and dependence on some nonopiate psychotropic drugs. Pharmacol. Rev., 23, 135-191.

Kalow, W. (1975). Genetics and psychoactive drugs. In E. M. Sellers (Ed.), Clinical Pharmacology of Psychoactive Drugs. Addict Res. Found., Toronto. pp. 105-115.

Kalow, W., and A. E. LeBlanc (1975). Implications of psychopharmacogenetic research. In B. E. Eleftheriou (Ed.), Psychopharmacogenetics. Plenum Press, New York. pp. 33-42.

Kampf, D., I. Roots, and A. G. Hildebrandt (1980). Urinary excretion of d-glucaric acid, an indicator of drug metabolizing enzyme activity, in patients with impaired renal function. Eur. J. Clin. Pharmacol., 18, 255-261.

Kangas, L., E. Ilsalo, J. Kanto, V. Lehtinen, S. Pynnöönens, I. Ruikka, J. Salminen, M. Sillanpää, and E. Syvalahli (1979). Human pharmacogenetics of nitrazepam: effect of age and disease. Eur. J. Clin. Pharmacol., 15, 163-170.

Kato, R. (1974). Sex related differences in drug metabolism. Drug Metab. Rev., 3, 1-32.

Kato, R., and J. R. Gillette (1965). Effects of starvation on NADPH-dependent enzymes in male and female rats. J. Pharmacol. Exp. Ther., 150, 279-284.

Kelly, E., J. G. Miller, D. G. Marquis, R. W. Gerard, and L. Uhr (1958). Personality differences and continued meprobamate and prochlorperazine administration. Arch. Neurol., 80, 241-246.

Klett, C. J., and E. C. Moseley (1965). The right drug for the right patient. J. Consult. Psychol., 29, 546-551.

Klinger, W. (1977). Development of drug metabolizing enzymes. In P. L. Morselli (Ed.), Drug Disposition and Development. Spectrum Publications, New York. pp. 71-88.

Klotz, U., G. R. Avant, A. Hoyumpa, S. Schenker, and G. R. Wilkinson (1975). The effect of age and liver disease on the disposition and elimination of diazepam in adult man. J. Clin. Invest., 55, 347-359.

Kohnen, R., G. A. Lienert, and F. I. Schmidt (1979). Klinisch-psychologische Schlaf- und Nachwirkungsspektren von Pentobarbital, Promazin und ihrer Kombination im Spiegel der Selbstbeurteilung junger und alter Versuchspersonen. Pharmakopsychiatr. Neuropsychopharmakol., 12, 261-268.

Kornetsky, C. (1960). Alterations in psychomotor functions and individual differences in responses produced by psychoactive drugs. In L. Uhr, and J. C. Miller (Eds.), Drugs and Behavior. Wiley, New York. pp. 297-312.

Koukkou, M., and D. Lehman (1979). Correlations between cannabis-induced psychopathology and EEG before and after drug ingestion. Pharmakopsychiatr. Neuropsychopharmakol., 11, 220-227.

Kretschmer, E. (1921). Körperbau und Charakter. Springer, Berlin.

Kuhlmann, K., M. Oduah, and H. Coper (1970). Über die Wirkung von Barbituraten bei Ratten verschiedenen Alters. Naunyn Schmiedebergs Arch. Pharmacol., 265, 310-320.

LaDu, B. N. (1974). Pharmacogenetics: Single gene effects. In T. Teorell R. L. Dedrick, and P. G. Condliffe (Eds.), Pharmacology and Pharmacokinetics. Plenum Press, New York. pp. 253-260.

Lasagna, L., V. A. Laties, and L. J. Dohan (1958). Further studies on the "pharmacology" of placebo administration. J. Clin. Invest., 37, 533-537.

Lemberger, L., and A. Rubin (1975). The physiologic disposition of marihuana in man. Life Sci., 17, 1637-1642.

Levi, A. J., S. Sherlock, and D. Walker (1968). Phenylbutazone and isoniazid metabolism in patients with liver disease in relation to previous drug therapy. Lancet, I, 1275-1279.

Liddle, D. E., F. M. Williams, and R. H. Briant (1975). Phenazone (antipyrine) metabolism and distribution in young and elderly adults. Clin. Exp. Pharmacol. Physiol., 2, 481-487.

Morselli, P. L. (1977). Psychotropic drugs. In P. L. Morselli (Ed.), Drug Disposition and Development. Spectrum Publ., New York. pp. 431-474.

Motulsky, A. G. (1957). Drug reactions, enzymes and biochemical genetics. J. Am. Med. Assoc., 165, 835-837.

Munkelt, P. (1965). Persönlichkeitsmerkmale (psychische Stabilität und Geschlecht) als Bedingungsfaktoren der psychotropen Arzneimittelwirkung. Psychol. Beitr., 8, 98-183.

Munkelt, P., and G. A. Lienert (1964). Blutalkoholspiegel und psycho-
    physische Konstitution. Arzneim.-Forsch. (Drug Res.), 14, 573-575.
Munkelt, P., and E. Othmer (1965). Der Einfluß der psychischen Stabi-
    lität und Labilität und der Körperkonstitution der Versuchspersonen
    auf die Wirkung des Psychotonikums 7-[2'-(1"-Methyl-2"-phenyl-
    aethylaminol-aethyl)]-theophyllin-HCl. Arzneim.-Forsch. (Drug Res.),
    15, 843-849.
Munkelt, P., G. A. Lienert, M. Frahm, and K. Soehring (1962). Ge-
    schlechtsspezifische Wirkungsunterschiede der Kombination von Alko-
    hol und Meprobamat auf psychisch stabile und labile Versuchspersonen.
    Arzneim.-Forsch. (Drug Res.), 12, 1059-1065.
Myrsten, A. L., C. Hollstedt, and L. Holmberg (1972). Alcohol - induced
    changes in mood and activation in males and females as related to
    catecholamine excretion and blood alcohol level. Reports from the
    Psychological Laboratories, No. 375. University of Stockholm.
Oduah, M. (1969). Effektivität und Wirkungsdauer von Thiopental beim
    Menschen in Abhängigkeit vom Alter. Der Anästhesist, 18, 308-310.
O'Malley, K. O., J. Crooks, E. Duke, and I. H. Stevenson (1971).
    Effect of age and sex on human drug metabolism. Br. Med. J., 3,
    607-609.
O'Malley, K. O., T. G. Judge, and J. Crooks (1980). Geriatric clinical
    pharmacology and therapeutics. In G. S. Avery (Ed.), Drug Treatment:
    Principles and Practice of Clinical Pharmacology and Therapeutics,
    2nd ed. Adis Press, New York. pp. 158-181.
Omenn, G. S., and A. G. Motulsky (1975). Pharmacogenetics: Clinical
    and experimental studies in man. In B. E. Eleftheriou (Ed.),
    Psychopharmacogenetics. Plenum Press, New York. pp. 183-228.
Oswald, W. D. (1979). Anxiolyse und subjektiv erlebte "Anpassungsän-
    derung" bei leichter kognitiver Belastung im Vergleich zwischen
    Betablockern und Tranquilizern. Vortrag auf der 21. Tagung experi-
    mentell arbeitender Psychologen. Heidelberg.
Pare, C. M. B., and J. W. Mack (1971). Differentiation of two genetic-
    ally specific types of depression by response to anti-depressant
    drug. J. Med. Genet., 8, 306-309.
Patwardhan, R. V., P. V. Desmond, R. F. Johnson, G. D. Dunn, D. H.
    Robertson, A. M. Hoyumpa, and S. Schenker (1980). Effects of
    caffeine on plasma free fatty acids urinary catecholamines and drug
    binding. Clin. Pharmacol. Ther., 28, 398-403.
Petrinovich, L. (1967). Drug facilitation of learning: strain differ-
    ences. Psychopharmacologia, 10, 375-378.
Prange, A. J., I. C. Wilson, A. M. Rabon, and M. A. Lipton (1969).
    Enhancement of imipramine antidepressant activity by thyroid hor-
    mone. Am. J. Psychiatry, 126, 457-469.
Propping, P., and M. Kopun (1973). Pharmacogenetic aspects of psycho-
    active drugs. Humangenetik, 20, 291-320.
Rapoport, J. L., M. S. Buchsbaum, T. P. Zahn, H. Weingartner, C.
    Ludlow, and E. J. Mikkelsen (1978). Dextroamphetamine: Cognitive
    and behavioral effects in normal prebuberal boys. Science, 199,
    560-563.
Raskin, A. (1974). Age-sex differences in response to antidepressant
    drugs. J. Nerv. Ment. Dis., 159, 120-130.
Raskin, A., and T. H. Crook (1975). Antidepressants in black and white in-
    patients. Differential response to a controlled trial of chlorpromazine
    and imipramine. Arch. Gen. Psychiatry, 32, 643-649.
Raskin, A., J. G. Schulterbrandt, and N. Reatig (1970). Differential
    response to chlorpromazine, imipramine and placebo: A study of sub-
    groups of hospitalized depressed patients. Arch. Gen. Psychiatry,
    23, 164-173.

Raskin, A., I. G. Schulterbrandt, N. Reatig, T. H. Crook, and D. Odle
    (1974). Depression subtypes and response to phenelzine, diazepam,
    and a placebo. Arch. Gen. Psychiatry, 30, 66-75.
Reidenberg, M. M., M. Levy, H. Warner, C. B. Coutinho, M. A. Schwartz,
    G. Yu, and J. Cheripko (1978). Relationship between diazepam dose,
    plasma level, age, and central nervous system depression. Clin.
    Pharmacol. Ther., 23, 371-374.
Reisby, N. (1972). The Influence of Alcohol and Meprobamate on Psycho-
    logical Processes in Man. Munksgaard, Copenhagen.
Riester, E. F., E. J. Pantuck, C. B. Pantuck, G. T. Passananti, E. S.
    Vesell, and A. H. Conney (1980). Antipyrine metabolism during the
    menstrual cycle. Clin. Pharmacol. Ther., 28, 384-391.
Rommelspacher, H., H. Coper, H. Lison, C. Fähndrich, and S. Strauß
    (1972). Über den Einfluß von Rezeptorenblockern und zentral wir-
    kenden Substanzen auf die Thermoregulation und den Katecholamin-
    haushalt bei erwachsenen und alten Ratten. Acta Gerontol., 1, 5-8.
Routledge, P. A., W. W. Stargel, B. B. Kitchell, A. Barchowsky, and
    D. G. Shand (1981). Sex-related differences in the plasma protein
    binding of lignocaine and diazepam. Br. J. Clin. Pharmacol., 11,
    245-250.
Salzman, C., R. I. Shader, J. S. Harmatz, and L. Robertson (1975). Psycho
    pharmacologic investigations in elderly volunteers: Effect of dia-
    zepam in males. J. Am. Geriatr. Soc., 23, 451-457.
Saunders, D. R., R. M. Paolino, W. F. Bousquet, T. S. Miya (1974).
    Age-related responsiveness of the rat to drugs affecting the central
    nervous system. Proc. Soc. Exp. Biol. Med., 147, 593-595.
Sellers, E. M., and M. R. Holloway (1978). Drug kinetics and alcohol
    ingestion. Clin. Pharmacokinet., 3, 440-452.
Sellers, E. M., C. A. Naranjo, H. G. Giles, R. C. Frecker, and M.
    Beeching (1980). Intravenous diazepam and oral ethanol interaction.
    Clin. Pharmacol. Ther., 28, 638-645.
Shapiro, A. K. (1964). Factors contributing to the placebo effect their
    implications for psychotherapy. Am. J. Psychother., 18 (Suppl. 1),
    73-88.
Sheldon, W. H., S. S. Stevens, and W. B. Tucker (1940). The Varieties
    of Human Physique. Harper, New York.
Sjöquist, F., B. Alexanderson, M. Asberg, L. Bertilsson, O. Borgä,
    B. Hamberger, and D. Tuck (1971). Pharmacokinetics and biological
    effects of nortriptyline in man. Acta Pharmacol., 29 (Suppl. 3),
    255-280.
Slanska, J., J. Plevová, O. Benešova, K. Tikal, and J. Hvizdošova
    (1974). Alteration of psychosomatic reactivity after a single thera-
    peutic dose of pentobarbital in relation to the sex of probands.
    Act. Nerv. Super., 16, 218-220.
Stevenson, I. H. (1973). The significance and determinants of drug
    metabolism in man. Digestion, 8, 80-86.
Storrie, M. C., and C. Eisdorfer (1978). Psychophysiological studies
    in aging: A ten year review. In M. A. Lipton, A. DiMascio, and K.
    F. Killam (Eds.), Psychopharmacology: A Generation of Progress.
    Raven Press, New York. pp. 1489-1492.
Taeuber, K., W. Rupp, H. F. Brettel, G. Gammel, and R. Bender (1976).
    Untersuchungen über Wechselwirkungen zwischen einem Psychopharmakon
    (Nomifensin) und Alkohol. Blutalkohol, 13, 3-18.
Thomson, P. D., M. Rowland, and K. L. Melmon (1971). The influence of
    heart failure, liver disease, and renal failure on the disposition
    of lidocaine in man. Am. Heart J., 82, 412-421.
Turner, P. (1978). Influence of age on drug metabolism in man. In
    J. W. Gorrod, and A. H. Beckett (Ed.), Drug Metabolism in Man.
    Taylor and Francis, London. pp. 119-125.

Uhlenhuth, E. H., R. S. Lipman, K. Rickels, S. Fisher, L. Coove, and
    L. C. Park (1968). Predicting the relief of anxiety with meprobamate:
    non-drug factors in the response of psychoneurotic outpatients.
    Arch. Gen. Psychiatry, 19, 619-630.
Vesell, E. S. (1972). Introduction: Genetic and environmental factors
    affecting drug response in man. Fed. Proc., 31, 1253-1269.
Vesell, E. S. (1973). Advances in pharmacogenetics. Progr. Med. Genet.,
    9, 291-367.
Vesell, E. S. (1974). Factors causing interindividual variations of
    drug concentrations in blood. Clin. Pharmacol. Ther., 16, 135-142.
Vesell, E. S., J. G. Page, and G. T. Passananti (1971). Genetic and
    environmental factors affecting ethanol metabolism in man. Clin.
    Pharmacol. Ther., 12, 192-201.
Vogel, F., and A. G. Motulsky (1979). Human Genetics. Springer, New
    York.
Wallgren, H. (1959). Sex differences in ethanol tolerance of rats.
    Nature, 184, 726-727.
Wender, P. H. (1978). Minimal brain dysfunction: An overview. In M. A.
    Lipton, A. DiMascio, and K. F. Killam (Eds.), Psychopharmacology:
    A Generation of Progress. Raven Press, New York. pp. 1429-1435.
Winsberg, B. G., J. M. Percel, M. J. Hurwic, and A. Klutsch (1974).
    Imipramine protein binding and pharmacokinetics in children. In
    I. S. Forrest, C. J. Carr, and E. Usdin (Eds.), The Phenothiazines
    and Structurally Related Drugs. Raven Press, New York. pp. 425-431.
Wolff, P. H. (1972). Ethnic differences in alcohol sensitivity.
    Science, 175, 449-450.
Worsham, E. D., E. P. Riley, N. Anandam, P. Lister, E. X. Freed, and
    D. Lester (1977). Selective breeding of rats for differences in re-
    activity to alcohol: An approach to an animal model of alcoholism.
    III. Some physical and behavioral measures. Adv. Exp. Med. Biol.,
    85a, 71-81.
Zerssen, D. von (1964). Dimensionen der morphologischen Habitusvaria-
    tionen und ihre biometrische Erfassung. Z. menschl. Vererb. u.
    Konstit. Lehre, 37, 611-625.
Ziem, M., H. Coper, I. Brovermann, and S. Strauss (1970). Vergleichen-
    de Untersuchungen über einige Wirkungen des Amphetamins bei Ratten
    verschiedenen Alters. Naunyn Schmiedebergs Arch. Pharmacol., 257,
    208-223.
Zubin, J., S. Sutton, K. Salzinger, S. Salzinger, E. J. Burdock, and
    D. Peretz (1961). A biometric approach to prognosis in schizo-
    phrenia. In P. H. Hoch, and J. Zubin (Eds.), Comparative Epidemio-
    logy of the Mental Disorders. Grune and Stratton, New York.
    pp. 28-39.

GENETIC AND EARLY ENVIRONMENTAL FACTORS IN RESPONSE VARIABILITY TO PSYCHOTROPIC DRUGS

Roger W. Russell

ABSTRACT

Drugs produce their effects by altering biochemical events already going on within the body. Many of the events affected, particularly those in the nervous system, are involved in the behavior of an organism as an integrated whole. In any individual organism the nature of these events is determined by interactions between genetic and environmental factors, interactions which are evidenced in intraindividual differences during development as well as in interindividual differences throughout the life span. It follows that genetic and environmental factors are involved in the variability of behavioral responses to psychotic drugs. In developing this theme, attention is given to the study of both human and other animal subjects. Examples of research involving experimental, clinical and "field" methodologies provide support for the basic concepts discussed.

KEYWORDS

Genetic factors; early environmental factors; behavioral phenotype; biochemical mechanisms of action; "systems" approach; psychopharmacogenetics; intraindividual differences; interindividual differences; pharmacokinetics; pharmacodynamics.

INTRODUCTION

A leader in the early development of neuropsychopharmacology once pointed to "... a very important principle in pharmacology...We cannot expect drugs to introduce anything new into the mind or into behavior, but merely to accentuate or to suppress functions in behavior which are already present (Kety, 1961)."The paragraphs which follow examine "functions" of living organisms which interact with chemicals (drugs) introduced into the body and which are involved in the variability of

an organism's subsequent responses. The ultimate responses of interest
to the present discussion are the behaviors of organisms as integrated
systems coping with the ever-changing physical and psychosocial environments within which they live. Drugs which affect behavior have come to
be called "psychoactive" or "psychotropic".

Accepting a literal definition, this category of chemicals is sometimes
limited to those agents which are perceived to have, in some sense,
"direct" effects on behavior. But in the complex internal environment
of an organism "direct" is difficult to define. The route to effects
on behavior of the total organism winds through many preceeding events
stimulated by the entry of a chemical into the body, through what bio-
chemists and pharmacologists call "mechanisms of action". The nature
of such events at any one time are dependent upon their past history
an their present status. Both genetic and environmental factors make
their contributions to the fact that people vary greatly in their sensitivity to drugs. What may be a safe and appropriate prescriptive
dosage for one person at one time may be an overdose for another -
and for the person himself at a different time. Both inter- and intra-
individual differences characterize responses to drugs generally
(Janke and others, 1979; Janke, 1980).

As the term itself suggests, "psychotropic" drugs are chemicals intended
to affect behavior. The term has often been identified with drugs used
in the treatment of psychiatric disorders, but it need not be so limited
In its broadest sense "psychotropic" may be taken to include all chemicals that may have changes in behavior among their effects: they are
"psychoactive". A "drug", broadly defined, is any chemical agent that
affects living processes. There are a great number that affect behavior.
Within the more limited definition, over 1500 compounds have been classi
fied as psychotropic agents (Usdin, 1978). However, behavior is sensitive to many more, including pollutants (e.g. pesticides, industrial
solvents, heavy metals such as lead and mercury) to which individuals
may be exposed in the workplace or in their native habitats (Russell,
1977a).

"Perhaps at this time there is no one who classifies behavior into two
categories, innate and learned. The dichotomy, carried to its logical
conclusion, would define innate behavior as that which appeared in the
absence of environment, and learned behavior as that which required
no organism (Fuller and Thompson, 1960)." It would be absurd (Verplanck,
1955) to assert that genetic and environmental factors are not involved
in all functions of living organisms. Information encoded in genetic
material determines the species to which an organism belongs. It interacts with environmental conditions to guide the development of those
particular characteristics which identify each individual. Environmental
factors - from intrauterine to the grand biosphere in which an individual lives from birth through senescence - affect that uniqueness, but
always within the constraints of genetic potential. It is not at all
strange that response variability of living organisms to psychotropic
drugs should be related in some way to such interactions between genetic
and environmental influences. "... the relationship between heredity
and behavior has turned out to be one of neither isomorphism nor independence. Isomorphism might justify an approach of naive reductionism,
independence a naive behaviorism. Neither one turns out to be adequate
(Hirsch, 1970)".

Hopefully the paragraphs which follow will throw some light on the
nature of such influences. They have significant implications both
for our basic knowledge about effects of chemicals on biological
systems and for the application of such knowledge for the benefits of
living organisms. To tell the story properly it is necessary to consider certain fundamental concepts about the modes of action of drugs
and about the nature of living organisms as integrated "systems".
Against this background it will then be possible to formulate questions
relating to genetic and environmental influences on behavioral response
variability to psychotropic drugs. Questions motivate the search for
answers, which, in turn, necessitates attention to methods by which
answers may best be obtained. By then we should be prepared to examine
evidence of the genetic and the environmental influences which are
the central concerns of the present discussion.

HOW DO DRUGS ACT?

"Logically all genetic effects on behavior involve biochemistry. There
is no other way for genes to act (Fuller and Thompson, 1978)". Effects
of a drug on a biological system arise from physicochemical interactions
between that drug and functionally important molecules in the living
organism. Interactions may involve combining with a small molecule or
ion, e.g. when an antacid neutralizes hydrochloric acid in the stomach.
However, in cases of the kind toward which we are now turning our attention, drugs are presumed to interact with large molecular components
of tissues. The particular components with which drugs combine are
called "receptors", the combination initiating biochemical processes
within the tissue.

Many processes are involved between the input of a drug and its effects
on the consequent behavioral output of the organism as a whole. A co-
ordinated output requires integration of the relevant functions. To
produce its characteristic effect(s), a drug must be present in appropriate concentrations at its site(s) of action, i.e. tissues and organs
react selectively to different drugs. Obviously the amount of drug administered affects the concentration at active sites, but concentrations are also dependent upon the extent and rate of the absorption
of a drug, its distribution in the body, binding or localization in
tissues, biotransformation and excretion. All of these processes are
dependent upon the biochemical, electrophysiological and morphological
properties of the organism, properties arising genetically but modified
by environmental conditions to which the organism is exposed during its
life span. The complexities of both genetic and environmental influences
are so great that the broad range of inter- and intra-individual differences in these properties found among members of the same species comes
as no surprise. "Our knowledge of the pathway from gene to behavior,
certainly a long and tortuous one, is as yet lettle understood (Shaw,
1976)".

A "SYSTEMS" APPROACH

How do molecular events affected by psychoactive drugs come to be reflected in molar changes in the organism's behavior? Systematic search
for answers to such questions requires some rational conceptual framework.

To find answers has been considered a vital endeavor since the earliest
beginnings of modern psychology. To Professor Wilhelm Wundt, founder
100 years ago of the first laboratory of experimental psychology, the
keystone of all total adjustments of living organisms is a psychophysiological process, an organic response approachable through both
physiology and psychology (Wundt, 1904). Even half a century later
Professor Clark Hull, one of the most important contributors of his
time to the "new" American psychology, commented that "... neuroana-
tomy and physiology have not yet developed to a point such that they
yield principles which may be employed as postulates in a system of
behavior theory ... (Hull, 1943)." Knowledge about events intervening
between the environment and on organism's success in coping with it
has undergone remarkable changes since then. New skills which make
possible new discoveries appear frequently and produce rewarding feelings of accomplishment that stimulate further search for information
about molecular events within the organism. This endeavor is very
praiseworthy. However, it would be tragic if, in the process, the fact
were overlooked that the organism as a whole is different from the
simple sum of its parts, that the molar function of the integrated
organism deserve equal attention.

The Organism as a System

The events which take place between the input of a drug and consequent
effects on behavior occur within an integrated organism, a total system
consisting of the organism in its biosphere (Russell, 1979). Within
that total system the organism receives inputs from the external environment and produces outputs to the environment, some of which may
alter the existing state of the organism. The multivariate and highly
integrated organization of living organisms has led to conceptualization in terms of hierarchies of "subsystems", e.g. the vascular, the
nervous. It is accepted that biochemical and electrophysiological
events in the nervous system are most directly related to behavior.
Chemicals (drugs) from the external environment transported to and
affecting neural tissue may produce effects in the overall behavior
of the organism. Behavioral effects may also be observed when changes
in other, non-neural subsystems are involved in ways which interact
with events in the neural subsystem. For example, genetically determined
individual differences in the hepatic biotransformation (inactivation
and elimination) of a drug which affects its time of action in the
body may have significant influences on the effects of the drug on
nervous tissue and hence on behavior.

Within limits the subsystems are self-regulatory, self-correcting.
Exposure to a drug which produces changes in one subsystem may lead
to subsequent compensatory changes in others. Relations within each
of them are reversible in the sense that alterations in one direction
may lead to compensatory changes in the opposite direction. These
processes of "homeostasis" have been shown by Claude Bernard,
Sherrington, Cannon and many others to be essential for adjustments
of living organisms to dynamic fluctuations in the external environment. Homeostatic processes may also involve such behavioral plasticities as habituation, tolerance development, and learning and memory.
All these plasticities show individual differences to which both genetic and environmental factors contribute. All have their limits
beyond which adverse effects appear.

It follows from the system concept that conditions which affect any subsystem may have effects on the integrity of the organism as a whole. Subsystems originate from the readout of information genetically coded. Their subsequent development is controlled by interactions between genetic and environmental factors, as is their functioning during the entire life span. Because drugs act by physicochemical interactions with molecules in various subsystems of the living organism it would be expected that their effects would also be under "control" of genetic and environmental influences.

Individual Differences

The study of individual differences in susceptibility of behavior to environmental changes is as old as experimental psychology. The early German psychophysicists discovered relations between magnitudes of sensory stimulation and consequent changes of behavior. Such relations may be described in terms of basal and terminal thresholds and of units, just noticeable differences, which characterize behavior as the magnitude of environmental change varies. In many instances this relation takes the form of ogival - of cumulative normal population - curves. Pharmacologists have found similar relations between drugs entering the body and subsequent changes in biochemical and electrophysiological events within the body. Psychopharmacologists have added measures of behavior to these variables. Both have discovered that the typical S-shaped dose-effect relation holds.

They have not only discovered that lawful relations exist between such parameters as the dose and the time of action of a drug, but also that the thresholds at which effects appear may vary from time to time within an individual. Such intraindividual differences are influenced by a variety of environmental conditions.

Interindividual differences in effects of drugs are also clearly apparent wherever one looks. Reactions to the same dose varies from person to person. In many instances the differences form themselves into a continuous series with the shapes of normal population curves. In some, however, the distribution is discontinuous, suggesting the existence of more than one population of individual "types."

"Pychopharmacogenetics"

Behavior genetics is concerned with questions about contributions of hereditory and environmental factors to the occurence of individual differences. What are the contributions of each factor to the total variance? What mechanisms are involved? From overlapping interests in behavior genetics and psychopharmacology has arisen a hybrid science of "psychopharmacogenetics," with the specific purpose of studying psychotropic drugs within the context of well-defined genetic systems. Effects on behavior produced by such drugs are the characteristics of the organism examined. The visible and measureable behavioral traits constitute an organism's behavioral phenotype. The systems approach discussed earlier emphasizes that behavioral phenotypes interact with morphological and biochemical phenotypes in the integrated organism.

In studying the origin and development of any phenotype, genetic and environmental determinants must both be considered. Within a population

the phenotypic variance, P, among individuals is closely associated
with differences in genetic determinats (G) and differences in non-
genetic (environmentalor acquired) determinants (E) and may be
influenced by interactions between the two: P = G + E + f(G,E). A
basic assumption of this analysis of variance model is that a population's total variance can be expressed as the sum of the variances
of independent determinants.

The complex nature of the living "system" becomes clearly apparent
when efforts are made to understand the bases for individual differences
in reactions to drugs. The number of potential determinants is great.
Some are characteristics of the organism: sex differences, age,
genetically-related susceptibility, nutritional condition, state of
biochemical processes especially within the nervous system. Others
relate to the characteristics of the drug: chemical structure, extent
and frequency or duration of exposure, route of entry into the body,
interaction with other chemicals present in the external environment
or already stored in body fluids or tissues. Others arise from the
structural integrity of the body, e.g. organisms with central nervous
system lesions may respond ideosyncratically. Still other determinants
are related to inter-individual differences in behavioral states:
attenuation of acute drug effects may be a specific consequence of
"learning to behave" in the drug state. Finally, there may be populations at special risk: in many instances these have been found to be
pregnant women, young children and workers subjected to occupational
exposures.

"We cannot understand the behavior of an organism without understanding
the organism not only as an integrated and coordinated system responsive
to its environment, but also as a member of a population with a unique
evolutionary history adapting it to the niche it presently occupies
(Hirsch, 1962)." To understand the nature of effects of psychotropic
drugs on individual differences in behavior we must search among
genetic factors which "control" biochemical events and behavior and
among environmental factors which modify them.

METHODOLOGICAL CONSIDERATIONS

Success in searching for genetic and early environmental factors
affecting individual differences in behavioral responses to psychotropic drugs depends on the ingenuity with which critical observations
are made. It requires strategies - research designs - for apportioning
the variation of behavioral responses to psychotropic drugs into
various genetic and environmental categories. To be implemented the
research designs must provide methods for varying the independent
variable: G, genetic or E, environmental similarity, or f(G,E),
interaction between the two. Techniques for measuring drug-behavior
interactions, the dependent variables, must be demonstrated to be
reliable and valid. The systemsapproach discussed above also suggests
the desirability of investigating mechanisms of action by which genes
or environmental conditions produce variations in drug response: this
requires a broad range of specialized techniques from biochemistry,
pharmacology and neurology. The discussion to follow is intended to
be a brief review of general approaches to researching the kinds of
questions considered above. It makes no pretense at specifying
procedures and techniques in detail. The general approaches arise from
the relation: P = G + E + f(G,E). "The genotypic approach starts with

a known difference in heredity and evaluates its influence on behavior.... In the phenotypic approach an attempt is made to discover the genetic factors (if any) responsible for observed variations in behavior (Fuller & Thompson, 1978)." In hypotheses of these two types, genetic determinants and behavioral phenotypes change places as independent variables. Both strategies have their advantages and their limitations. Both have been applied to research on human subjects and on animal models.

Human Subjects

Social and ethical considerations place strict restraints on experimental manipulations and control of important variables when human subjects are involved, including limitations on administration of psychotropic drugs for research purposes. This means that 1) situations must be sought where desired differences in independent variables already occur and that 2) heavy demands are placed on statistical control over differences in environmental and mating variables that may interact with genetic determinants. Put in another way, the research calls for a general strategy of finding subsets of individuals in whom genetic and environmental similarities are imperfectly correlated and studying their respective reactions to the drugs (Loehlin, 1975). Fuller and Thompson (1978) have proposed a useful classification for special methods based upon whether we are dealing with discrete, unitary traits or with continuous (or quasi-continuous) complex characters. The specific rationales and procedures in each case need to be outlined before we proceed further.

Perhaps the oldest of approaches to testing hypotheses that some unitary behavioral trait is inherited is by determining its occurence and nonoccurence in family pedigrees. Pedigree analysis may provide evidence of inherited patterns when a particular drug effect occurs significantly more frequently in one lineage than in others. A second approach to the study of unitary traits has involved population surveys. Predictions from a hypothesis providing an expected incidence in occurrence of particular behavioral effects of a psychotropic drug are compared with the observed incidence in a random sample of the population. The operation of genetic factors is suggested when discontinuities in effects are observed - when subgroups within the population sampled are found to have significantly different frequencies of drug reaction.

Many behavioral effects of psychotropic drugs are continuous rather than dichotamous in their manifestations and a more extensive array of approaches to studying them has been developed. Perhaps the best known among them is the study of identical genotypes using sets of twins. Comparisons may be made between monogygotic and digygotic twins for rates of concordance in reactions to drugs. Comparisons of twins reared together and apart may provide cues about possible involvement of environmental variables. In theory adoption studies make it possible to test either genetic or environmental hypotheses about determinants of drug-behavior interactions. It is possible to make predictions about the biological and adopting parents from the drug reactions of the adoptees or to make predictions about the latter from reactions of the former. Approaches using other subsets of persons with such varying extents of familiar resemblance as half siblings, i.e.individuals with only one biological parent in common, are becoming of increasing interest.

Animal Models

The use of animal models of human conditions has long been a feature
of research in the biomedical sciences. Their usefulness in experimental studies in behavioral genetics has long been recognized (e.g.
Hall, 1951; Russell, 1953). Critical reviews of this approach (e.g.
Serban & Kling, 1976) have discussed the advantages and the conceptual
problems associated with their various uses. In searching for factors
affecting response variability to psychotropic drugs animal models
can usefully supplement research on human subjects, particularly in
research in two very important areas where the latter cannot be used.
One of these areas involves experimental studies of conditions internal to the subject that require sampling or manipulation of tissues
in order, for example, to carry out neurochemical assays or to investigate interactions between effects of a drug and a tissue lesion.
The second area is one in which mating techniques such as selective
breeding are involved.

Various degrees of genetic similarity may be achieved when mating is
controlled. During the past quarter century increasing availability
of genetic stocks has led to a wealth of experimentation. Among the
most used stocks are those in which genetic homogeneity has been
achieved by carefully controlled programs of inbreeding, i.e. inbred
lines. Heterogenic stocks deliberately bred for high genetic variability and natural populations, heterogeneous by natural selection,
serve their purposes in research designed to study ranges of phenotypic variation, as backgrounds, "controls", for comparisons with
selectively-bred lines, and for studies of genetic relationships
between behavioral and somatic traits. Selected lines, developed
through procedures for assortative mating, have been developed for
several behavioral traits and for somatic traits, e.g. brain weight,
brain enzyme activity, believed to be involved in the mechanisms of
action related to behavioral traits.

It is well recognized that problems arise when attempts are made to
generalize principles established in one species to another. Although
there are means for testing how well a sample represents the population
within a species, there is no equivalent statistic to ensure that a
phenomenon in one species is in fact equivalent to what may appear
to be the same phenomenon in another, i.e. analogies may be mistaken
for homologies. Caution is required in generalizing from animal models
to human systems. However, the advantages of experimental procedures
to the development of a systematic body of basic principles makes
the use of animal models attractive for many purposes.

The conclusions and insights arising from any set of observations
are dependent upon both the theoretical model within which an investigation is planned and the operation by which it is carried out.
Darwin once commented: "How odd it is that anyone should not see that
all observation must be for or against some view if it is to be of
any service (Stone, 1980)." The preceding sections of the present
paper have been devoted to setting the background - the conceptual
framework, the hypotheses and the procedures by which predictions'
may be tested - against which the search for genetic and early environmental factors in response variability to psychotropic drugs is
carried out. We may now proceed to examine typical results of the
search.

GENETIC FACTORS IN RESPONSE VARIABILITY

"Different organisms respond differently to their environments because
of different genetic endowments. Since drugs are part of the human
environment, it is natural to encounter hereditary factors that affect
the responsiveness of the human organism to drugs, and one should find
these factors in all forms of life which are appropriately studied
(Kalow, 1968)." This statement by one of its pioneers writing on
"Pharmacogenetics in Animals and Man" sets the broad boundaries of
the search for genetic factors in response variability to psychotropic
drugs.

Animal Models

There is a kind of value in starting an examination of what the research literature has to offer on the subject by looking at animal
models: "... experimental behavior genetics has developed to the
point that it can illuminate problems that cannot be studied experimentally in human beings (Fuller and Thompson, 1978).""Experimental"
has an aura of greater control over the circumstances in which observations are made than does "non-experimental", although the latter
may be even more powerful for answering some kinds of questions.
"In man, any approach to the problem of the nature of gene function
is necessarily rather indirect (Meier, 1963)."

Drug-behavior interactions: line differences. Despite the obvious
potential value to psychopharmacogenetics of comparisons between
subjects with different genotypes, studies of line differences in
reactions to drugs have only relatively recently come into vogue.
However, already the number from which to select examples for purposes of the present discussion is sufficiently large to cause some
conflict in choosing. Those described below have been selected for
particular points they illustrate. A full review of the literature
would contain many more references.

A report by Ray and Barrett (1975) of research on two behaviorally
very different lines of rats illustrates both the use of genetic
differences to analyze behavioral and biochemical traits and also
the use of the latter to study mechanisms of action by which the
former are reflected in behavior. The research program began by demonstrating significant line differences in conditional avoidance
behavior, indicating genetic influences of some kind. The next step
was to examine various parameters of the behavior in order to pin-
point more precisely the one(s) under genetic control, leading to
the conclusion that "... differences in shuttle box avoidance acquisition is genetic and is based on their activity response to
shock stress rather than to a difference in general learning ability
(Ray and Barrett, 1975)." Having established that genotypic differences
were associated with differences in the behavioral phenotype the investigators then sought information about neurochemical mechanisms
underlying the relationship. Drugs known to affect avoidance learning
(e.g. amphetamine, parachloramphetamine) and with known neurochemical
actions were administered and effects on the criterion behavior
measured, with results which suggested that the behavioral differences
were related to differences in brain monoamine responses to shock
stress. Finally, biochemical studies showed that turnover in the

brain neurotransmitter substances, serotonin, norepinephrine and dopamine,followed exposure to the shock stress used to motivate subjects during conditioned avoidance training.

Most studies using line differences as means for varying genotypes
are more fully focussed on genetic relationships. For example, studies
by Oliverio and co-workers (Oliverio and others, 1973; Oliverio, 1974)
have sought to use "stain distribution patterns (SDP)" to assess the
probable location of a new gene related to behavior by matching its
SDP with those of other genes among a set of inbred lines. Short-term
exploratory activity was found to be significantly higher in one line
than in a second line. Administration of the drug, scopolamine, reversed the activity levels in the two lines. Basal activity levels
and effects of scopolamine were then assessed in the two original
lines, their reciprocal F hybrids, their recombinant inbred lines
and three congenic lines. Results suggested the characterization of
a gene exerting the main influence on the behavioral phenotype and
also a gene modulating drug effect of scopolamine on the behavior.
The opposite behavioral effects were produced by administration of
amphetamine, the results suggesting a polygenic basis for that drug's
action. Physostigmine exerted a suppressing effect on exploratory
behavior in all genotypes. The findings with the cholinergic drugs,
scopolamine and physostigmine, suggest involvement of the cholinergic
neurotransmitter system in the behavioral phenotype, the differences
in their effects being understandable in that the former is an anta-
gonist and the latter an indirect agonist in that system.

A similar study (van Abeelen, 1974), worthy of special note, used a
psychopharmacogenetic approach to investigate cholinergic regulation
of exploratory behavior in two inbred mouse strains, and in two lines
derived from a cross between the strains. The results were interpreted as "... compatible with the idea of a genotype-dependent
cholinergic mechanism, probably located in the hippocampus, which
controls the response of mice to novelty. A functionally optimal
ACh/AChE ratio will guarantee efficient synaptic transmission and
thereby facilitate exploration. Any genetically-determined imbalances
... may be restored by administration of an anticholinergic drug"
(van Abeelen, 1974). These conclusions have interesting implications
in light of increasing attention being given the cholinergic system
in cases of human behavioral abnormalities.

Reports on effects of some of the most widely used psychotropic drugs
have further documented the existence of genetic influences. Strain
differences have been noted in effects of chlorpromazine and chlordiazepoxide on active and passive avoidance responding, with "...
relative invariance of strain rankings in activity regardless of
experimental conditions (Fuller, 1970)." Bovet and co-workers (1967)
have referred to tobacco as representing "... one of the oldest and
most widely used psychotropic drugs" in discussing their research
on effects of nicotine on spontaneous and acquired behavior in rats
and mice. Nicotine had a facilitating effect on the behavioral phenotype in six of nine inbred strains of mice studied; it had less
effect on one strain and impaired performance in two.It was of
particular interest that three strains belonging to the same "strain
family" showed strikingly different reactions: two were low in performance and one, high. A final example focusses an another commonly
used psychotropic drug, ethyl alcohol. MacPhail and Elsmore (1980)
have reported results which suggest that genetic variables may determi

the extent to which toxicant-induced conditioned aversions can be
established in mice.

These and many other studies are consistent in demonstrating genetic
influences on responses to psychotropic drugs. They also illustrate
how, when properly used, the "line differences" approach can provide
basic information about behavioral phenotype-genotype relations and
the discovery of mechanisms of action underlying them.

Drug-Behavior Interactions: Selected Lines

Clear evidence for the influence of genetic factors on behavior has
also come from research using assortative mating procedures. Samples
of animals from a general population have been tested for individual
differences in some behavioral phenotype. Males and females at each
end of the distribution have then been mated, high performers with
high and low with low. Several studies have reported success in
breeding lines of animals which differ significantly in the target
behavior: emotionally (Broadhurst, 1960; Hall, 1938), general activity (De Fries and Hegmann,1970), maze (Tryon, 1940) and conditioned
avoidance learning (Bignami, 1965).

It has also been possible to use the assortive mating approach to
breed lines of animals with significantly different neurochemical
phenotypes.Selection for high and low levels of activity of the enzyme, cholinesterase, in the rat cerebral cortex has been reported
(Roderick, 1960). Large phenotypic differences between inbred strains
of mice in cholinesterase activity has also been noted (Pryor and
others, 1966).

That genetic influences on <u>interactions</u> between the behavioral and
neurochemical phenotypes may be significant determinants of individual
differences in responses to psychotropic drugs is suggested by studies
of both human and animal subjects. Evidence has been presented that
elevated plasma cholinesterase activity may be a genetic variant in
humans (Neitlick, 1966) which could influence the effects of certain
classes of psychoactive drugs. A research program in our own laboratory has been designed specificially to study such possibilities
using the assortative mating approach (Overstreet and others, 1979a).
Male and female rats of the original parental generation were continuously distributed in terms of measures of several physiological
and behavioral measures when administered a standard dose of the
anticholinesterase agent, diisopropyl fluorophosphate (DFP). DFP
has been shown to have differential effects on a wide variety of
behaviors, affecting some and not others (Russell, 1977b). Its primary
action is to lower the level of activity of the enzyme cholinesterase
which has a key role in maintaining normal functioning of the cholinergic neurotransmitter system in brain. By inter-mating males and
females who were least reactive to DFP and also mating those most
reactive it was possible to develop two new lines of animals, a
resistant R-line and a sensitive S-line which began to differ from
each other by the second filial generation. The differences have
been maintained through 14 generations. Challenging animals from the
two lines with various psychotropic drugs has shown that they differ
in their responses and that they differ in the rates at which they
develop tolerance to chronic administration of DFP. The possibility
that genetic influences may also be involved in the variability of

human reactions to psychotropic drugs affecting the cholinergic system
has a particular present significance when increasing attention is
being given to that system in the pharmacotherapy of behavioral disorders. It is a reasonable hypothesis that interactions between other
neurochemical systems and behavior may also be subject to similar
genetic influences. "Success in changing a behavioral phenotype by
means of genetic selection is a priori evidence for heritability of
the criterion character, provided precautions have been taken to rule
out effects due to environmental factors and genetic drift (Fuller
and Thompson, 1978)."

A question not yet answered by the work in our laboratory concerns
the specificity of the linkage between genotype and behavioral phenotype. Is the relation so specific that selective breeding affects
only one behavior pattern? Or, will selective breeding for a particular
behavioral phenotype generalize to related behaviors - analogous,
perhaps, to the phenomenon of cross-tolerance which characterizes
chronic treatment with many drugs? A recent report on hypnotic sus-
ceptability to various depressant drugs in rats selectively bred for
differential sensitivity to ethyl alcohol suggests that there may not
be a simple answer to those questions (Riley and others, 1979). Sleep
time was used as the behavioral measure. Animals from the selectively-
bred lines were challenged with doses of three central depressants:
ethyl alcohol, chloral hydrate and phenobarbital. The lines showed
disparate reactions to the drugs: some differed in sensitivity to
alcohol, others on the more general phenotype of differential sensitivity to depressants generally.

A program of assortative mating designed to produce selected lines
of animals calls for a significant commitment in research effort and
laboratory costs. There also is the spectre of relative small payoff
for effort expended. These concerns may account for the relative
dirth of projects using this approach despite the contributions such
research may make to establishing basic principles underlying genetic
influences on variability of responses to psychotropic drugs.

Drug-Behavior Interactions: Sex Differences

In the search for genetic influences on behavior it is surprising
that more attention has not been given to male-female differences.
Studies of behavior have tended to eliminate such differences as
"confounding variables". Yet the unique role of the sex chromosomes
to determine sex and the existence of well known human sex-linked
traits (e.g. color blindness, hemophilia) suggests that the study
of sex differences in behavior has promise of providing another
approach to the discovery of principles underlying response variability to drug action. "In fact, one of the especially timely questions
about human behavior is the issue of male/female differences and the
extent to which they reflect cultural impact of the assigned sex
role or biological impact of the sex chromosomes and sex hormones"
(Omenn, 1975).

A series of experiments designed to study sex differences in reactions
to psychoactive drugs may serve as an example of the directions in
which such research may lead (Overstreet and others, 1979b). During
the course of our laboratory's selective breeding experiments described above it was found that female rats were more resistant thar

males to physiological and behavioral effects of the drug, DFP.
A series of experiments finally led to the mechanism underlying the
difference. The first showed that the phenotypic effects were related
to less inhibition of the brain enzyme, acetylcholinesterase (AChE),
following administration of the same dose of DFP in females than in
males. Examination of the five isoenzymes of AChE separated from
homogenates of brain demonstrated that all were more inhibited in
male animals. The possibility that the differences might depend upon
decreased sensitivity of postsynaptic receptors in females was dis-
carded when they were found to be supersensitive to the cholinergic
agonist agent, pilocarpine. Measurement of radioactivity in brain
homogenates following peripheral administration of radiolabelled DFP
indicated that the uptake of DFP into brain was less for females than
for males. A final experiment confirmed that the females had higher
normal levels of serum cholinesterase activity than males and that
DFP produced greater inhibition of the enzyme in females. Thus, the
differential psychoactive effects of the drug were found to be dependent upon sex differences in peripheral tissues which affected the
distribution of the drug to its target sites in the brain.

Human Subjects

A search of the literature leads to relatively few studies specifically designed to examine genetic factors in human responses to psychotropic drugs. Discussions with those who work in the even broader
field of human behavior genetics suggest that the present social
climate is not prepared to accept the possibility that there may be
genotypic constraints on human plasticities involved in coping with
the psychosocial, as well as the physical environment. "Suffice it
to say at this point that human behavior genetics, of all disciplines
in science, is always in danger of edging into the political domain
(Fuller and Thompson, 1978)". Despite limitations in directly relevant
reports, attention can be called to certain modal points of special
interest to human psychopharmacogenetics.

Studies of twins. The most frequently used research approach has been
through the study of identical genotypes and comparisons with less
closely related subjects. Results of such studies indicate much greater
similarity between identical than between fraternal twins. That control
is polygenic is suggested by the unimodal distribution curves obtained
when the results are plotted graphically (Vesell, 1975).

Empirical evidence from twin studies in support of the conclusion that
effects of commonly used drugs are under genetic control has come
from research on a range of agents, some of which may be considered
as primarily, and others only indirectly, psychotropic. For example,
Vesell and Page (1968a, 1968b, 1968c) have reported results of studies
of genetic control of metabolism of antipyretic, analgesic and anti-
coagulant drugs which have shown that large differences found among
unrelated individuals disappeared almost completely in identical
twins but appeared to some extent in fraternal twins. "The results
obtained were surprising to pharmacologists familiar with the multiple
environmental factors capable of altering rates of drug elimination
in animals. In our twins, large individual differences in rates of
elimination of ethanol (twofold), antipyrine (threefold), phenylbutazone (sixfold), and dicumarol (tenfold) were almost exclusively

under genetic control and under "basal" conditions were influenced negligibly by environmental factors (Vesell and others, 1971)".

An example more specifically related to psychotropic drugs is research into influences of genetic factors and drug therapy on reactions to nortriptyline, a tricyclic antidepressant which blocks reuptake of biogenic amines (Alexanderson and others, 1969). The investigation involved 19 sets of monozygotic and 20 of dizygotic twins. Nortrptyline was administered orally in doses of 0.2 mg/kg three times daily for eight days. The steady-state plasma levels of the drug served as a measure of its presence in the body. Healthy adults showed individual differences in steady-state plasma concentrations when treated with the same dose. Comparisons showed a much smaller interpair difference for monozygotic than for dizygotic twins, indicating that genetic factors played a major role in the variability of reaction to the drug. That environmental influences were also operative is indicated by the fact that exposures to other drugs influenced the steady-state plasma concentrations of nortriptyline, and consequently the variability of its effects.

A small number of experiments carried out using animal models to study individual differences in the effects of opiates have suggested that genetic mechanisms are involved in reactions to morphine (Broadhurst, 1978). Despite the importance of such a finding to an understanding of processes involved in drug abuse, the first genetic study of morphine in humans has only recently been completed (Liston and others, in press). Ten pairs of male monozygotic twins aged 21 to 28 years were given a battery of physiological and psychological tests once before and twice after intramuscular injection of a placebo on one day and of morphine on a second day, the two experimental periods separated by one to three weeks. Analyses of results suggested intrapair similarities both prior to and following administration of morphine for many of the variables measured, including pain tolerance, self-reports of hostility and anxiety, timed motor behavior, and several psychiatric ratings. Twin pairs were completely concordant for nausea and vomiting following injection of the drug. Although the lack of comparison groups leads the authors to consider their conclusions as preliminary, these results are consistent with a concept of strong genetic influences underlying individual differences in responses to psychiatric drugs.

Another study completed very recently (Jarvik, personal communication) provides evidence for genetic mediation of a variety of behavioral effects of amphetamines. Six pairs of male monozygotic twins were tested before and after administration of d- or l-amphetamine or placebo. Cognitive, psychomotor, personality, mood and pain variables were measured. The subjects responded similarly under placebo on many of the measures, indicating genetic influences. Although their behavior was affected by the drug conditions, they tended again to respond in similar ways in cognitive functioning, pain thresholds and several of the mood and personality variables.

Normal monozygotic twins and euthymic patients with bipolar affective disorders have participated in research designed to study effects of "pharmacogenetic probes" on individual differences in patient and normal human affective responses (Nurnberger and others, 1980): "Twin studies of pharmacologic responses may identify heritable neurochemical variations in man. Vulnerability to affective illness may be

uncovered by pharmacologic challenges of patients in the well state."
Challenges with d-amphetamine, a monoaminergic agonist, prolactin
and growth hormones produced responses which were highly concordant
in twins, but did not distinguish well-state patients from controls.
Bipolar patients in the well state and drug-free did differ from
controls by two responses to cholinergic agonists: more rapid development of REM sleep and greater pupillary conscription. The results
suggest the possibility that the influences of genetic and environmental factors on individual differences in responses to psychoactive
drugs may involve balancesbetween neurotransmitter systems, rather
than differences in one alone.

Studies of pedigrees. Results from family studies are in close agreement with those from twin studies in showing significant genetic influence on the large individual differences which characterize responses to drugs. Application of the pedigree approach in research on
genetic effects on the actions of psychotropic drugs is illustrated
in a study of the kinetics of the antidepressant drug, nortriptyline,
in relatives of persons with extremely high plasma concentrations
following administration of the drug. Twenty-nine relatives and 20
randomly selected subjects were given eight daily oral doses (Åsberg
and others, 1971). There was no tendency toward bimodality in the
distribution of plasma concentrations of the combined subjects, including all relatives and all full siblings. These results suggest
that the manner of inheritance of nortriptyline kinetics is probably
polygenic.

One of the problems of long term administration of antipsychotic drugs
is the appearance of movement disorders, "drug-induced parkinsonism"
or "tardive dyskinesia". Research using the pedigree approach has
provided evidence of a genetic influence on development of these disorders. One study (Myrianthopoulos and others, 1962) surveyed 728
relatives of 59 propositi (individuals from whom pedigrees were
traced) who had developed symptoms of parkinsonism (akinesia, rigidity,
tremor) when receiving phenothiazine drugs. Also included in the study
were 777 relatives of 67 control subjects resistant to parkinsonian
effects of the same drugs. Parkinson's disease was found significantly more frequently among relatives of the propositi than among relatives
of the control subjects. "The findings suggest that there may be a
hereditory susceptibility to parkinsonism produced by ataraxic drugs
(Myrianthropoulos and others, 1962)". A contrasting study (Myrianthropoulos and others, 1969) showed that individuals who have a relative
with naturally occurring parkinson's disease appear to have a greater
susceptibility for the drug induced condition.

An example of the use of "pharmacogenetic probes" to identify heritable
neurochemical variations in studies of twins was described above. A
similar approach has been employed in research designed to study
effects of LSD - 25 on relatives of schizophrenic patients (Anasta-
sopoulos and Photeades, 1962). The hypothesis was that relatives of
schizophrenics might reveal common specific symptoms during the intoxication. Members of families of schizophrenic patients, none of
whom had even shown psychiatric features, served as subjects. LSD
was administered orally. "Pathological manifestations" (paranoid
features, delerious ideas, severe depression, fear, visual and auditory
hallucinations) appeared in at least one parent of 18 of the 20
participating families; only two pairs of parents showed no abnormal-

ities. Of 44 of the patients' siblings, 19 showed the pathological
signs, signs which were not common during LSD intoxication of non-
psychiatric comparison subjects.

These and similar studies provide further evidence, based upon the
frequency of occurrence of particular reactions within families as
compared to unrelated individuals, that genetic factors influence effects of psychotropic drugs and thereby contribute to response variability in the general population.

Population surveys. "What has become quite clear from recent molecular
genetics is that whatever genes do, and however many of them operate
in the designation of behavior, a large proportion of the total genes
... vary within any natural population. Their variation provides the
genetic basis for the wide and complex differences in behavior ...
(Shaw, 1976)." The basic point as it applies to individual differences
in reactions to psychotropic drugs has been stated as a "pharmacological
principle" "... the normal dose for one patient may be toxic for a
second patient or ineffective for a third" (Vesell, 1972). The principle
implies that there exist within a general population individual differences in the thresholds at which a drug will produce its effects.
Population surveys can reveal the nature and stability of the distribution of such differences. Comparisons of different populations can
provide cues about genetic and environmental factors which may underlie the differences. Studies within a population can furnish expectancy
rates for the occurrence of particular reactions to drugs which can
serve as bases for comparisons with expectancy figures obtained from
investigations of twins and of pedigrees.

Despite the potential usefulness of the approach, "... there is very
little information on most of the world's populations concerning behavioral variety that is likely to be of value to geneticists (Harrison
1975)." Information collected by anthropologists and psychologists
has tended to focus more on central tendencies than on individual
variation. The questions they have posed for investigation have not
been of a form suitable for formal genetic analysis.

The preceding paragraphs have been oriented toward examining evidence
that genetic factors influence response variability to psychotropic
drugs. This emphasis may appear in some way to overshadow one of the
assumptions with which the discussion began: phenotypic variance (P)
among individuals is closely associated with differences in genetic
determinants (G) and environmental determinants (E), and may be influenced by interactions between the two: $P = G + E + f(G,E)$. It is
now appropriate to examine the influence exerted by environmental
factors, to look at examples of their contributions to response variability. For present purposes attention will be focussed on conditions
during early development when the organism's ultimate structures and
functions are unfolding.

EARLY ENVIRONMENTAL FACTORS IN RESPONSE VARIABILITY

The systems view of living organisms provides for several "environments", any or all of which may have influences on responses to psychotropic drugs. Intraindividual differences in responses may be expected during the course of normal development, when intracellular
processes are undergoing change (e.g. transport of precursor materials
to sites within a cell where syntheses of substances upon which drugs
act occur). Developmental trends involving changes in dynamic relationships between cells, tissues, and organs are also reflected in responses
to drugs. These are involved in the normal development of an organism's
internal environment and, as earlier discussion has pointed out, are
normally under primary genetic control (Vesell, 1972).

From the time of zygosis the organism is exposed to external environments which vary in their complexities and provide increasingly broad
opportunities for interindividual differences to appear. For purposes
of convenience the present discussion will classify external environments into three main categories: gestation environment, postnatal
environment, and postweaning environment. It must be kept in mind
that these are continuous and not discrete categories. However, each
has special features which influence effects of exposure to drugs.
Organogenesis continues to change substrates with which drugs interact and new routes appear by which drugs may enter the body.

Early environmental influences on drug-behavior relations are clearly
illustrated by age-dependent individual differences in reactions to
psychotropic agents. It has long been recognized that the young of
humans and of other animal species may be more sensitive to drugs than
are adults. A summary of median lethal doses in newborn and adult
animals (Goldenthal, 1971) has shown that central nervous system (CNS)
depressant drugs are 6 to 20 times more toxic in the young than in
adults. On the other hand, CNS stimulants may be more toxic to the
latter than to the former. Drug-induced malfunctions in behavior may
also vary with age. Considerable evidence is accumulating that children constitute populations at special risk from relatively low level
exposures to a wide variety of chemicals.

Gestation Environment

The gestation or prenatal environment in human and other more highly
evolved organisms is sufficiently complex to provide at least the
opportunities for nonheritable factors to contribute to the development of individual variability in those characteristics which influence drug action (Joffe, 1969). In humans the embryo and fetus
develop within an amniotic sub-environment which: 1) prevents adhe-
sions of the sticky embryonic body; 2) equalizes pressure; 3) absorbs
shocks; 4) maintains a constant temperature "acquarium"; and 5) allows
freedom of movement. The amniotic fluid is not stagnant, being completely replaced about every three hours. Constituents of the fluid
change as development progresses: early contributions come from the
amnion cells; later, from fetal kidneys, lungs and skin. The fetus
is able to swallow its own amniotic fluid and, later, respiratory-
like movements cause the fluid to be drawn into the fetal lungs.
Critical exchanges go on continuously in the fetal-placental unit
between fetal fluid compartments and the maternal circulation. Alterations in any of these events may produce lasting changes in structural

and/or functional characteristics of the developing organism that
will be reflected in ideosyncratic reactions to drugs at some later
time.

The long held belief that this delicately balanced environment is
protected by the placental barrier is not well founded. The concept
of lipid barriers applies, i.e. the rate of transfer through the
blood-placental barrier is governed chiefly by the lipid solubility
of molecules (Moya and Smith, 1965). Such molecules as drugs commonly in use in anesthesia and analgesia transverse the placenta easily
either by simple diffusion or by some type of active transport system.
The consequence is to alter the chemical nature of the normal intrauterine environment, with the possibility of affecting the developing
embryo or fetus. It is important to appreciate that chemicals which
may induce such effects are not limited to drugs alone, but are to
be found in the air, water and soil. They may be found among foods,
food additives, pesticides, among the great variety of pollutants
now being recognized as constituting the "ecological traps" of a
technological society (Russell, 1977a). Finally, human congenital
anomalies may also arise from the entrance of infections and toxins
into the gestation environment. Effects of chemicals from any of
these sources are confounded by the fact that the fetus has not yet
developed mechanisms to detoxify and to excrete them.

Effects on postnatal reactions to psychotropic drugs after experimental intervention in the gestation environment are illustrated in
a study reported by Hughes and Sparber (1978). Pregnant female rats
were given various doses of methyl mercury (MM) at three stages of
gestation (0, 7 or 14 days). Measures of general exploratory behavior
and of operant conditioning revealed effects of the treatments when
the postnatal offspring were challenged by administration of psychoactive drugs: "... early prenatal exposure to low doses of MM can
result in behavioral consequences subtle enough to require unmasking
of the effects with psychotropic drugs" (Hughes and Sparber, 1978).
It is tempting - and not unrealistic - to generalize that exposures
to many chemicals may affect the gestation environment in subtle
ways, altering biochemical processes in the developing organism which
extend into postnatal life to influence the variability of the organism's responses to psychotropic drugs.

That prenatal drug administration can have significant behavioral
effects in later life is not a new discovery. An early experiment
illustrates the kind of reasoning involved some twenty years ago
(Werhoff and others, 1961). Psychoactive drugs (reserpine, iproniazid,
5-hydroxytryptophane, the benzyl analog of serotonin) and a sterile
water control were injected intraperitoneally in daily doses during
days 8 to 14 of gestation. The investigators reported that there were
no observably uniform effects on the pregnant females. However, very
significant consequences of the changes induced by the drugs in the
gestation environment were clearly apparent in the offspring: neonatal mortality was highest for iproniazid; all drugs were associated
with decreased body weight, increased activity and emotionality; and,
susceptibility to audiogenic seizures increased. No defects were found
in learning, either in maze or conditioned avoidance response situations.

The concern aroused by tragic instances of structural abnormalities induced by effects of drugs on the gestation environment has encouraged a number of studies designed to search for possible effects on behavior. The term "behavioral teratology" has begun to appear. With the new interest has come more sophisticated approaches to research techniques for cross-fostering (to permit evaluation of effects of different nutrition and type of maternal care) and regulation of litter size (to control the nature of early experience and extent of intralitter competition) are illustrated in a study of effects of fetal and neonatal exposure to methadone (pharmacological actions similar to morphine) (Grove and others, 1979). Twenty-two female rats were exposed to methadone or served as prenatal controls througout gestation. Within 48 hours after birth 129 pups were cross-fostered. Litters were standardized at four males and four females. The offspring were weaned at 23 days. In addition to an increase of still births in the prenatally treated litters "... the effect of methadone on growth, emotionality and activity level was mild compared with the effects of drug-induced maternal disorganization" (Grove and others, 1979). The cross-fostering procedure made it possible to differentiate drug-induced effects on maternal care, a dominant feature in the early postnatal environment, from other factors affecting behavioral development.

As a final example of changes induced in the gestation environment it will be useful to note behavioral effects of commonly used psychotropic agents themselves. In an experiment by Vorhees and his colleagues (Vorhees and others, 1979) three different types of psychotropic drugs were studied which have been shown to produce little or no morphological teratogenicity: prochlorperazine (a phenothiazine); fenfluramine (a sympathomimetic drug); and, propoxyphene (an analgesic agent). The date of conception was determined on the basis of expelled vaginal plugs. Daily on days 7 and 20 pregnant females were administered (by stomach tube) one of the drugs, with saline or with Vitamin A as controls. Directly after parturition litters were standardized, behavioral testing being carried out on 4 males and 4 females from each litter. Effects of the various treatments may be summarized as follows: prochlorperazine had the most disruptive effects on reproduction and growth, with the least on behavior; propoxyphene had no effect on reproduction or growth, but induced a variety of behavioral anomalies; effects of fenfluramine on reproduction and growth were intermediate between the other two drugs and produced behavioral effects during preweaning development.

The results of this sample of experimental studies clearly show that psychotropic drugs may produce changes in the gestation environment which significantly affect response variabilities of organisms at birth and during later life. Knowledge about the "behavioral teratogenicity" of exposure to an increasing number of chemicals is being obtained not only by controlled laboratory investigations, but also by clinical and epidemiological studies of human subjects. Studies of mothers treated with various drugs during pregnancy are leading investigators to suggest that specific phenotypes, "syndromes", can be identified which include both behavioral (e.g. mental deficiency, speech difficulties) and morphological abnormalities (Hanson and Smith, 1975; Jones and Smith, 1973; Streissguth and others, 1980).

Postnatal Environment

"... the process of birth itself is merely an incident in the development of a human being, with development, and all that implies, continuing in the postnatal period" (Harrison, 1978). Effects of events
occurring during the gestation period would be expected to influence
the functioning of the organism in its postnatal environment. Added
to this is the opportunity for new factors to exert their influence,
factors which are very much greater in variety than those with access
to the highly controlled gestation environment. Organogenesis is still
underway, to be influenced by the viscissitudes of external physical
and psychosocial environments. Because of the close affiliations between behavior and the nervous system effects on the latter are of
particular interest when our concern is with "psychotropic" drugs.

One reasonable hypothesis is that genetic and environmental factors
may control the rate of development of enzyme systems affected by or
acting to detoxify (inactivate) a psychotropic drug. In general, most
neuronal function in the neonate is incompletely developed. There is
evidence that synthesis, storage and release of transmitter substances
involved in functioning of the nervous system are less well developed
compared with the adult. So also is the capacity to inactivate neurotransmitters once they have been released during nerve conduction.
The blood brain barrier is generally not so effective in the developing
brain, allowing penetration of chemicals that might only act peripherally in the adult. A more detailed example may illustrate the steps
by which the neonatal state matures.

During recent years the ontogeny of the cholinergic neurotransmitter
system has received special attention, in part because of the increasing
use in therapy of drugs to alter the state of that system. Very recent
research (Butcher and Jenden, personal communication) has shown that
levels of the transmitter, acetylcholine (ACh) increase only slightly
in certain areas of the rat brain during the first postnatal week.
Rapid increase follows during the second and third weeks. The synthesis of ACh is poorly developed during the first two weeks. Adult
levels of ACh are reached between the third and fourth weeks. These
states are paralleled by changes in the activity of the synthetic
enzyme (Coyle and Yamamura, 1976). During the first three weeks of
life levels of endogenous choline, one of the precursors in the synthesis of ACh, are slightly higher than adult levels, some of which
may be involved in the formation of synapses basic to the functioning
nervous system. These evidences of the immaturity of the early postnatal cholinergic system are compatible with reports that cholinergic
drugs produce no responses in the rat until 15 days postpartum. Other
neurotransmitter systems and interactions between them also show onto-
genetic development (Coyle and Campochiaro, 1976).

Emphasis in the above example was on age-dependent differences in the
internal environment of the CNS that influence effects of psychotropic
drugs. Other subsystems within the body may also be involved. Increased
susceptibility has been shown to be related to deficient hepatic degradation of psychoactive drugs (Gagne and Brodeur, 1972). Tissues of
the fetus and the newborn of mammals lack the enzyme systems which
metabolize several common therapeutic drugs (Jondorf and others, 1958;
Driscoll and Hsia, 1958). Biotransformation capacity, low initially,
increases during the early postnatal weeks, although the rate of increase varies with different enzymes (Mayer and others, 1980). In

summary, "... the fetus and the infant... (are) ... metabolically and phenotypically different than older established organisms of the same species..." (Kretchmer, 1970). Some of the variation among individuals in response to psychotropic drugs arises from age-dependent developmental changes in the internal environment affecting biochemical events with which drugs interact.

Postweaning Environment

The postweaning period provides a still broader variety of environmental conditions which may contribute to response variability to psychotropic drugs. The postweaning organism is still deficient in mechanisms for degrading chemical substances entering the body and the postweaning brain is still more sensitive to at least some drugs than the adult brain. Age dependent differences related to interactions between continuing organic development and expanded environmental influences are illustrated by the variability of reactions to the psychoactive drug, dextroamphetamine. This drug is used as an adjunctive therapy to other remedial measures in treatment of children suffering from minimum brain dysfunction (MBD). Among the characteristic signs of MBD are a chronic history of impulsivity and moderate to severe hyperactivity. Treatment with dextroamphetamine suppresses these signs in some but not all children. By contrast, the same drug in the human adult has the contrasting effects of increasing motor and speech activity, alertness, and physical performance.

There is evidence that the variations in postweaning reactions to drugs do not follow a monotonic progression. For example, behavioral effects of psychotropic drugs on postweaning rats at approximately 35 to 42 days postnatal age ("peri-adolescent") differ markedly from effects on animals even slightly younger or older (Spear, 1979). Drugs which potentiate the catecholaminergic transmitter system are associated with decreased responsiveness during this relatively brief period in development, whereas they produce marked age-dependent effects in younger and older animals (Reinstein and Isaacson, 1977). Peri-adolescent animals also show increased sensitivity to other drugs that decrease the functional activity of the catecholaminergic system (Spear and others, 1980). Other transmitter systems show similar discontinuities during development.

These examples indicate that the internal milieu upon which drugs act show systematic changes during early development which are reflected in response variability to the drugs. The changes themselves are primarily under initial genetic control. By affecting the nature of the internal environment the changes appear as differences in reactions of the same individual at various times during development and of different individuals at the same time postpartum.

Psychosocial Factors

It would be an incomplete picture were effects of factors in the psychosocial environment not given due attention. Only under unusual circumstances are individuals in contact only with their physical environments, isolated from other living organisms. The fact that different observers have different perceptions of the same objective realities produces effects which interact with psychotropic drugs to

produce response variabilities. Some twenty years ago an innovative
series of experiments stimulated a direction of research which still
continues. The experiments demonstrated that the substrates with
which drugs act may be modified significantly by the nature of the
psychosocial environment. Animals exposed to environments "enriched"
by group living and by learning experiences had greater brain weights,
higher levels of activity in enzymes involved in neurotransmission
and performed tasks more readily than animals living in isolation
(Rosenzweig and others, 1960).

That the task or situation in which individuals are engaged may affect
responses to psychotropic agents is clearly illustrated in reports of
experiments on effects of acetaldehyde. Considerable evidence has accumulated in support of genotypic influences on alcohol preferences of
mice. Acetaldehyde is a major metabolite of ethyl alcohol, with pharmacological effects of stimulating catecholamine release, depression
of oxygen consumption, and other effects of chronic alcoholism. Results of experiments on mice "... have shown that genotypic influences
on reactivity of acetyldehyde depend on the task used to evaluate the
drug effect" (Dudek and Fuller, 1978). "Task" is a psychological term
implying relations between an organism and its environment. In these
experiments effects of a drug were contingent upon an organism's perception of its environment. Such task dependency may be viewed as an
example of genotype x environment interaction.

Aggregation of individuals has been shown to be a significant factor
in toxicity of drugs with nervous system actions. Subcutaneous injection of adrenaline doubles its toxicity in grouped mice when compared
with mice living in isolation; amphetamine raises toxicity by tenfold;
methedrine and ephedrine have intermediate effects (Chance, 1946).
Toxicity may also be increased by environmental noise and by confine-
ment. That interactions can occur between variables of the psychosocial
and physical environments is evident, for example, in experiments in
which toxicity increased with aggregation at normal ambient temperature
(25°C) but was less affected at lower temperatures (10°C) (Höhn and
Lasagna, 1960).

The clinical use of monoamine oxidase (MAO) inhibitors in treatment of
affective disorders has given prominance to the influence on behavior
of the enzyme's roles in the catecholaminergic and serotonergic neurotransmitter systems. There is evidence that MAO activity in brain may
be affected by social interactions between members of a species. Such
effects could be expected to influence responses to psychotropic drugs
acting on the enzyme. In a novel series of experiments Eleftheriou and
Boehlke (1967) studied MAO activity in the hypothalamus, amygdala and
frontal cortex of mice after exposure to aggression and defeat. Un-
trained animals were exposed to repeated defeat by trained fighters
for two five minute periods a day, different groups being exposed for
different numbers of days from one to 20. MAO activity in the hypothalamus was elevated significantly during the first two days, the
other areas being essentially unchanged. After eight days activity
in all three areas decreased; after 14 days it was normal, followed
by decreases in all areas after 20 days. Psychotropic drugs (MAO inhibitors) administered during this period would act upon quite different substrates.

Biochemical substrates upon which psychotropic drugs act also show both intra- and inter-individual variabilities in humans as functions of changes in the psychosocial environments. For example, results of experimental and field research have concluded that: 1) a quantitatively close positive relationship exists between degree of subjective stress and amount of adrenaline secreted; 2) adrenaline secretion rises when a new situation or unfamiliar environment is encountered, habituation occurring with familiarity; 3) adrenaline production rises both in monotonous, unstimulating environments and those characterized by time pressure and overstimulation; 4) increased control over the immediate environment is an effective means of counteracting the increased output of adrenaline which accompanies exposure to new stresses. Other biochemical events are altered by conditions of the psychosocial environment and thereby add to the variabilities in effects produced by psychotropic drugs which act upon them.

    IN CONCLUSION

The preceding discussion may have appeared at times to wander from its title: Genetic and Early Developmental Factors in Response Variability to Psychotropic Drugs. Hopefully the basic theme has been sufficiently clear to make any divergences from it meaningful. The basic theme may be stated quite simply. Drugs produce their effects by altering biochemical events already going on within the body. Many of the events affected, particularly those in the nervous system, are involved in the behavior of an organism as an integrated whole. In any individual organism the nature of these events is determined by interactions between genetic and environmental factors, which differ within as well as between species. It follows that genetic and environmental factors are involved in the variability of responses to psychotropic drugs.

Within an organism's complex internal environment the variety of events which may participate in the effects of drugs on behavior is great. Included are processes involved in the "pharmacokinetics" (absorption, distribution, biotransformation and excretion) and in the "pharmacodynamices" (biochemical and physiological effects and mechanisms of action) of the drugs. Examples of evidence showing involvement of genetic and environmental influences in these processes have been discussed above. Many more could be considered. However, it is doubtful that expanding the details would alter very much the general theme which has already emerged.

In developing the theme, attention has been given to the study of both human and other animal subjects. Contributions by the latter to the development of the biomedical sciences have been many. Within our present frame of reference it is interesting to point out that the first fully documented evidence of a heritable modification of a pharmacological effect came from observations of rabbits (Kalow, 1962). Although reports that rabbits could thrive on belladonna leaves, which contain antimuscarinic agents (e.g. atropine) with psychoactive properties, had been reported by the mid-19th century, considerable controversy existed until it was recognized that there are pharmacogenetic differences between various lines of the animals. The serum and liver of some lines contain an enzyme (atropinesterase) that inactivates atropine, providing protection against untoward effects of the drug. Further investigation of the occurrence of the enzyme established that its inheritance followed a simple pattern. This example illustrates the overall search for genetic influences in the variability of responses to psychotropic drugs: from recognition of the involvement of a hereditable component to specification of a mechanism of action to identification of the genotypic basis of the variability.

Such an example has a kind of precision that tempts overgeneralization about the rigidity of the influences genetic factors play, a conclusion inconsistent with a number of examples explored earlier in the present discussion. Further evidence of the involvement of environmental factors in response variability to psychotropic drugs comes from the fact that genetic faults which would lead to behavioral abnormalities may be counteracted by environmental controls. "... a genetically determined predisposition rarely signifies the inevitable development of a trait. There are instances already where we can intervene to prevent the noxious consequences of a given genetic constituion and, if not prevent them, ameliorate them or cure the ensuing disease ... there is every reason to believe that in those disorders where intervention and prevention are not yet feasible they will become so in the not too far distant future"(Jarvik, 1976). Phenylketanuria (PKU), transmitted as an autosomal recessive characteristic, is an often quoted example. The genetic fault is failure to produce an enzyme (phenylalanine hydroxylase) essential for the normal process within the body of converting phenylalanine, a constituent of food, to tyrosine. One effect of this genetic abnormality is mental retardation, which can be prevented by early diagnosis and by manipulation of the neonatal environment, i.e. maintenance on a low phenylalanine diet continuing for several years. The intimate interrelation between genetic and environmental factors is here evidenced in yet another way: were it not for certain environmental conditions (i.e. the fact that phenylalanine is a component in normal food) the existence of the genetic fault might not be known.

And so we return to the assertion made early in the present discussion: $P = G + E + f(G,E)$. Because genotypes and environments vary among different individuals, phenotypes would also be expected to vary, including phenotypic responses to psychotropic drugs. Reasons have been given above for believing that this expection is supported by facts. The facts are also revealing ways in which genetic and environmental factors influence the mechanisms of action by which psychotropic drugs produce their behavioral and physiological effects, influences which are reflected in variations in reactions to the drugs during the life spans of individuals as well as in variations between individuals.

ACKNOWLEDGEMENTS

I am indebted to Dr. Donald J. Jenden, Chairman of the Department of Pharmacology at the University of California, for the opportunity to carry on research into neuropsychopharmacological effects of psychotropic drugs under USPHS grant MH-17691. Research at the Flinders' University of South Australia in psychopharmacogenetics supported by the Australian Research Grants Committee and the University's research funds has encouraged my long-standing interest in that area of behavioral biology. I am also appreciative of the editorial assistance provided by Flo Comes during preparation of this manuscript.

REFERENCES

Alexanderson, B., D. A. Price-Evans, and F. Sjoqvist (1969). Steady
    state plasma levels of nortriptyline in twins. Influence of genetic
    factors and drug therapy. Br. Med. J., 4, 764-768.
Anastasopoulis, G., and H. Photeades (1962). Effects of LSD-25 on re-
    latives of schizophrenic patients. J. Ment. Sci., 108, 95-98.
Åsberg, M., D. A. Price-Evans, and F. Sjoqvist (1971). Genetic control
    of nortriptyline kinetics in man: a study of relatives of propositi
    with high plasma concentrations. J. Med. Genet., 8, 129-135.
Bignami, G. (1965). Selection for high rates and low rates of condi-
    tioning in the rat. Anim. Behav., 13, 221-227.
Bovet, D., F. Bovet-Nitti, and A. Oliverio (1967). Action of nicotine
    on spontaneous and acquired behavior in rats and mice. Ann. NY
    Acad. Sci., 142, 261-267.
Broadhurst, P.L. (1960). Experiments in psychogenetics: applications
    of biometrical genetics to the inheritance of behavior. In H. J.
    Eysenck (Ed.), Experiments in Personality, Vol. 1, Psychogenetics
    and Psychopharmacology. Routledge & Kegan Paul, London. pp. 3-102.
Broadhurst, P.L. (1978). Drugs and the Inheritance of Behavior.
    Plenum Press, New York.
Chance, M. A. (1946). Aggregation as a factor influencing the toxicity
    of sympathomimetic amines in mice. J. Pharmacol. Exp. Ther., 87,
    214-219.
Coyle, J. T., and P. Campochiaro (1976). Autogenesis of dopaminergic-
    cholinergic interactions in the rat striatum: a neurochemical study.
    J. Neurochem., 27, 673-678.
Coyle, J. T., and H. I. Yamamura (1976). Neurochemical aspects of the
    ontogenesis of cholinergic neurons in the rat brain. Brain Res.,
    118,429-440.
DeFries, J. C., and J. P. Hegmann (1970). Genetic analysis of open-
    field behavior. In G. Lindzey, and D. D. Thiessen (Eds.), Contri-
    butions to Behavior-Genetic Analysis: the Mouse as a Prototype.
    Irvington Publ., New York. pp. 23-56.
Driscoll, S. G., and D. Y. Hsia (1958). The development of enzyme
    systems during early infancy. Pediatrics, 22, 785-845.
Dudek, B. C., and J. L. Fuller (1978). Task-dependent genetic influ-
    ences on behavioral responses of mice (Mus musculus) to acetyldehyde.
    J. Comp. Physiol. Psychol., 92, 749-758.
Eleftheriou, B. E., and K. W. Boehlke (1967). Brain monoamine oxidase
    in mice after exposure to aggression and defeat. Science, 155,
    1693-1694.
Fuller, J. L. (1970). Strain differences in the effects of chlorpro-
    mazine and chlordiazepoxide upon active and passive avoidance in
    mice. Psychopharmacologia, 16, 268.
Fuller, J. L., and W. R. Thompson (1960). Behavior Genetics. Wiley,
    New York. p. 3.
Fuller, J. L., and W. R. Thompson (1978). In Foundations of Behavior
    Genetics. C.V. Mosby, St. Louis. p. 75, p. 81, p. 225.
Gagne, J., and J. Brodeur (1972). Metabolic studies on the mechanisms
    of increased susceptibility of weanling rats to parathion. Can. J.
    Physiol. Pharmacol., 50, 902-915.
Goldenthal, E. I. (1971). A compilation of LD_{50} values in newborn and
    adult animals. Toxicol. Appl. Pharmacol., 18, 185-207.
Grove, L. V., M. K. Etkin, and J. A. Rosecrans (1979). Behavioral
    effects of fetal and neonatal exposure to methadone in the rat.
    Neurobehav. Toxicol., 1, 87-95.
Hall, C. S. (1938). The inheritance of emotionality. Sigma Xi Q., 26,
    17-27.

Hall, C. S. (1951). The genetics of behavior. In S. S. Stevens (Ed.),
    Handbook of Experimental Psychology. Wiley, New York. pp. 304-329.
Hanson, J. W., and D. W. Smith (1975). The fetal hydantoin syndrome.
    J. Pediatr., 87, 285-290.
Harrison, G. A. (1975). Populations for the study of behavior traits.
    In K. W. Schaie, V. E. Anderson, G. E. McClearn, and J. Money (Eds.),
    Developmental Human Behavior Genetics. Lexington Books, Lexington.
    p. 65.
Harrison, R. G. (1978). Clinical Embryology. Academic Press, London.
    p. 2.
Hirsch, J. (1962). The contribution of behavior genetics to the study
    of behavior. In F. J. Kallman (Ed.), Expanding Goals of Genetics
    in Psychiatry. Gruen & Stratton, New York. p. 30.
Hirsch, J. (1970). Behavior-genetic analysis and its biosocial conse-
    quences. Semin. Psychiatr., 2, 103.
Hohn, R., and L. Lasagna (1960). Effects of aggregation and temperature
    on amphetamine toxicity in mice. Psychopharmacolgia, 1, 210-220.
Hughes, J. A., and S. B. Sparber (1978). D-Amphetamine unmasks post-
    natal consequences of exposure to methylmercury in utero: methods
    for study behavioral teratogenesis. Pharmacol. Biochem. Behav., 8,
    365.
Hull, C. L. (1943). The problem of intervening variables in molar be-
    havior theory. Psychol. Rev., 50, 273-291.
Janke, W. (1980). Psychometric and psychophysiological actions of
    antipsychotics in man. In F. Hoffmeister, and G. Stille (Eds.),
    Handbook of Experimental Pharmacology, Vol. 55/I. Springer, Berlin.
    pp. 305-336.
Janke, W., G. Debus, and N. Longo (1979). Differential psychopharmaco-
    logy of tranquilizing and sedating drugs. In Th. A. Ban et al. (Eds.
    Modern Problems in Pharmacopsychiatry, Vol. 14. Karger, Basel.
    pp. 13-98.
Jarvik, L. F. (1976). Genetic modes of transmission relevant to psycho-
    pathology. In M. A. Sparber, and L. F. Jarvik (Eds.), Psychiatry
    and Genetics: Psychosocial, Ethical, and Legal Considerations.
    Basic Books, New York. p. 36.
Joffe, J. M. (1969). Prenatal Determinants of Behavior. Pergamon Press,
    London.
Jondorf, W. R., R. P. Maickel, and B. B. Brodie (1958). Inability of
    newborn mice and guinea pigs to metabolize drugs. Biochem. Pharmacol
    1, 352-354.
Jones, K. L., and D. W. Smith (1973). Recognition of the fetal alcohol
    syndrome in early infancy. Lancet, 2, 999-1001.
Kalow, W. (1962). Pharmacogenetics: Heredity and the Response to Drugs
    Saunders, Philadelphia. p. 231.
Kalow, W. (1968). Pharmacogenetics in animals and man. Ann. NY Acad.
    Sci., 151, 694.
Kety, S. S. (1961). Chemical boundaries of psychopharmacology. In
    S. M. Farber, and R. H. L. Wilson (Eds.), Control of the Mind.
    McGraw-Hill, New York. p. 79.
Kretchmer, N. (1970). Developmental biochemistry - a relevant endeavor
    Pediatrics, 46, 179.
Liston, E. H., J. H. Simpson, L. F. Jarvik, and D. Guthrie (1981).
    Morphine and experimental pain in identical twins. Adv. Twin Res.
    (in press).
Loehlin, J. C. (1975). Empirical methods in quantitative human be-
    havior genetics. In K. W. Schaie, V. E. Anderson, G. E. McClearn,
    and J. Money (Eds.), Developmental Human Behavior Genetics.
    Lexington Books, Lexington. pp. 41-54.

MacPhail, R. C., and T. F. Elsmore (1980). Ethanol-induced flavor aversions in mice: a behavior-genetic analysis. Neurotoxicology, 1, 625-634.

Mayer, S. E., K. L. Melmon, and A. G. Gilman (1980). Introduction: the dynamics of drug absorption, distribution, and elimination. In A.G. Gilman, L. S. Goodman, and A. Gilman (Eds.), The Pharmacological Basis of Therapeutics, 6th ed. Macmillan, New York. pp. 1-27.

Meier, H. (1963). Experimental Pharmacogenetics. Academic Press, New York. p. 165.

Moya, F., and B. E. Smith (1965). Distribution and placental transport of drugs and anesthetics. Anesthaesiology, 26, 465-476.

Myrianthopoulos, N. C., A. A. Kurland, and L. T. Kurland (1962). Hereditary predisposition in drug-induced parkinsonism. Arch. Neurol., 6, 9.

Myrianthopoulos, N. C., F. N. Waldrop, and B. L. Vincent (1969). A repeat study of hereditary predisposition in drug-induced parkinsonism. In A. Barbeau, and J. R. Brunette (Eds.), Progress in Neuro-Genetics. Excerpta Medica Foundation, Amsterdam. pp. 486-491.

Neitlick, H. W. (1966). Increased plasma cholinesterase activity and succinylcholine resistance: a genetic variant. J. Clin. Invest., 45, 380-387.

Nurnberger, J. I. Jr., E. S. Gerson, N. Sitaram, J. C. Gillin, G. Brown, M. Ebert, P. Gold, D. C. Jimerson, and L. R. Kessler (1980). Pharmacogenetic probes of affective illness and normal human affective response. Annual Meeting: American College Neuropsychopharmacology, San Juan.

Oliverio, A. (1974). Genetic factors in the control of drug effects on the behavior of mice. In J. H. F. van Abeelen (Ed.), The Genetics of Behavior. North-Holland Publ., Amsterdam. pp. 375-395.

Oliverio, A., B. E. Eleftheriou, and D. W. Bailey (1973). Exploratory activity. Genetic analysis of its modification by scopolamine and amphetamine. Physiol. Behav., 10, 893-899.

Omenn, G. S. (1975). Genetic mechanisms in human behavioral development. In K. W. Schaie, V. E. Anderson, G. E. McClearn, and J. Money (Eds.), Developmental Human Behavior Genetics. Lexington Books, Lexington. p. 104.

Omenn, G. S., and A. G. Motulsky (1976). Psychopharmacogenetics. In A. R. Kaplan (Ed.), Human Behavior Genetics. Thomas, Springfield. p. 479.

Overstreet, D. H., R. W. Russell, S. C. Helps, and M. Messenger (1979a). Selective breeding for sensitivity to the anticholinesterase DFP. Psychopharmacology, 65, 15-20.

Overstreet, D. H., R. W. Russell, S. C. Helps, P. Runge, and A. M. Prescott (1979b). Sex differences following pharmacological manipulation of the cholinergic system by DFP and pilocarpine. Psychopharmacology, 61, 49-58.

Pryor, G. T., K. Schlesinger, and W. H. Calhoun (1966). Differences in brain enzymes among five inbred strains of mice. Life Sci., 5, 2105-2111.

Ray, O.S., and R. J. Barrett (1975). Behavioral, pharmacological, and biochemical analysis of genetic differences in rats. Behav. Biol., 15, 391-417.

Reinstein, I. K., and R. L. Isaacson (1977). Clonidine sensitivity in the developing rat. Brain Res., 135, 378-382.

Riley, E. P., N. R. Shapiro, and E. A. Lochry (1979). Hypnotic susceptibility to various depressants in rats selected for differential ethanol sensitivity. Psychopharmacology, 60, 311-312.

Roderick, T. H. (1960). Selection for cholinesterase activity in the
    cerebral cortex of the rat. Genetics, 45, 1123-1140.
Rosenzweig, M. R., D. Krech, and E. L. Bennett (1960). A search for
    relations between brain chemistry and behavior. Psychol. Bull.,
    57, 476-492.
Russell, R. W. (1953). Experimental studies of hereditary influences
    on behavior. Eugenics Rev., 45, 19-30.
Russell, R. W. (1977a). The psychochemistry of pollutants. In J. O. M.
    Bockris (Ed.), Environmental Chemistry. Plenum Press, New York.
    pp. 33-52.
Russell, R. W. (1977b). Cholinergic substrates of behavior. In D. J.
    Jenden (Ed.), Cholinergic Mechanisms and Psychopharmacology. Plenum
    Press, New York. pp.709-731.
Russell, R. W. (1979). Neurotoxins: a systems approach. In J. Chubb,
    and L. B. Geffen (Eds.), Neurotoxins: Fundamental and Clinical
    Advances. University of Adelaide Press, Adelaide. pp. 1-7.
Serban, G., and A. Kling (1976). Animal Models in Human Psychobiology.
    Plenum Press, New York. p. 297.
Shaw, C. R. (1976). Human biochemical variation. In A. R. Kaplan (Ed.),
    Human Behavior Genetics. Thomas,Springfield. p. 393.
Spear, L. P. (1979). The use of psychopharmacological procedures to
    analyse the ontogeny of learning and retention: issues and concerns.
    In N. E. Spear, and B. A. Campbell (Eds.), Ontogeny of Learning and
    Retention. Lawrence Associates, Hillsdale. pp. 135-156.
Spear, L. P., I. A. Shalaby, and J. Brick (1980). Chronic administra-
    tion of haloperidol during development: behavioral and psychopharma-
    cological effects. Psychopharmacology, 70, 47-58.
Stone, I. (1980). A Biographical Novel of Charles Darwin. Doubleday,
    New York. p. 538.
Streissguth, A. P., S. Landesman-Dwyer, J. C. Martin, and D. W. Smith
    (1980). Teratogenic effects of alcohol in humans and laboratory
    animals. Science, 209,353-361.
Tryon, R. C. (1940). Genetic differences in maze-learning ability in
    rats. Yearbook Nat. Soc. Study Educ., 39, 111-119.
Usdin, E. (1978). Classification of psychotropic drugs. In W. G. Clark,
    J. del Guidice (Eds.), Principles of Psychopharmacology. Academic
    Press, New York. pp. 193-246.
van Abeelen, J. H. F. (1974). Genotype and the cholinergic control of
    exploratory behavior in mice. In J. H. F. Abeelen (Ed.), The Gene-
    tics of Behavior. North-Holland Publ., Amsterdam. p. 371.
Verplanck, W. S. (1955). Since learned behavior is innate, and vice
    versa, what now? Psychol. Rev., 62, 139-144.
Vesell, E. S. (1972). Genetic and environmental factors affecting drug
    response in man. Fed. Proc., 31, 1253.
Vesell, E. S. (1975). Pharmacogenetics. Biochem. Pharmacol., 24, 445-
    450.
Vesell, E. S., and J. G. Page (1968a). Genetic control of dicumarol
    levels in man. J. Clin. Invest., 47, 2657-2663.
Vesell, E. S., and J. G. Page (1968b). Genetic control of drug levels
    in man: phenylbutazone. Science, 159, 1479-1480.
Vesell, E. S., and J. G. Page (1968c). Genetic control of drug levels
    in man: antipyrine. Science, 161, 72-73.
Vesell, E. S., T. Passananti, F. Greene, and J. G. Page (1971). Gene-
    tic control of drug levels and induction of drug-metabolizing
    enzymes in man. Ann. NY Acad. Sci., 179, 771-772.
Vorhees, C. V., R. L. Brunner, and R. E. Butcher (1979). Psychotropic
    drugs as behavioral teratogens. Science, 205, 1220-1225.
Werhoff, J., J. S. Gottlieb, J. Havlena, and T. J. Word (1961). Beha-
    vioral effects of prenatal drug administration in the white rat.
    Pediatrics, 27, 318-324.

Part III

**DRUG RESPONSE VARIABILITY AND
PERSONALITY**

PSYCHOPHARMACOLOGY AND PERSONALITY

Hans J. Eysenck

ABSTRACT

In this paper an effort is made to state in some detail the Drug
Postulate, linking personality and the effect of certain drugs. It is
suggested that a rational scheme for drug action can be achieved by
grouping them according to their action on the major physiological
and hormonal systems causally related to the three major dimensions
of personality. The system is testable because the general personality
theory predicts the effects of drugs on everyday-life behaviour, and
also on laboratory tasks. Of particular interest in this connection
is the role played by Pavlov's postulate of "transmarginal inhibition",
which is important in relating personality to performance, and is
equally important in predicting the effects of drugs. There are many
complications of this kind in testing the system, and some of these
are pointed out in detail. It is concluded that there is a good deal
of supporting evidence for the theory, and that many of the criticisms
arise because of faulty deductions, experimental designs and statistical evaluations.

KEYWORDS

Drugs; personality; drug-personality interaction.

DRUG ACTION AND PERSONALITY DIMENSIONS

There is much agreement on the following propositions: (1) Pharmaca
can have a strong influence on human behaviour, in the laboratory or
in everyday-life situations. (2) These influences can be beneficial
(improve performance), or detrimental (worsen performance). (3) There
is no good, agreed and scientifically supported scheme for classifying
pharmaca, particularly as regards their effects on human performance.
(4) Effects of pharmaca on animals and humans are often contradictory;
the same dose of a given drug, even corrected for weight and other
factors, may improve the performance of one organism, worsen that of
another. (5) Differential effects of pharmaca are often related to
constitutional factors (such as strain of animal).

RVPD - E*

(6) Differential effects of pharmaca are often related to personality factors in humans; these in turn have a strong genetic basis (Fulker, 1981).

Based on these well-known facts, I ventured to suggest a scheme linking psychopharmacology and personality, in order to provide a proper classification of pharmaca, and their psychological effects, and in order to provide a system of prediction and explanation of apparently contradictory effects of drugs on different types of organism, but in particular on human beings (Eysenck, 1963). There is now a great deal of evidence relating to this system and the drug postulates it contains, much of it positive, but some negative; it is not the purpose of this paper to review in detail the various findings. It is intended, rather, to explain the principles on which the system is built, to cite some illustrative researches to document the different methods of testing and verification open to experimentalists, and to discuss certain theoretical points relating to choice of parameter values and other details of experimentation, neglect of which has often led to the failure of predictions to be verified.

The scheme takes its inception from the fact that large numbers of empirical investigations are agreed in finding three major dimensions of personality; these are called by various names, but we shall here refer to them as extraversion-introversion (E), neuroticism-stability (N), and psychoticism-superego (P). Evidence for the widespread occurrence of these major factors in personality research can be found in Royce (1973), Eysenck and Eysenck (1969), and Eysenck and Eysenck (1976). We will not here argue the point; it is discussed in great detail in Eysenck (1981a).

These three major dimensions of personality have a strong genetic basis (Eysenck, 1976; Fulker, 1981), the architecture of which is reasonably well understood. Of the true variance, approximately 2/3 to 3/4 is due to additive genetic factors; assortative mating and dominance play little if any role in the genetic transmission of these three personality dimensions (unlike intelligence, where both these non-additive genetic factors can be shown to play an important role - Eysenck, 1979); environmental influences are nearly all within-family, and not between-family (again unlike intelligence, where between-family environmental influences are twice as important as within-family environmental variance - Eysenck, 1979). The strong genetic determination of P, E and N suggests that there must be some physiological, anatomical, or biochemical-hormonal factors underlying the observed behaviour patterns, and the theory suggests that these factors are related to certain well-known bodily systems (Eysenck, 1967, Eysenck and Eysenck, 1976).

It has been suggested (and there is much empirical evidence to support this view) that individual differences in N are associated with the limbic system (visceral brain), which coordinates and regulates the activities of the sympathetic and parasympathetic branches of the autonomic nervous system. Differences in E appear to be related to high (introversion) or low (extraversion) states of arousal in the cortex, mediated probably by the reticular formation; these are differences in the resting state (i.e. they would be washed out in states of high tension, excitement or stress), and can be studied along psychophysiological or laboratory experimental lines (Stelmack, 1981). Differences in P appear to be related to male hormones (androgens), although serotonin metabolites (e.g. 5-HIAA), monoamine oxidase platelets, and a leucocyte antigen (HLA-B27) have also been found correlated with it in unpublished studies. It is not suggested that the evidence definitively establishes the correctness of the theories associated with these major dimensions of personality; all that can be said is that at present there is good evidence in favour, but also some negative studies, and some anomalies. A thorough review is presented in Eysenck (1981a), with different chapters contributed by experts in the various areas in question.

These major dimensions of personality, being solidly based on genetic predispositions, and having an equally firm biological background, would be expected to be relatively immune to cultural and other environmental factors. That this is so has been repeatedly demonstrated (Eysenck and Eysenck, 1981). Replication of the original factor analytic studies which gave rise to the Eysenck Personality Questionnaire (Eysenck and Eysenck, 1975) have been carried out in many different countries (e.g. Japan, Hong Kong, Nigeria, India, Yugoslavia, France, Brazil, etc.), and factors emerging from the analysis compared by means of indices of factor comparison. Nearly all the coefficients were in excess of .95, with most in excess of .98. The factors in question may therefore be said to have trans-cultural validity, and to be truly fundamental principles of personality differentiation.

Starting with these three orthogonal (independent) factors, dimensions or axes, we next note that for each factor there appear to be drugs which seem to push a given person in one direction or other. Thus stimulant and depressant drugs would appear to have introverting and extraverting effects; dexamphetamine sulfate might be an example of the former, and amobarbital sodium of the latter. Ethanol is another good example of a depressant drug, nicotine (in small doses) of a stimulant one. Similarly, minor tranquilizers (and nicotine in larger doses) have the effect of reducing neuroticism, while adrenalin would appear to have the opposite effect. As regards psychoticism, phenothiazine and other anti-psychotic drugs would appear to push a person towards the P- end of the continuum, while L.S.D. and similar drugs would appear to have the opposite effect. It might thus be suggested that a possible method for constructing a scientifically meaningful and useful scheme for the classification of drugs could be based on their action in pushing people (and animals!) in one or other direction along these three major dimensions of personality. Thus we would have E+ and E- drugs, N+ and N- drugs, and P+ and P- drugs. It is not required that all drugs should be part of such a scheme (some drugs have effects not related to these personality factors), and it is not required that all relevant drugs would have effects only on one dimension; it is perfectly possible to have drugs in the quadrants or octants generated by the three axes (Eysenck, 1963).

EXPERIMENTAL METHODOLOGY: SEDATION THRESHOLDS

There are essentially two ways along which we can test specific hypotheses derived from this scheme. For the purpose of illustration I shall use the E dimension, but of course the discussion can easily be generalized to all three dimensions. Figure 1 shows the two major methodologies in question. Let us consider first of all method A. We take a random sample of the population, i.e. one containing equal numbers of extraverts and introverts, with a large number of ambiverts

in the middle; we then test each person under conditions of placebo,
stimulant or depressant drug administration. Our prediction would be
that the stimulant drug would displace the subject's performance on
a given test known to correlate with E in the direction of E-, i.e.
greater introversion, while the depressant drug would have the opposite effect. The placebo treatment would produce scores intermediate
between the other two groups. For certain types of test where repeti-
tion is impossible or difficult (e.g. conditioning or learning tests),
it may be necessary to divide the original group into three, on a random basis, and administer a different drug to each group. It may also
be permissible to leave out the placebo group, and rely for evidence
on the observed difference between the other two groups, although such
a design would clearly be inferior to the complete design.

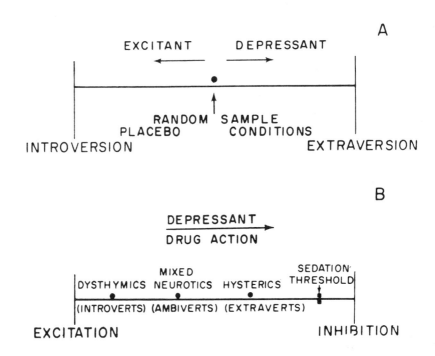

Fig. 1.   Two methodological paradigms for investigating
          the drug postulate. (From Eysenck, 1963)

Consider now method B. Here we again start with a continuum of personality types, ranging from introverts, high on arousal-excitation according to the theory, to extraverts, low on excitation (or high on
inhibition, according to the theory), with ambiverts, intermediate
according to the theory, in the middle. (In the diagram, there is also
reference to dysthymics, i.e. neurotic introverts, and hysterics, i.e.
neurotic extraverts - Eysenck, 1947). We now define a test, such as
the sedation threshold, which measures in some sort of absolute sense
a particular high degree of inhibition. Sedation threshold tests were
originally introduced by Shagass (1954, 1957), using the onset of
speeach slurring and certain EEG changes as his criterion; the score
on the test is the amount of depressant drug (often sodium amytal)

required by a given person to reach this _terminus ad quem_. As will be clear from the Fig., extraverts (and hysterics) should reach this point earlier than ambiverts and introverts, being from the beginning nearer to it on the continuum; hence the prediction is that extraverts need less drug to reach the threshold than introverts.[1]

Much more work has been done on method A than on method B, and hence we will briefly discuss the sedation threshold method before turning to a more detailed discussion of method A. The work of Shagass and others (1955, 1956, 1958, 1959) tends on the whole to support the hypothesis, although some confounding influence of N seems to be apparent in some of the studies. Claridge and Herrington (1963) give a good review of the methods and results of sedation threshold work, as well as recording their own results; they point out that the use of speech slurring and EEG changes has many difficulties, and that these difficulties may account for some of the failures reported by other workers trying to replicate Shagass' work. They prefer a procedure using a simple task of attention. The stimulus material consisted of a tape recording of random digits, and while receiving a continuous intravenous infusion of sodium amytal at the rate of 0.1 g/min, the subject was required to respond by doubling the digits, which were presented at a rate of 1 every 2 sec. The sedation threshold was defined in terms of weight-corrected dosage at a point characterised by suddenly increasing number of errors on this task. Typical sedation threshold curves are given in Fig. 2, for a hysteric, a normal, and a dysthymic subject. Mean threshold values for groups of hysterics (6.43), normals (7.86) and dysthymics (10.18) were all significantly different from each other. For the normal group the sedation threshold correlated - .52 with extraversion, but for the neurotic groups N confounded the picture. This is not unexpected in view of the stressful nature of the experiment; such stress in high N subjects would be expected to influence arousal levels (Eysenck, 1967).

---

[1] A third method, not dealt with in this chapter, relates to the effects of drugs as expressed in choice or preference judgements, as for instance in smoking, drinking, drug addiction, and so forth. Drug-taking has been found related to extraversion, neuroticism and psychoticism, with minor differences according to type of drug (Eysenck, 1980; Schenk, 1979; Sieber, in press). The motivation to use drugs, whether common (alcohol, nicotine, caffeine, etc.) or illicit (L.S.D., marijuana, heroin) appears to be derived from, and related to personality factors, and hence the personality - drug-taking relation is of considerable interest in throwing light on the effects of drugs on different personality types.

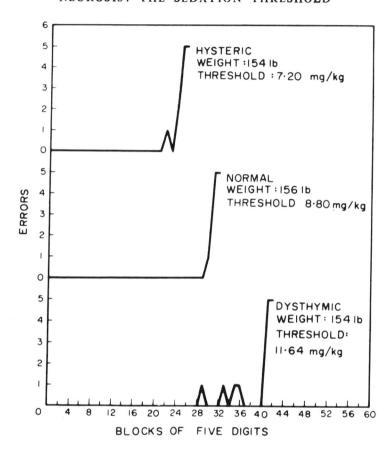

NEUROSIS: THE SEDATION THRESHOLD

Fig. 2.   Typical sedation threshold curves: one subject
          from each group. (From Claridge and Herrington,
                                                    1963)

Claridge and Herrington also studied the relation between sedation threshold and a laboratory test of extraversion, namely the rotating spiral after-effect (Claridge, 1960; Holland, 1960). The test not only relates to E, but also responds, in a manner consistent with this to stimulant and depressant drugs (Costello, 1960; Eysenck and others, 1957). The sedation threshold in the Claridge and Herrington experiment correlated .46 with duration of rotating spiral after-effect; details are given in Fig. 3. The results are fully significant. Many other experiments are described by Claridge and Herrington, who also give an extended theoretical account of methods and results; their paper should be consulted for further details. Other methods of measuring sedation thresholds are described by Rodnight and Gooch (1963).

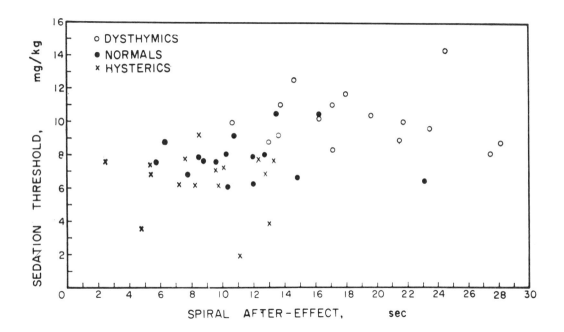

Fig. 3.   Sedation threshold and spiral after effect.
(From Claridge and Herrington, 1963)

The method holds out considerable promise, and it is to be regretted that it has not been much used by psychologists. One important extension might be the discovery of a suitable method for measuring "arousal threshold", i.e. a test which showed sudden and clearly observable changes after administration of a stimulant drug. No such test seems to have appeared in the literature. If one could be found, we would of course predict that extraverts would require larger dosages of the drug in question to reach the sedation point. This would constitute a perfect control experiment to sedation threshold experiments. In

a sense, the method of drug-modulated thresholds presupposes data
acquired by method A; we must know that the tests used to define the
threshold (e.g. the vigilance/attention task used by Claridge and
Herrington) is in fact a measure of inhibition before being able to
use it for that purpose. However, our knowledge in this field is by
now sufficient to create no difficulties in this respect. Some of the
possible difficulties which may arise with this method are similar to
those arising in connection with method A, and will be discussed later
on, in connection with the other method.

EXPERIMENTAL METHODOLOGY: LABORATORY TESTS

We will now turn to method A, and discuss one or two examples of its
use, before turning to a discussion of the difficulties and complexities of the whole approach. Let us consider the relationship between
Pavlovian conditioning (eyeblink conditioning) and personality. Much
evidence has accumulated to show that with relatively weak UCSs at
least introverts condition more readily and more strongly than extraverts (Levey and Martin, 1981). (With strong UCSs the position is
reversed - Eysenck and Levey, 1972. The reasons for this reversal will
be discussed later on; they are related to Pavlov's concept of
"transmarginal inhibition".) According to our drug postulate, stimulant drugs should facilitate conditioning, depressant drugs should
inhibit it, provided UCSs of reasonable strength were used. The first
study to use this paradigm was done by Franks and Laverty (1955),
using sodium amytal; a placebo injection constituted the control.
The drug was found to reduce the number of conditioned responses
during both acquisition and extinction. Despite the high correlation
between acquisition and extinction measures, the data suggested that
as far as eyeblink conditioning is concerned, resistance to extinction appears to be a more sensitive measure of the effects of sodium
amytal that is the number of acquisition conditioned responses. No
stimulant drug was used in this experiment: this lack was remedied in
a later paper by Franks and Trouton (1958). Using amobarbital sodium,
placebo, or dexamphetamine sulfate, the authors found that the dexamphetamine sulfate group conditioned more readily than the placebo
group, whereas the amobarbital sulfate group conditioned less readily.
Figure 4 shows the detailed results. In a third experiment, Willett
(1960) found that two depressant drugs, doriden and meprobamate, decreased conditioning scores, with the former (in the doses given) more
effective. There seems to be little doubt that as far as eyeblink conditioning is concerned, predictions can be made successfully from personality correlations and theory to drug effects. Many other experiments are discussed by Eysenck (1960, 1963, 1967, 1981), and the outcome on the whole encourages us to believe that this approach can be
used with advantage for the purpose intended.

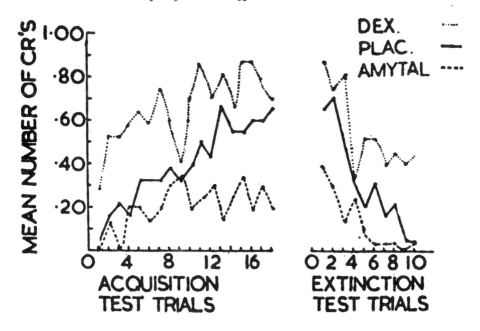

Fig. 4. The mean number of CRs given on each test trial,
         under three drug conditions.
         (From Franks and Trouton, 1958)

Instead of reviewing this large literature, we may be better advised
to turn to an extension of the paradigm which introduces a new methodology. Let us consider two depressant drugs, such as those used by
Willett in the experiment described above. If we assume that these
drugs differ only in the degree to which they reduce arousal (or produce inhibition), then certain testable consequences follow. These
consequences are deduced from the assumption that the two drugs lie
at different points of a single continuum, namely the excitation-
inhibition continuum.

We can test this hypothesis by experimentally creating three groups
of subjects, i.e. those tested under doriden, those tested under
meprobamate and those tested under placebo or no-drug conditions.
It would be possible to have different people in these three groups,
and if tests were used scores on which changed considerably due to
practice or learning, this would be the only experimental design open
to us. However, in view of the great individual differences on test
scores even under no-drug conditions, this design would be wasteful
and would require large numbers of subjects; consequently a design
seems preferable in which the three groups are made up of the same
people tested under the three conditions in question. This is the
design which was used by various collaborators in Eysenck's (1960)
book Experiments in Personality, and data from these experiments will
be used to illustrate the method of analysis. Five tests in all were
used for the analysis, each of which had been employed in experiments
involving these three conditions - nonsense syllable learning, reaction times, level of skin resistance, flicker fusion, and perimeter
threshold differences (Eysenck and Eysenck, 1960).

The choice of the five tests from a much larger battery depended on the total effectiveness of the separation of the groups achieved, and on the necessity of maintaining experimental independence between the tests. A canonical variate analysis of the test scores gave results which are shown in Table 1. It will be seen that the first of the latent roots is significant at the 0.001 level, whereas the second latent root fails to be significant even at the 5% level. The results therefore bear out the hypothesis and show that both meprobmate and doriden lie on a continuum with respect to their psychological effects, and do not differ from each other in mode of action. (The term "mode of action" does not of course, refer to the biochemical and physiological type of action, but merely to the behavioural effects of these drugs.) It is clearly possible that had other tests been used, results might have been different, but the experiment will suffice to illustrate the method.

TABLE 1   Canonical Variate Analysis of Five Tests,
           Showing Effects of Two Drugs
           (From Eysenck and Eysenck, 1960)

Latent vectors

		X_1	X_2
1.	Nonsense syllable learning	-0.040971	-0.014399
2.	Reaction time	-0.013625	-0.161517
3.	Level of skin resistance	-0.080835	-0.013827
4.	Flicker fusion	1.000000	1.000000
5.	Perimeter threshold difference	-0.475330	0.147773

Latent roots

$$\lambda_1 = 0.453220 = 90.03\% \qquad \lambda_2 = 0.050205 = 9.97\%$$

$$\text{Diagonal entries of matrix } G^{-1} B = 0.503425$$

Significance of roots

$$R_1^2 = \lambda_1 : x^2 = 40.446 : P < 0.001$$
$$R_2^2 = \lambda_2 : x^2 = 3.450 : \text{n.s.}$$

Scores were computed for each subject on both canonical variates, and the means of these scores were used to calculate what might be called the percentile of correct classification, i.e. given that we only know the canonical variate scores of a person, could we correctly identify him as a person who had been tested under no-drug condition, under meprobamate or under doriden? Results of applying this method are shown in Table 2; it will be seen that over 70% of accurate classification could be made under these conditions, which is a remarkable achievement considering (a) the very slight amount of drug administered, and (b) the fact that both drugs had the same effect, and were only differentiated by __strength__ of the effect. (Nearly all the discrimination is of course contributed by the first value; the second one might have been omitted without much change in the number of misclassifications.)

TABLE 2   Number of Correct Classifications of Control, Meprobamate and Doriden Conditions (From Eysenck and Eysenck, 1960)

	C	M	D
C	20	6	1
M	1	14	6
D	3	4	17
Total:	24	24	24

70.8% correct classification

This approach could of course have been greatly enlarged by having stimulant as well as depressant drugs, by having further tests, and finally by extending it to other dimensions as well, either in separate or in identical designs. It is suggested that the drug postulate mentioned at the beginning of this paper could thus be quantified very much more extensively and accurately than is possible with single experiments employing only one laboratory measure. Such a task clearly lies in the future. However, it may be suggested that this method constitutes one way of getting over the difficulties pointed out by Debus and Janke (1978) which arise in comparing different drugs thrown together into identical pharmacological categories.

INTERACTION EFFECTS AND THE YERKES-DODSON LAW

So far we have dealt exclusively with __main effects__, i.e. with general and monotonic predictions of drug effects on people in general. It might be expected on theoretical grounds, and it has been demonstrated empirically, that while such main effects can sometimes be predicted, nevertheless in many cases it is __interaction__ effects which are much more pronounced. To take but one example, Debus and Janke (1978) give a long list of experimental investigations which show that when tranquilizers, neuroleptics and sedatives are administered to normal subjects varying in their N scores, the effects on high and low N subjects are entirely different and contradictory. Subjects with high N scores show a __lessening__ of tension and anxiety, and perform __better__ on many tasks, while subjects with low N scores either show __no__ positive effects, or may even show __negative__ effects and a __worsening__ of performance. Debus and Janke (1978) summarise their discussion along the following lines: "In healthy subjects neuroticism seems to be associated with reactions to tranquilizers mainly in the sense that highly neurotic subjects show a lessening of anxiety and excitement, whereas non-neurotic subjects often show a paradoxical increase in excitement after administration of sedatives, tranquilizers and neuro-leptics." (p. 2188)

There are probably many reasons for this, but the main one, leading to the present writer's prediction of such interactions, is the so-called Yerkes-Dodson Law (1908), which has two parts. According to this law, the relationship between motivation or drive on the one hand, and learning or performance on the other, is curvilinear, the optimal drive level usually lying below the highest level used in the experiment and above the lowest level. Further, the level at which the drive is most effective depends on the complexity of the task; the more complex the task, the lower the optimal drive level (Broadhurst, 1957, 1959). A review of this law, and modern theories relating to it, particularly that of K. Spence, will be found else-where (Eysenck, 1973). Here we would merely wish to state that the well-established facts summarised in this law make it mandatory to include situational factors in any prediction, as clearly behaviour depends on the amount of anxiety or other drive experienced, and the degree to which the situation is complex (requiring relatively low anxiety-drive) or simple (requiring high anxiety-drive for optimal motivation). Note also that the dimension complexity-simplicity may not be the correct one in relation to the Yerkes-Dodson Law; Spence has made other suggestions better in line with modern learning theory. According to him the contradictory influence of anxiety as a drive stems from the habit levels existing pre-learning, and their relation-ship to the habits required to be learned. If the two are contradic-tory, then strong anxiety, multiplying with the existing habits, will make learning more difficult;this accounts for the descending limb of the Yerkes-Dodson curvilinear regression. If, however, the material to be learned is in line with existing habits, then strong anxiety-drive will have a facilitating effect, accounting for the ascending limb. There is much support for Spence's hypothesis, although there are also some anomalies and difficulties (Eysenck, 1973).

This is not the point to go into these complexities and theories; let it be sufficient at this moment to state merely that the existence of such curvilinear regressions, whatever their cause, must bring into any prediction not only situational factors, but also personality ones. Under identical stimulation, and in identical situations, high N scorers are likely to be in a higher state of anxiety than low N scorers, and consequently will have optimal levels of learning and performance (in situations producing anxiety) well below the optimum for low N scorers. This inevitably means that the influence of phar-macological agents on high and low N scorers will often be far from identical, and may be contradictory. If high N scorers are beyond the optimum on the Yerkes-Dodson curve, and low N scorers below it, then the administration of tranquilizing drugs will take the high N scorers up to a better level of performance, and may easily reduce the low scorers to a lower level than before. As it is difficult to measure indepently the various parts of this complex equation, it will be clear that verification of falsification of specific predictions may be difficult to achieve.[2]

---

[2] Another problem is presented by the Law of Initial Value, as it is sometimes known, namely the fact that for high N scorers in parti-cular the state of sympathetic activation is already quite high at the beginning of the experiment, i.e. prior to the administration of the experimental stimuli. This leads to possible ceiling and in-cremental effects which make comparisons difficult. For a discussion of this "Law", see Myrtek (1980).

TRANSMARGINAL INHIBITION

What has been said of neuroticism and the Yerkes-Dodson Law is equally
true of extraversion-introversion, where Pavlov already pointed out
the existence of curvilinear regressions. Pavlov postulated his "law
of strength" on the basis of his findings that as he increased the
strength of the UCS, so the strength of the conditioned response increased also. However, he was forced to introduce his "law of transmarginal inhibition" when he found that beyond a certain optimal point
further increases in strength of the UCS led to a reduction in the
strength of the CR. He attributed this to "protective inhibition",
i.e. a property of the brain cells which reacted with inhibition to
possibly injurious strong stimulation. This explanatory hypothesis has
found no support in modern physiological research, but the facts of a
curvilinear regression of performance on cortical arousal is indis-
putable.

A few examples of this pression may be illustrative of the general
law. These are associated with extraversion-introversion in the same
way that neuroticism is associated with the Yerkes-Dodson Law. Extraverts and introverts, by virtue of their differential degree of arousal,
will be found at different points of the curvilinear regression line,
and changes in stimulation (or the effects of drug administration)
may change their behaviour in different and opposite directions. One
example, already mentioned, is that of eyeblink conditioning, where
as Fig. 5 and 6 show introverts condition more readily under weak UCS
and other unfavourable conditions, whereas extraverts condition better
under strong UCS and other favourable conditions (Eysenck and Levey,
1972).

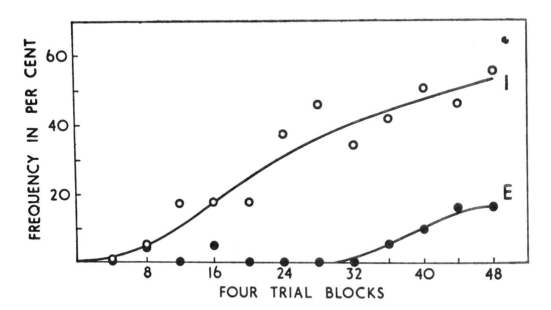

Fig. 5. Acquisition of eyeblink conditioned responses
         of introverts and extraverts under conditions
         theoretically considered favourable to intro-
         verts. (From Eysenck and Levey, 1972)

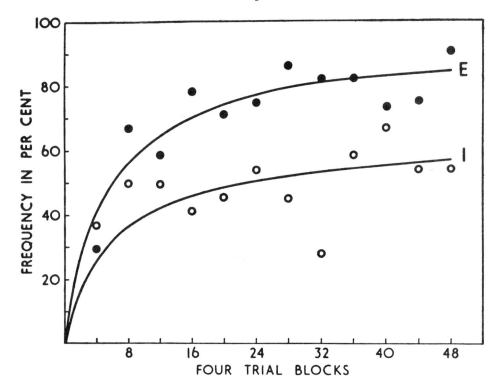

Fig. 6. Acquisition of eyeblink conditioned responses
         of introverts and extraverts under conditions
         considered theoretically favourable to extra-
         verts. (From Eysenck and Levey, 1972)

Another interesting example of the application of the concept of
transmarginal inhibition, and its relation to personality, is the work
of Shigehisa and Symons (1973a, 1973b). Their work was concerned with
the hypothesis that thresholds in one modality (say the auditory modality) are lowered by increases in the intensity of stimulation in
another modality (say the visual modality). This hypothesis rests on
the belief that increasing the intensity of ambient illumination would
increase arousal, and hence lower thresholds in general. They argue
that the failure of many studies to give replicable results may have
been due to the fact that transmarginal inhibition would reverse the
predicted effect, and that this inhibition would set in earlier for
introverts than for ambiverts, and for ambiverts than for extraverts.
Figure 7 shows in diagrammatic form the predictions made from the
hypothesis; results were in full agreement with the theory, and it
was also reported that they could be reversed; in other words, measuring visual stimuli in response to differences in the strength of auditory backgrounds.

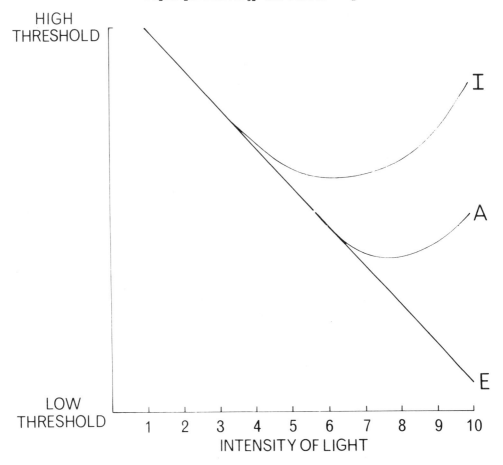

Fig. 7.   Auditory thresholds as a function of intensity
          modulation of ambient light, for introverts,
          ambiverts and extraverts.

Another example, again from quite a different field, is reported by
Zuckerman and others (1974). These authors measured the mean amplitude
of the averaged evoked potential at different levels of stimulus intensity, and found that while subjects high on their disinhibition scale
(extraverts) followed the predictions of the law of strength, subjects
low on disinhibition (introverts) showed a curvilinear regression indicating the presence of transmarginal inhibition. The correlation of
the slope with extraversion-disinhibition was found to be .59, thus
indicating the importance of personality variables in respect to the
effects of the stimulation.

A fourth example comes from the work of Eysenck and Eysenck (1967),
on the so-called "lemon-test". In this test, salivary secretion rate
is measured under resting conditions, and then again after 4 drops of
lemon juice have been deposited on the tongue of the subject. As required by theory, introverts show a very much greater increase in the
rate of salivary flow after the stimulation than extraverts, correla-

lations in the 70s having been reported in the literature, and found
in this study also. It would seem to follow from the law of transmarginal inhibition that if the strength of the stimulus could be increased, then the correlation should reverse, and this has been found
by S.B.G. Eysenck and H.J. Eysenck (1967); when subjects were asked
to swallow the drops of lemon juice, thus increasing considerably
the strength of the stimulus, the correlation between introversion
and the increment in salivary rate flow turns from positive to negative.

Another interesting example is found in the work of Fowles and others
(1977) which also demonstrates again the importance of situational
factors. These authors carried out a number of experiments in an effort to investigate the influence of introversion-extraversion on the
skin conductance response to stress and stimulus intensity. In the
first two experiments they found that when a stressful task preceded
presentation of a series of tones, extraverts showed an increase in
skin conductance level as a function of an increased intensity of the
tones, but introverts did not. As a result, for the stress subjects,
103 dB condition (the most arousing in the experiment), skin conductance levels were higher for extraverts than for introverts. At the
other end of the arousal continuum, they found that in two experiments
in which there was no task or other stressors, skin conductance level
was higher for introverts than for extraverts, at least for the lower
intensity tones (75 dB and 83 dB). They conclude that "the empirical
generalisation seems warranted that at low to moderate levels of stimulation SCL is greater for introverts but that the reverse is true
at higher levels, while no differences are to be found in intermediate
levels of stimulation ..." (p. 141-142).

A last and final experiment relating to transmarginal inhibition and
personality is one reported by Eysenck and O'Connor (1979), and
O'Connor (1980) (see also Eysenck, 1980). They used the CNV (contingent negative variation) as a measure of arousal, and the smoking of
one cigarette as the experimental variable chosen to increase arousal
potential. The hypothesis under investigation is shown in Fig. 8,
where E and I stand for extraversion and introversion, S.S. for sham-
smoking (manipulation by subject of an unlit cigarette), and R.S. for
real-smoking, i.e. the smoking of a cigarette under carefully controlled conditions.

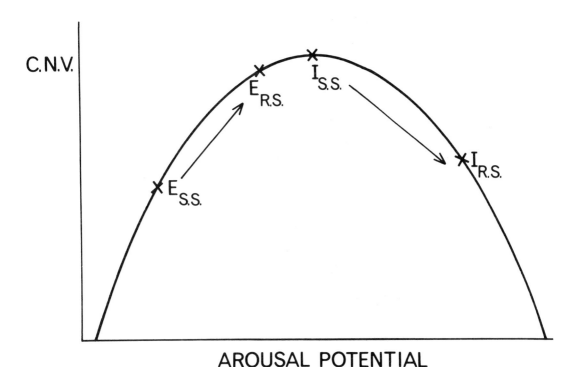

Fig. 8.   Curvilinear regression of CNV on arousal potential,
          showing effects of smoking one cigarette on extra-
          verts and introverts. (From Eysenck, 1980)

The hypotheses investigated were that extraverts would be at a low
level of arousal potential, and that the nicotine contained in the
cigarette would increase this arousal, whereas introverts would be
at a optimum or high level of arousal potential, and that smoking
a cigarette would decrease their arousal as monitored by the CNV.
Figure 9 shows the actual result, and it will be clear that both for
short (1.25 sec) and long (4 sec) inter-stimulus intervals the predicted cross-over does in fact take place. The results of this experiment are exceptionally clear and significant and indicate again the
interaction between personality, transmarginal inhibition and situation.

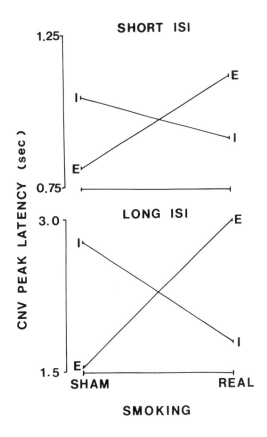

Fig. 9.   Effects of smoking on extraverts and intro-
          verts under two I.S.I. conditions.
          (From Eysenck, 1980)

As Eysenck (1981) has pointed out, there are certain difficulties associated with the whole conception of an inverse-U relation which must
be kept in mind. In the first place, these laws and rules tell us that
at some place the regression of stimulus intensity on response will
cease to be monotonic, and reverse itself, but the rules do not tell
us precisely at what point this should occur. As already pointed out,
Pavlov's conception of protective inhibition is physiologically mean-
ingless and practically useless - surely the smoking of one cigarette
cannot be regarded as a serious physiological threat to the intact
nerve cells in the brain! If, however, we cannot predict at what point
the reversal of regression will occur, then we are at the mercy of
ad hoc investigations, which require us to discover this point separately for each particular experiment that we carry out. What is
urgently needed, clearly, is some clarification of this point, and
some theoretical rationale which will enable us to make predictions
before the event, rather than simply noting what happens. Perhaps
this can only be done after a much larger number of studies in many

different fields has been carried out, but at the moment this certainly is a weakness that should be noted. It does not detract essentially
from the force of the demonstration that wherever a point of reversal
may occur, it occurs earlier for introverts than for extraverts. That
is the prediction made from the theory, and that is the prediction
borne out by a large number of different studies. Nevertheless, we
would feel most certain of our ground if we could only have a better
understanding of the reason for the reversal; the notion of "intensity modulation" is a very acceptable one, but it does not tell us at
what level of intensity different people begin to react differentially.

Another very real problem is that clearly the law of transmarginal
inhibition refers to many different types of experiments, and different concepts. Fowles and others (1977), in comparing the dimension of
extraversion-introversion to the Russian concepts of a weak and strong
nervous system, point out "that as index of arousal, SCL bears on an
important difference between Russian and Western theorising. In Russian theorising transmarginal inhibition reduces the central exicta-
tory process as well as peripheral responsiveness, whereas in arousal
theory as formulated by Westerners "... central arousal continues to
increase even though efficiency of performance decreases"(p. 142).
The experiment by Eysenck and O'Connor just quoted fits in with the
Russian conception, but there is also ample evidence for the Western
view, as noted by Fowles and others. Possibly both may be right and
apply under different circumstances, and in relation to different
experimental designs. Clearly, there are still many doubtful areas to
be cleared up in the field before we can rest content that our concep-
tions are adequate to account for the observed phenomena.

PROBLEMS AND DIFFICULTIES

In addition to those mentioned already, there are many additional
difficulties and complexities which are not usually taken into account
when hypotheses such as those contained in the drug postulate are
tested. Thus for instance extraverts and introverts appear to perform
differentially depending on whether they are tested alone or in groups;
introverts do better alone, extraverts in groups (Eysenck, 1967).
Thus control over situational factors involving the number of people
present is obviously necessary, and this may extend to the presence
of the experimenter in the same room as the subject, as opposed to
the experimenter's presence in an adjacent room.

Another, possibly more important item is the time of day at which
testing takes place. Biological rhythms, and their influence on human
performance, have been well documented, as has the interrelation of
these with personality (Colquhoun, 1971). It would appear that, relative to extraverts, introverts have higher arousal levels in the morning and early afternoon, and lower arousal levels late at night. This
produces interaction effects which also appear to be involved in the
study of drug effects (Revelle and others, 1980). Thus for instance
caffeine was found to have a _favourable_ effect on the performance of
impulsive extraverts during morning testing, but a _depressing_ effect
during evening testing, with the effects reversed for introverts. In
fact, the situation was even more complicated because the effects
changed from the first day of testing to the second day of testing
(Revelle and others, 1980). No simple hypothesis to explain these
findings seems tenable (Eysenck and Folkard, 1980; but see Humphreys

and others, 1980), but there seems to be no doubt that time of day is
a variable that must be taken into account in drug experiments involving stimulants and depressants, and the extraversion-introversion
dimension. The drug postulate may easily seem to be disproved when
diurnal rhythms of this kind are not controlled in the experimental
design, even though the data may agree perfectly with prediction when
attention is paid to these additional factors.

Additionally, it is not always realized that in making any specific
prediction with respect to laboratory tasks and their relation with
personality (and hence with drug effects), much care must be taken to
incorporate relevant laws in the prediction. Thus it might seem obvious that introverts should remember better material which they learned to an equal criterion with extraverts; yet such a prediction would
fail to take into account Walker's theorem which states that high
arousal results in slower but more permanent consolidation of the
memory trace, and that while the trace is consolidating, it is not
readily available for retrieval. This law led Howarth and Eysenck
(1968) to predict that introverts would show reminiscence during the
24-hour period following paired associate learning, while extraverts
would show forgetting, leading to a cross-over result. Figure 10
shows the outcome of an experiment carried out to investigate this
hypothesis; the results clearly agree with prediction. The effect of
drugs on this experimental paradigm could only be predicted if the
investigator included Walker's law as part of his theoretical background.

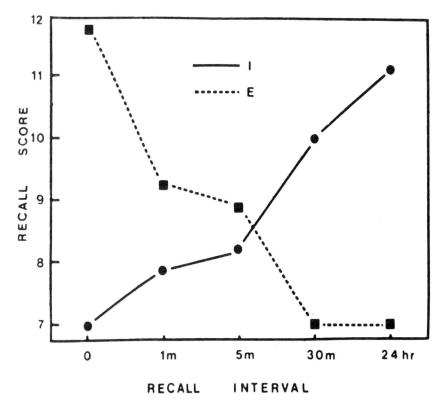

RECALL   INTERVAL

Fig. 10.   Recall of paired associates by extraverts and intro-
           verts as a function of interval from learning to recall.
           (From Howarth and Eysenck, 1968)

Finally, it must be said that the usual univariate approach to the
problem of testing the drug postulate is inadequate; what is needed
is not only the multivariate statistical approach suggested in relation to the discriminant function type of analysis used by Eysenck
and Eysenck (1960), but a more fundamental systems theory approach.
This concept, introduced into science by Bertalanffy (1968), applies
to systems, i.e. sets of elements related in such a manner that a
change in the state of any element induces changes in the state of
other elements. Related to the personality and drug postulates, this
means that a person's reaction to a given situation often depends not
only on his position on one dimension, but also on other dimensions;
high extraversion issues in quite different behaviour when found in
an N+ or an N- personality (Eysenck, 1967). The ideal experiment,
therefore, would start with a population of subjects embodying all
the different combinations of high, average and low P, E, N values
as a minimum, i.e. 27 groups; this would enable us to study not only
main personality effects, but also interactions. Practical considerations may make such a choice impossible, but it must remain an ideal
to be aimed at.

In this chapter I have been concerned to discuss an approach to the
psychological effects of drugs which not only takes into account personality variables, but also situational factors, and their relation
to drug effects. In doing so I would not wish to countenance the extreme views of some modern situationalists who have almost denied the
existence of stable and measurable personality dimensions; these views
have been criticized in detail by Eysenck and Eysenck (1980). It is
clear that a given personality trait (e.g. conditionability) immediately implies a situation, namely one which presents the subject with
a CS and a UCS in close association. Thus the concept of "situation"
is implied in the concept of personality trait, and almost synonymous
with it. What I wish to stress, and what may seem to be a quite different use of the term "situation" to that adopted by Mischel and others,
is simply the control of stimulus parameters, such as the strength of
the UCS in a conditioning situation. As I see it, it is the task of
personality theory to specify the parameter values which would produce correlations of a given kind between personality and experimental outcome; in the case of conditioning the prediction relates such
factors as strength of the UCS, duration of CS-UCS interval, and the
partial or complete nature of reinforcement to the personality variable extraversion-introversion (Eysenck and Levey, 1972). Unless the
theory can do that, it cannot make predictions in the proper sense,
and it is only when such predictions can be made that proper tests
of the hypothesis become feasible.[3]

---

[3] The term "situation" is often misused, and the implication is usually that the term refers in some objective manner to a given set of
stimuli. This is clearly erroneous; the physical situation is one
thing, the psychological situation is another, and the two cannot be
equated. A written or oral examination constitutes an objectively
identical situation for the pupils or students subjected to it, but
for one student it will be an anxiety provoking situation, for another indifferent, and for a third a joyful chance to prove his ability. It is this reaction, which is dependent on personality, past
history, intelligence, and many other factors which constitutes the
psychological situation, and it is this psychological situation that
is interacting with drug effects. Description and definition of the
objective situation as such is barren from the point of view of psychological experimentation, and the apparent objectivity does nothing
to make it relevant to the kind of experiments considered in this
chapter.

VERIFICATION AND FALSIFICATION

It follows from what has been said that many of the studies purporting
to test the drug postulate advanced here, and which fail to agree with
prediction, are of doubtful value in falsifying the theory. Falsification would only be assumed if the correct parameters had been chosen
for the experiment; as parameter choices are often arbitrary, results
may or may not bear out prediction, depending on accident. This is a
considerable criticism of much of the work reported in the literature,
yet it will be seen that the insistence on proper choice of parameter
values is absolutely essential if negative results are to be taken
seriously as falsifications of the theory.

It may be asked whether, if falsification is almost impossible because
of the complexity of the facts, the theory here considered can be regarded as scientific at all; it will be recalled that Popper and other
modern philosophers of science have chosen falsification as the demarcation point of truly scientific theories. There is indeed much discussion among philosophers of science about the demarcation question
(Suppe, 1974), and it may be worthwhile to state my own view. Briefly,
it would seem that there are four different points of view in this
field. There is the original Baconian theory of induction, according
to which scientists collect facts, and then base hunches or hypotheses
on these facts. Next we have the theories of the Viennese School of
logical positivism, which prefers to start with theories, and relies on
experimental verification of these theories. Next we have Popper, who
put forward the view that theories can never be verified in this sense
because we can never test all the possible deductions from a theory;
he prefers the criterion of falsification. If a theory can be experimentally falsified in principle, then it is scientific. Last we have
Kuhn's theory about revolutionary science; ordinary science works
away at problem solving within the context of an existing paradigm;
anomalies accumulate until a revolutionary new theory or law is proposed.

My own view would be that all four criteria are useful in deciding on
the scientific status of a given theory or hypothesis; they mark
different evolutionary stages during the progress of a given scientific discipline. Thus astronomy and physics passed through an inductive
phase at the time of the early Mesopotamian cultures, and when
Stonehenge and other partly religious, partly astronomical markers
were constructed. A verification phase came later, at the time of
Ptolemy, and extending up to the time of Copernicus and Keppler.
Newton introduced the falsification stage, and finally Einstein provided the revolutionary impetus for a complete change in the nature
of the laws involved.

The philosophical views involved, therefore, are not antithetical or
alternative, but sequential; they mark the stages of development of
scientific theories. I would suggest that the hypotheses, theories
and facts associated with the drug postulate have not reached the falsification stage, but are still "weak theories" in the sense in which
I have used this term elsewhere (Eysenck, 1960). To put it slightly
differently, at this stage it is so easy to falsify a theory (because
precise parameter values to test it properly are not known, because
there are many unknown external factors influencing performance, and
because much needed knowledge of details about the biochemical nature
of pharmaca, etc. is missing), that experimental failures to support
theoretical predictions are of comparatively little value. Much more

important at this stage is verification; if predictions which at first
sight might seem unlikely in this field are in fact verified then
clearly the theory in question has some scientific value. Thus we consider that the work of Gupta and Kaur on the effects of dextroamphetamine on kinesthetic figural after effects (1978), the work of Revelle
and others (1976) on the effects of time stress and caffeine on verbal
performance, the work of Gibson and others (1977) on hypnotic susceptibility, personality and sex, the work of Janssen and others (1978)
on the contingent negative variation, the work of McManis and others
(1978) on the effects of a stimulant drug on extraversion level in
hyperactive children, and the work of many others too numerous to
mention in such widely different fields as conditioning, sedation
threshold, vigilance, rotating spiral after effect, suppression of
the primary visual stimulus, nonsense syllable learning, motor responses, time perception, pupillary responsiveness, static ataxia,
palmar skin resistance adaptation, critical flicker fusion thresholds,
alternation behaviour, after-image duration, visual fields sensitivity, pursuit rotor performance, apparent movement thresholds, visual
masking effects, set, resk taking, performance accuracy, retroactive
interference, and CERs (Eysenck, 1963), establishes the validity of
the theory over a wide range. The admitted presence of negative and
anomalous results is of course not unexpected when we are dealing with
a weak theory, and even strong theories are constantly plagued by such
failures of verification and replication. Newton's theory of gravita-
tion, a prime example of a strong theory for many years, was constantly under pressure because of failures of prediction and the occurence
of anomalies; when these were studied in detail it was usually found
that adequate explanations could be given which did not contradict
the general theory. Hopefully we may expect the same to occure in relation to the drug postulate, although of course there is no guarantee
that this will in fact be so. In any case, the main upshot of this ex-
cursion into the philosophy of science is that theories in an early
stage of development should not be judged by the criteria appropriate
at a later stage; unless we accept this restriction we will make impossible the development of scientific theories in this field altogether. (This point, in different contexts, has been made by many
writers - Beveridge, 1980; **Krebs and Shelley, 1975;**
Kuhn, 1970; Nossal, 1975.)

What, one might ask, is the alternative to a provisional acceptance
of the drug postulate, at least as a heuristic guide to further research? It must surely be the elaboration of a better, more comprehensive, more accurate, more predictive theory, which would at the
same time embrace all the existing facts and data. Science generally
prefers an imcomplete, partly successful theory to no theory at all,
and it would seem that at the moment at least no alternative theory
is being put forward which could take the place of the drug postulates.
Until such a theory elaborated, it may be suggested that efforts to
improve, update, and generally increase the predictive accurary of
the drug postulate may be the best method of increasing our scientific
understanding of these very complex and difficult areas.

CONCLUSIONS

I would like to conclude with a general statement which I believe to be true, and which I believe explains a great deal of the failure of psychological experiments in this field, as in many others, to lead to consistent and replicable advances in knowledge. Psychologists on the whole seem to lack the discipline of physicists and other "hard" scientists, who realise that a solid body of knowledge can only be built up by careful, large-scale, co-ordinated studies within a given field, following up a given theory, and mutually reinforcing the conclusions derived from these various studies. Psychologists are much given to doing "one off" investigations, clever, often brilliant, but not the kind of bricks that can be used to good purpose in erecting a strong and durable building. There is little attempt to try and build according to some plan; each man is his own architect, and consequently no consensus and no great final product is achieved.

Different people try their hands at using concepts like the Yerkes-Dodson Law, the inverse-U relationship, or Pavlovian transmarginal inhibition, in relation to one or other of the many possible experimental paradigms that could be used for the purpose. The results are of course useful to some extent, and they are all we have, but what is missing is the detailed, long-continued study of these paradigms involving changes in parameter values, relation of results to personality variables, and similar integrative attempts to try and link together the disparate and widely different experiments that are all that we have so far. Until such unification is achieved, and until we can elaborate general laws which at present can only be hinted at, we will find it difficult to make use of these concepts to explain and predict the effects of drugs on individual human beings, in particular situations, given particular parameter values.
It is of course possible, and it may even be likely, that the attempt here made to try and organise the interaction between drugs, people and situations is in error, but I doubt if the theory can easily be falsified at the present stage of knowledge. Much the same must be true of other, alternative theories. It will need a much more determined effort on the part of experimental psychologists to render quantitative the largely qualitative concepts we have inherited from our predecessors, and with which we have to work at the moment. It is to be hoped that when this effort is made, those who make it will bear in mind the various hypotheses, theories, complexities and anomalies discussed in this chapter; the possibility still exists that the general concept of an overall relationship between the variables involved outlined here may be along the right lines, and may lead us to a better understanding of the relationship between personality and drug effects.

It has often seemed to me that one of the reasons why the present state of affairs in psychopharmacology is relatively unsatisfactory is simply that we have been more concerned with practical issues and with therapeutic effectiveness of drugs, rather with the simple scientific question of drug-person-situation interactions. This is of course understandable, because our main reason for looking at drugs is inevitably their use in the improvement of the human condition, and as therapeutic agents. Nevertheless, this may not be the best way of improving our scientific understanding of these relations, and until our interest shifts at least to some extent in the direction of strictly academic, scientific investigations, with practical application only a secondary consideration, we are unlikely to acquire a proper understanding of the intricacies of psychopharmacology.

REFERENCES

Bertalanffy, L. von (1968). General System Theory. Brazillier, New York.

Beveridge, W. T. (1980). Seeds of Discovery. Heinemann, London.

Broadhurst, P. L. (1957). Emotionality and the Yerkes-Dodson Law. J. Exp. Psychol., 54, 345-352.

Broadhurst, P. L. (1959). The interaction of task difficulty and motivation: the Yerkes-Dodson Law revisited. Acta Psychol., 16, 321-338.

Claridge, G. S. (1960). The excitation-inhibition balance in neurotics. In H. J. Eysenck (Ed.), Experiments in Personality, Vol. 2. Routledge & Kegan Paul, London. pp. 107-156.

Claridge, G. S., and R. N. Herrington (1963). Excitation-inhibition and the theory of neurosis: A study of the sedation threshold. In H. J. Eysenck (Ed.), Experiments with Drugs. Pergamon Press, London. pp. 131-168.

Colquhoun, W. P. (Ed.) (1971). Biological Rhythms and Human Performance. Academic Press, New York.

Costello, C. G. (1960). The effects of meprobamate on perception. III. The spiral after-effect. J. Ment. Sci., 106, 331-336.

Debus, G., and W. Janke (1978). Psychologische Aspekte der Psychopharmakotherapie. In L. Pongratz (Ed.), Handbuch der Psychologie, Band 8(1). Hogrefe, Göttingen. pp. 2161-2227.

Eysenck, H. J. (1947). Dimensions of Personality. Routledge & Kegan Paul, London.

Eysenck, H. J. (Ed.) (1960a). Experiments in Personality. Routledge & Kegan Paul, London.

Eysenck, H. J. (1960b). The place of theory in psychology. In H. J. Eysenck (Ed.), Experiments in Personality, Vol. 2. Routledge & Kegan Paul, London. pp. 303-315.

Eysenck, H. J. (Ed.) (1963). Experiments with Drugs. Pergamon Press, London.

Eysenck, H. J. (1967). The Biological Basis of Personality. Thomas, Springfield, Ill.

Eysenck, H. J. (1973). Personality, learning, and "anxiety". In H. J. Eysenck (Ed.), Handbook of Abnormal Psychology. Pitman, London. pp. 390-419.

Eysenck, H. J. (1976). Genetic factors in personality development. In A. R. Kaplan (Ed.), Human Behaviour Genetics. Thomas, Springfield, Ill. pp. 198-229.

Eysenck, H. J. (1979). The Structure and Measurement of Intelligence. Springer, New York.

Eysenck, H. J. (1980). The Causes and Effects of Smoking. Maurice Temple Smith, London.

Eysenck, H. J. (1981a). A Model for Personality. Springer, London.

Eysenck, H. J. (1981b). Arousal, intrinsic motivation, and personality. In H. I. Day (Ed.), Advances in Intrinsic Motivation and Aesthetics. Plenum Press, New York. pp. 131-147.

Eysenck, H. J., and J. A. Easterbrook (1960). Drugs and personality. VIII. The effects of stimulant and depressant drugs on visual after-effects of a rotating spiral. J. Ment. Sci., 106, 842-844.

Eysenck, H. J., and S. B. G. Eysenck (1960). The classification of drugs according to their behavioural effects: A new method. In

H. J. Eysenck (Ed.), Experiments in Personality, Vol. 1. Routledge
  & Kegan Paul, London. pp. 225-233.
Eysenck, H. J., and S. B. G. Eysenck (1967). On the unitary nature of
  extraversion. Acta Psychol., 26, 383-390.
Eysenck, H. J., and S. B. G. Eysenck (1969). Personality Structure
  and Measurement. Routledge & Kegan Paul, London. (San Diego, Edits).
Eysenck, H. J., and S. B. G. Eysenck (1975). The Eysenck Personality
  Questionnaire. Hodder & Stoughton, London.
Eysenck, H. J., and S. B. G. Eysenck (1976). Psychoticism as a Dimen-
  sion of Personality. Hodder & Stoughton, London.
Eysenck, H. J., and S. B. G. Eysenck (1981). Culture and personality
  abnormalities. In I. Al-Issa (Ed.), Culture and Psychopathology.
  University Park Press, New York.
Eysenck, H. J., and A. Levey (1972). Conditioning, introversion-extra-
  version and the strength of the nervous system. In V. D. Nebylitsyn
  and J. A. Gray (Eds.), Biological Bases of Individual Behaviour.
  Academic Press, London. pp. 206-220.
Eysenck, H. J., and K. O'Connor (1979). Smoking, arousal, and person-
  ality. In A. Remond and C. Izard (Eds.), Electro-physiological
  Effects of Nicotine. Elsevier, Amsterdam.
Eysenck, H. J., H. Holland, and D. S. Trouton (1957). Drugs and per-
  sonality: III. The effects of stimulant and depressant drugs on
  visual after-effects. J. Ment. Sci., 103, 650-655.
Eysenck, M. W. (1977). Human Memory. Pergamon Press, London.
Eysenck, M. W., and H. J. Eysenck (1980). Mischel and the concept of
  personality. Br. J. Psychol., 71, 191-204.
Eysenck, M. W., and S. Folkard (1980). Personality, time of day, and
  caffeine: Some theoretical and conceptual problems in Revelle et
  al. J. Exp. Psychol. (General), 109, 32-41.
Eysenck, S. B. G., and H. J. Eysenck (1967). Physiological reactivity
  to sensory stimulation as a measure of personality. Psychol. Rep.,
  20, 45-46.
Fowles, D. C., R. Roberts, and K. E. Nagel (1977). The influence of
  introversion-extraversion on the skin conductance response to
  stress and stimulus intensity. J. Res. Pers., 11, 129-146.
Franks, C. M., and S. G. Laverty (1955). Sodium amytal and eyelid
  conditioning. J. Ment. Sci., 101, 654-663.
Franks, C. M., and D. Trouton (1958). Effects of amobarbital sodium
  and dexamphetamine sulphate on the conditioning of the eyeblink
  response. J. Comp. Physiol. Psychol., 51, 220-222.
Fulker, D. (1981). The genetic and environmental architecture of
  psychoticism. In H. J. Eysenck (Ed.), A Model for Personality.
  Springer, New York.
Gibson, H. B., M. E. Corcoran, and J. D. Curran (1977). Hypnotic susceptibility and personality: The consequences of diazepam and the
  sex of the subjects. Br. J. Psychol., 68, 51-59.
Gupta, B. S., and S. Kaur (1978). The effects of dextroamphetamine
  on kinesthetic after effects. Psychopharmacology, 56, 199-204.
Holland, H. C. (1960). The effects of depressant drugs on some perceptual processes. In H. J. Eysenck (Ed.), Experiments in Personality, Vol. 1. Routledge & Kegan Paul, London. pp. 138-158.
Howarth, E., and H. J. Eysenck (1968). Extraversion, arousal, and
  paired-associate recall. J. Exp. Res. Pers., 3, 114-116.
Humphreys, M. S., W. Revelle, L. Simon, and K. Gilliland (1980). Individual differences in diurnal rhythms and multiple activation
  states: A reply to M.W. Eysenck and Folkard. J. Exp. Psychol.
  (General), 109, 42-48.

Janssen, R., H. Mattie, P. Plooig van Gorsel, and P. F. Werre (1978). The effects of a depressant and a stimulant drug on the contingent negative variation. Biol. Psychol., 6, 209-218.

Krebs, H. A., and J. H. Shelley (Eds.) (1975). The Creative Process in Science and Medicine. American Elsevier Publ. Co., New York.

Kuhn, T. S. (1970). The Structure of Scientific Revolutions. University of Chicago Press, Chicago.

Levey, A., and I. Martin (1981). Personality and conditioning. In H. J. Eysenck (Ed.), A Model for Personality. Springer, New York.

McManis, D. L., H. McCarthy, and R. Koval (1978). Effects of a stimulant drug on extraversion level in hyperactive children. Perc. Mot. Skills, 46, 88-90.

Martin, I. (1960a). The effects of depressant drugs on palmar skin resistance and adaptation. In H. J. Eysenck (Ed.), Experiments in Personality, Vol. 1. Routledge & Kegan Paul, London. pp. 197-220.

Martin, I. (1960b). The effects of depressant drugs on reaction times and "set". In H. J. Eysenck (Ed.), Experiments in Personality, Vol. 1. Routledge & Kegan Paul, London. pp. 221-224.

Myrtek, M. (1980). Psychophysiologische Konstitutionsforschung. Hogrefe, Göttingen.

Nossal, G. (1975). Medical Science and Human Goals. Arnold, Melbourne.

O'Connor, K. (1980). The contingent negative variation and individual differences in smoking behaviour. Pers. Ind. Diff., 1, 57-72.

Revelle, W., P. Amaral, and S. Turriff (1976). Introversion/extraversion, time stress, and caffeine: Effect of verbal performance. Science, 192, 149-150.

Revelle, W., S. Humphreys, L. Simon, and K. Gilliland (1980). The interactive effect of personality, time of day and caffeine: A test of the arousal model. J. Exp. Psychol. (General), 109, 1-31.

Rodnight, E., and R. N. Gooch (1963). A new method for the determination of individual differences in susceptibility to a depressant drug. In H. J. Eysenck (Ed.), Experiments with Drugs. Pergamon Press, London. pp. 169-193.

Royce, J.R. (1973). The conceptual framework for a multi-factor theory of individuality. In J. R. Royce (Ed.), Multivariate Analysis and Psychological Theory. Academic Press, London. pp. 305-407.

Schenk, J. (1979). Die Persönlichkeit des Drogen Konsumenten. Hogrefe, Göttingen.

Shagass, C. A. (1954). The sedation threshold. A method for estimating tension in psychiatric patients. EEG Clin. Neurophysiol., 6, 221-233.

Shagass, C. A. (1957). A measurable neurophysiological factor of psychiatric significance. EEG Clin. Neurophysiol., 9, 101-108.

Shagass, C., and A. L. Jones (1958). A neurophysiological test for psychiatric diagnosis: results in 750 patients. Am. J. Psychiat., 114, 1002-1009.

Shagass, C., and A. B. Kerenyi (1958). Neurophysiologic studies of personality. J. Nerv. Ment. Dis., 126, 141-147.

Shagass, C., and J. Naiman (1955). The sedation threshold, manifest anxiety and some aspects of ego function. A.M.A. Arch. Neurol. Psychiat., 74, 397-406.

Shagass, C., and J. Naiman (1956). The sedation threshold as an objective index of manifest anxiety. J. Psychosom. Res., 1, 49-57.

Shagass, C., H. Azima, and H. Sangowicz (1959). Effect of meprobamate in sustained high dosage on the electroencephalogram sedation threshold. EEG Clin. Neurophysiol., 11, 275-283.

Shigehisa, T., and J. R. Symons (1973a). Effect of intensity of visual stimulation on auditory sensitivity in relation to personality. Br. J. Psychol., 64, 205-213.

Shigehisa, T., and J. R. Symons (1973b). Reliability of auditory re-
    sponses under increasing intensity of visual stimulation in rela-
    tion to personality. Br. J. Psychol., 64, 375-381.
Sieber, M. F. (in press). Personality scores and licit and illicit
    substance use. Pers. Ind. Diff.
Stelmack, R. M. (1981). The psychophysiology of extraversion and
    neuroticism. In H. J. Eysenck (Ed.), A Model for Personality.
    Springer, New York.
Suppe, F. (Ed.) (1974). The Structure of Scientific Theories.
    University of Illinois Press, London.
Treadwell, E. (1960). The effects of depressant drugs on vigilance
    and psychomotor performance. In H. J. Eysenck (Ed.), Experiments
    in Personality, Vol. 1. Routledge & Kegan Paul. pp. 159-196.
Willett, R. A. (1960). The effects of depressant drugs on learning
    and conditioning. In H. J. Eysenck (Ed.), Experiments in Persona-
    lity, Vol. 1. Routledge & Kegan Paul, London, pp. 110-137.
Yerkes, R. M., and J. D. Dodson (1908). The relation of strength of
    stimulus to rapidity of habit formation. J. Comp. Neurol., 18,
    459-482.
Zuckerman, M., T. Murtaugh, and J. Siegal (1974). Sensation seeking
    and cortical augmenting - reducing. Psychophysiology, 11, 535-542.

SEDATION THRESHOLD AND PERSONALITY DIFFERENCES

Gordon Claridge

ABSTRACT

Earlier studies of individual differences in drug tolerance, using the 'sedation threshold' technique, demonstrated that, although, as predicted, the Eysenckian dimensions of extraversion (E) and neuroticism (N) appear to have a major influence on drug response, neither characteristic alone can account for the observed variation. Sedation threshold differences seem, instead, to be the result of an interaction between both dimensions, 'zone analyses' of data from three separate experiments suggesting that both neurotic introversion and non-neurotic extraversion are associated with raised sedative drug tolerance; low tolerance is found in non-neurotic introverts as well as in neurotic extraverts. The present report describes the results of a more elaborate analysis in which comparisons were made of the drug tolerance scores of nine subgroups of subjects showing different combinations of high, moderate, and low E and N; this was done by combining the data from several samples of normal subjects in whom sedation thresholds had been obtained using either thiopentone or amylobarbitone sodium. Findings broadly confirmed those of the previous, smaller analyses, though some new trends were observed. The very highest tolerance was found in introverts with moderate, rather than high, degrees of neuroticism; this reflected a tendency for introversion-extraversion to be most clearly related to drug tolerance in the mid-range of N and for high levels of N in extraverts, or its absence in introverts, to be associated with very low sedation thresholds. The results are discussed with reference to Eysenck's biological theory of personality and the modifications to it suggested by the present author and by Gray.

KEYWORDS

Sedation threshold; drug tolerance; introversion - extraversion; neuroticism.

Most current research attempting to relate drug effects to personality adopts the strategy of giving subjects a small standard dose of the chosen drug and then examining how people differ in their reactions on some behavioural or physiological measure. An alternative strategy is to administer varying amounts of the drug to the subjects, continuing until they reach some pre-determined criterion of response; the dose received then becomes the measure of the drug's effect and can be related across individuals to personality or other variables. This second strategy is the basis of the drug threshold procedures, of which the most well-known is the sedation threshold. Introduced nearly thirty years ago by Shagass (1954), the latter involved determining the amount of amylobarbitone sodium required to bring about a defined change in the amplitude of fast frontal EEG activity.

In the decade following Shagass' 1954 paper there was a flurry of interest in drug threshold procedures, partly motivated by an attempt to find simpler, more reliable, or merely interesting, alternatives to his original technique. One group of workers (Giberti and Rossi, 1962) developed a daring stimulant drug equivalent, the 'stimulation threshold' for methamphetamine. Most researchers, however, continued to concentrate on sedative drugs, usually barbiturates, though two unique studies, one of nitrous oxide (Rodnight and Gooch, 1963) and the other of ethyl alcohol (Kawi, 1958), were also reported. As alternatives to EEG change, other criteria for deciding when the individual was sedated were also adopted; these included lateral gaze nystagmus (Fink, 1958), suppression of the GSR (Perez-Reyes and others, 1962), and behavioural unresponsiveness to various kinds of stimuli (Claridge and Herrington, 1960; Rodnight and Gooch, 1963; Shagass and Kerenyi, 1958).

Because the sedation threshold[1] was initially introduced and subsequently mainly investigated as a potentially useful tool for psychiatric diagnosis, much of the research conducted on it during its heyday involved the use of patient samples and had the simple empirical aim of trying to distinguish individuals according to clinical status; the ability of the procedure to diagnose different forms of depression is a good example (Perez-Reyes and Cochrane, 1967; Shagass and others, 1956). Research having a more theoretical basis and concerned with individual differences in drug response per se was less common. An exception was work having its origins in Eysenck's biological theory of personality. Early on, Eysenck (1957) had formulated a drug postulate leading to the prediction that introverted individuals should have higher sedation thresholds, that is greater sedative drug tolerance, than extraverted individuals. Furthermore, he had already (Eysenck, 1947) postulated differences in the degree of introversion-extraversion to be found among various neurotic types, proposing specifically that dysthymic neurotics were more introverted than hysterical neurotics. It followed that dysthymics, because of their greater introversion, should have higher sedation thresholds than hysterics. That prediction was amply confirmed (Claridge, 1967; Claridge and Herrington, 1960; Shagass and Jones, 1958).

---

[1] Although the term 'sedation threshold' strictly refers to Shagass' original EEG-based technique, it has through usage come to refer to sedative drug threshold procedures in general. Unless the context requires otherwise, I shall use the term here in that generic sense.

The conclusion usually drawn from these early studies of psychiatric patients has been that introverts are indeed more tolerant of sedative drugs than extraverts. There are difficulties, however, with such a simple equation of drug tolerance with introversion-extraversion. Direct studies of Eysenck's original drug postulate in normal subjects, as distinct from psychiatric patients, have generally failed to show any consistent relationship between sedation threshold and question-naire measures of extraversion. The first authors to comment on this were Rodnight and Gooch (1963) who, following their own study of nitrous oxide tolerance in normal volunteers, noted that there was no correlation with extraversion - or, indeed, with neuroticism, the other personality dimension they examined. Neither personality char-acteristic alone seemed capable of predicting individual differences in drug response. However, Rodnight and Gooch then unearthed an inter-esting set of relationships. They carried out on their data what even-tually came to be known as 'zone analysis' (Eysenck, 1967); that is, they examined drug tolerance scores in individuals selected according to different combinations of extraversion and neuroticism. Using this method they found that there was a systematic relationship between personality and the tolerance of nitrous oxide, but that the relation-ship involved a complex interaction between introversion-extraversion and neuroticism. It is with the further analysis of that interaction, and with its possible biological basis, that the present paper is concerned. First, however, it is necessary to look in more detail at the results reported by Rodnight and Gooch and at subsequent attempts to replicate them.

The appearance of Rodnight and Gooch's report coincided with the be-ginning of a decline of interest in the sedation threshold as a tech-nique for examining drug response differences, especially among normal subjects, and as far as I can tell there have since then only been two other studies in which similar data have been subjected to zone analysis. Both of these were conducted by my colleagues and myself, in two separate experiments. One was an investigation of sedation threshold for amylobarbitone sodium in a sample of normal twins (Claridge and Ross, 1973); the other was a more recent study of thio-pentone by Claridge and others (1981) who obtained sedation threshold measurements on a group of surgical patients just prior to operation.

The zone analyses of the results from these three experiments - in-cluding the original Rodnight and Gooch data - are shown in Table 1.

TABLE 1

(a)   E and Drug Tolerance in High and Low N Scorers

	High N		Low N	
	r	p	r	p
Nitrous oxide	-0.40	NS	+0.72	.05
Amylobarbitone sodium	-0.45	NS	+0.65	.05
Thiopentone	-0.71	.01	+0.38	NS

(b)   N and Drug Tolerance in High and Low E Scorers

	High E		Low E	
	r	p	r	p
Nitrous oxide	-0.80	.01	+0.42	NS
Amylobarbitone sodium	-0.65	.02	+0.34	NS
Thiopentone	-0.64	.01	+0.07	NS

Data from: Rodnight and Gooch (1963) - Nitrous oxide
            Claridge and Ross (1973) - Amylobarbitone sodium
            Claridge and others (1981) - Thiopentone

It should be noted that in each case two zone analyses were carried out. First the samples were divided into subjects with high neuroticism scores and those with low neuroticism scores; then within each of these two subgroups sedation threshold was correlated with extraversion. In the second set of zone analyses the samples were divided according to extraversion and separate correlations calculated between sedation threshold and neuroticsm. The exact cut-off points used to define high and low extraversion and high and low neuroticism are given in the original reports of the three studies.

Referring to Table 1, and considering first the division according to neuroticism it can be seen that, in all three experiments, the correlations between extraversion and sedation threshold are opposite in direction in Low N subjects compared with High N subjects. In the latter, sedation threshold is negatively correlated with extraversion; that is, introverts have greater drug tolerance than extraverts. But in Low N subjects the opposite is true: extraverts tend to have greater drug tolerance than introverts. It can also be seen that a similar reversal of correlation was found when the samples were divided according to extraversion and sedation threshold related to neuroticsm: in all three cases neuroticism leads to decreased tolerance in extraverts but increased tolerance in introverts.

It is true that some of the correlations shown in Table 1 are fairly low and are not significant. However, bearing in mind that different drugs were used in each experiment, the pattern of relationships across the three studies is remarkably similar and the results for the two sets of zone analysis quite consistent with each other. Taken together, they suggest that very poor tolerance of depressant drugs is likely to be found in subjects showing a combination of high neuroticism and high extraversion whereas neuroticism combined with extreme introversion is likely to be associated with raised tolerance. Looked at from the point of view of Eysenck's theory relating drug response to personality and personality to neurosis, this part of the results would be consistent with the findings of those studies, already mentioned, in which sedation threshold differences have been examined in samples of psychiatric patients. There, it will be recalled, patients assumed to represent extremes of introversion and neuroticism (dysthymics) have also been found to have higher sedation thresholds than patients considered to be extraverted and neurotic (hysterics). Eysenck's original drug postulate is therefore supported if the analysis is confined to individuals who are high in 'neuroticism' - whether judged by personality questionnaire or on the basis of clinical diagnosis. However, in individuals especially lacking in neuroticism the postulate fails completely; indeed there the relationship between drug response and extraversion is actually opposite to prediction.

This reversal of prediction in Low N subjects is puzzling, but the consistency with which it has appeared suggests that it is a real phenomenon warranting further investigation. Unfortunately, more detailed examination of the apparently interacting effect of neuroticism and extraversion on drug tolerance faces two, related, problems. One is that the method of zone analysis used to do so requires a relatively large number of subjects because of the need to subdivide the sample in order to arrive at subgroups for the appropriate comparisons to be made. The other is that collection of an adequately large amount of data is, if not precluded, at least made difficult by the nature of the sedation threshold test, involving as it does the administration of a large quantity of drug, usually by injection. Thus, each of the three examples of zone analysis given in Table 1 was based on relatively small samples, ruling out any further manipulation of the individual sets of data.

An alternative strategy, and one we have recently used, is to combine the data from several experiments. Apart from merely increasing the total sample size available, this method has a further advantage. As we shall see in a moment, it allows a more detailed breakdown of the sample to be made in terms of the two personality dimensions of interest. Previous zone analyses have been confined to simple two-way comparisons of High and Low E or High and Low N scorers, respectively. But it would clearly be more informative if a rather larger number of combinations of extraversion and neuroticism could be arrived at in order to determine more exactly how their interaction influences drug response.

The results to be described, using this procedure, were obtained by combining three sets of sedation threshold data on barbiturates (the Rodnight and Gooch nitrous oxide data were unfortunately not available to us). The two main sources of data were the experiments on amylobarbitone sodium and thiopentone referred to in Table 1. To these were added a further small amount of data on amylobarbitone,

collected earlier by my colleagues and myself (Claridge, 1967). A complete account of the method and results of this 'composite' zone analysis has been published elsewhere (Claridge and others, 1981) and
here I shall confine myself to giving essential details.

The sedation thresholds had in all cases been obtained using the
'digit-doubling' method developed by Claridge and Herrington (1960);
it involved determining the amount of drug (amylobarbitone sodium or
thiopentone) required to suppress the subject's performance on a
simple task in which he was required to double aloud each of a succes-
sive series of digits. Personality measures of extraversion and neuroticism had been obtained using one of Eysenck's questionnaires -
either the Maudsley Personality Inventory (MPI) or the Eysenck Personality Inventory (EPI). Because different questionnaires, and different
drugs, had been used in the original experiments the raw scores were,
of course, not comparable and in this form could not be combined to
produce a single sample. This was overcome by converting both the sedation threshold and the personality measures for each subject to
standard scores, based on the standard deviations of the sample to
which he or she originally belonged.

The total number of subjects available for zone analysis was 126,
80 of whom were male and 46 female; the mean age was 27.92, SD 9.92
years. This sample was subdivided, according to their extraversion
and neuroticism scores, into nine subgroups to give various combinations of Low, Medium, and High E and Low, Medium, and High N, the
cut-off points used to define high and low scores on the two dimensions being half a standard deviation above or below the mean in each
case.

Figure 1 shows, in graphical form, the mean drug tolerance scores for
each of the nine different combinations of extraversion and neuroticism.
Analysis of variance of the data in this form demonstrated that extraversion alone had no significant overall influence on tolerance, while
neuroticism had the small effect - significant at the .05 level - of
slightly raising drug tolerance scores. However, the most striking
result was a highly significant interaction term in the analysis of
variance (p < .001), an effect which is clearly illustrated in Fig. 1.
It can be seen there that the nature of the interaction is complex
and, although largely mirroring the relationships described earlier,
shows some trends not previously evident. Most obvious is the fact
that the highest drug tolerance is found in individuals who, while
certainly introverted, have moderate, rather than very high neuroticism scores; indeed t-test comparisons showed that this group had
significantly greater drug tolerance than all other groups, with the
marginal exception of the MedE/HiN combination. Using a three-way
breakdown of this larger sample suggested, therefore, that very high
neuroticism combined with introversion is associated with a relative
lowering of drug tolerance, an effect presumably masked in the
simpler zone analyses discussed previously. However, it can be seen
in Fig. 1 that, as predicted from the earlier analyses, LoE/LoN subjects continue to show poor drug tolerance, in that respect being
similar to, though not as extreme as, neurotic extraverts; the latter
show the lowest tolerance scores of all.

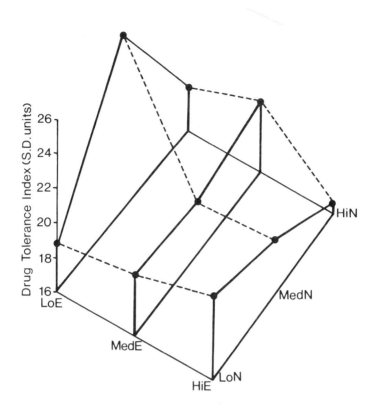

Fig. 1. Diagram showing the plotted mean drug tolerance
         index scores for different combinations of
         extraversion and neuroticism.

The overall picture that seems to emerge from this more elaborate zone
analysis is that in the middle, and perhaps to a lesser extent in the
upper, range of neuroticism introversion does, as Eysenck predicts,
lead to gradually increasing tolerance of depressant drugs. However,
the relationship is much more evident among individuals with moderate
degrees of neuroticism, any correlation that exists at higher levels
being more due to the very reduced tolerance of extraverts than to a
particularly high tolerance in introverts. Clearly, in the absence
of neuroticism a straightforward relationship between introversion
and tolerance is even less evident; indeed it disappears entirely,
non-neurotic introverts being actually more sensitive to the effects
of depressant drugs than extraverts. It seems therefore as though
any departure from moderate degrees of neuroticism - whether an increase or a decrease - leads to a distortion of the originally predicted relationship between introversion-extraversion and drug
response.

Paralleling the complexity of these empirical findings, any attempt
at a physiological explanation of them must be extremely speculative,

though elsewhere (Claridge and others, 1981) I have offered a possible, tentative, explanation. This relies on combining certain features of two modifications to Eysenck's original biological model of personality: that described by Gray (1970) as an alternative account of extraversion and my own suggestion for a possible causal basis for 'neuroticism' and 'psychoticism' (Claridge, 1967). Although Gray's model is more 'physiological', both he and I have arrived at similar conceptual nervous systems for personality; each of these incorporates the notion of a feedback arrangement between arousal, on the one hand, and an excitatory - inhibitory mechanism regulating arousal, on the other. Gray has specifically identified the relevant neural structures with, respectively, the ascending reticular formation and the septo-hippocampal system. My own proposal was for two hypothetical systems - 'tonic arousal' and 'arousal modulation' - which might, however, be tentatively considered to refer to that same circuitry. Applying his model to personality, Gray has emphasized the <u>negative</u> feedback nature of the relationship between the ARAS and the septo-hippocampal system, mainly because he has been concerned with variations in normal introversion-extraversion; or, more correctly, with variations cutting across Eysenck's dimensions of extraversion and neuroticism and identified by him as a major continuum of anxiety, defined at the high end by neurotic introversion. Some years ago I made a not dissimilar suggestion for a continuum of 'dysthymia-hysteria', reflecting variations in - to use my own terminology - the level of tonic arousal, together with a negative feedback relationship between the latter and arousal modulation. My own model went further, however, in proposing that a state of <u>positive</u> feedback could also prevail in the circuit, this being responsible for variations along a second major continuum of 'psychoticism'. With these points in mind, let us now consider a possible explanation of the present findings.

Put in the most general terms it seems reasonable to suppose that, in any given individual, the sedation threshold represents an end-state in which the administered drug overcomes the various excitatory and inhibitory influences that are maintaining consciousness. Indeed, this was precisely the conclusion reached by Perez-Reyes and Cochrane (1967), following an investigation, in cats, of the possible physiological basis of the 'GSR-inhibition threshold', their version of the sedation threshold. Combining injections of thiopentone with lesions at different levels in the nervous system they concluded that the progressive administration of barbiturates is really like a serial downward transection of the CNS, the final sedation threshold representing the point at which inhibitory influences prevail. In this respect it is also worth noting that, as Gray and his colleagues have shown (Gray and Ball, 1970), an early effect of barbiturates is on the septo-hippocampal system, altering its inhibitory properties; however, in larger doses, corresponding more to those used in sedation threshold procedures, the ascending reticular formation is a major site of action (Killam, 1962).

Returning to the present data, my suggestion, therefore, is that during determination of the sedation threshold the administered drug progressively alters the sensitivity of the various elements in the neural circuit identified by Gray, the final end-point in any given subject being decided by the excitability of the element ultimately affected, namely the ascending reticular activating system. However, I would further propose that this end-point will only reflect ARAS activity in a simple manner in those individuals in whom a negative feedback

arrangement between the different parts of the Gray circuit is maintained throughout the sedation threshold procedure; these should be
individuals located by Gray along his dimension of 'anxiety', and considered by myself to have a 'balanced' or 'neurotic' type of nervous
system organisation (Claridge, 1967). They would also be people in
whom the relationship between drug tolerance predicted by Eysenck
would obtain.[2]

The effect of continuous administration of barbiturates in those individuals who, it is proposed, show a positive feedback arrangement
between - to use my own terminology - arousal and arousal modulation
might be quite different. Certainly it would be expected that excitatory or inhibitory mechanisms that are intrinsically weak or strong
relative to each other would be thrown further out of balance by drugs;
the sedation threshold is then unlikely to relate in a simple fashion
to dimensions like introversion or neuroticism. My own suggestion is
that such individuals represent a part of the personality domain not
tapped directly by the E and N scales but instead are high in 'psychotic' traits.

There are several reasons for this emphasis on psychoticism. First,
although admittedly there are difficulties with the questionnaire
measurement of psychotic traits in normal people (Claridge, 1981),
the existence of psychoticism as a third major dimension of personality seems to be beyond doubt (Eysenck and Eysenck, 1976). Given that
that is so it seems inconceivable that variations along such a dimension should not be reflected in some way in the response to drugs;
certainly in other ways individuals high in psychoticism appear to be
psychophysiologically distinct (Claridge and Birchall, 1978). Secondly,
it is clear that the E and N scales used in studies of the kind reported here were not 'pure' measures of extraversion and neuroticism, in
the sense that they are known to tap some characteristics such as impulsivity, which currently would be referred to psychoticism (Eysenck
and Eysenck, 1975). It is therefore likely that correlations between
biological measures like the sedation threshold and personality scores
derived from the earlier MPI and EPI scales actually reflect, in part,
some covariation due to psychotic traits. Thirdly, there is some evidence from our own psychiatric studies of sedation threshold (Claridge,
1967) that, among psychotic patients, extraverted and introverted characteristics do relate to drug tolerance in the opposite direction
from that found in other people. That evidence included one finding -
directly relevant here - that in a group of schizophrenics there was
a small positive correlation between the sedation threshold and a
measure of extraversion derived from the MPI. Indeed, it was on the
basis of this and other clinical correlates of the sedation threshold
that I was led to propose two major 'styles' of normal central nervous organisation, one 'neurotic' and one 'psychotic'; the latter,
characterised by a positive feedback arrangement between 'tonic arousal'
and 'arousal modulation', would be expected to show a fundamentally
different pattern of relationships from that predicted by Eysenck
between extraversion and biological measures, including drug response.

---

[2] The fact, however, that the closest alignment between tolerance and
introversion occurs along the axis of moderate neuroticism (see Fig.1)
should not be overlooked. This is possibly because, as will be discussed later, the personality scales used in this study are not un-
contaminated measures of neuroticism.

To summarise, then, the empirical findings are clear, namely that drug
response, at least as indexed by the sedation threshold, is related to
introversion-extraversion as originally predicted only in certain individuals. These could be said to be people with a certain kind of
'neurotic' central nervous organisation, of the form emphasised by
Gray and now perhaps identifiable with the psychophysiological continuum which I previously argued underlies the descriptive dimension
of 'dysthymia-hysteria'. The relationship between sedation threshold
and introversion-extraversion is, however, quite opposite in some
other individuals who, less certainly, might be identified as high in
psychotic traits and therefore forming a psychophysiologically distinct
'nervous type'. Direct support for this latter conclusion is, at present, less strong partly because studies using the sedation threshold
procedure have so far been confined to the manipulation of only the
two dimensions of extraversion and neuroticism. It seems likely that
such data do in fact hide other sources of variation. What is required
is zone analysis in which the interactions between extraversion, neuroticism, and psychoticism are investigated simultaneously. Such an
analysis would obviously require a very large sample - even larger
than that available here - and the prospects are gloomy, given the
nature of the sedation threshold and the ethical problems associated
with its use, particularly in normal subjects. However, one strategy
that could be adopted is that used in our most recent study (Claridge
and others, 1981), namely to exploit the fact that many people undergoing minor dental or surgical treatments receive intravenous barbiturates prior to operation. In our experience it is fairly easy to
arrange for the anaesthetist to standardise his injection routine and
so obtain an accurate measure of the patient's sedation threshold. By
administering, in addition, appropriate questionnaires, it should then
be possible to collect the large amounts of data which would allow us
to disentangle even further some of the relationships which clearly
exist between drug tolerance and personality. Alternatively, of course,
the hypothesis suggested by the evidence described here could be tested
in experiments which involve the administration of small oral doses
of drugs. In my view, this is less satisfactory, compared with the
already established powerful advantages of the sedation threshold as
a research tool for investigating the differential response to central-
ly acting drugs.

REFERENCES

Claridge, G. S. (1967). Personality and Arousal. Pergamon Press,
   Oxford.
Claridge, G. S. (1981). Psychoticism. In R. Lynn (Ed.), Dimensions of
   Personality. Papers in Honour of H. J. Eysenck. Pergamon Press,
   Oxford.
Claridge, G. S., and P. M. A. Birchall (1978). Bishop, Eysenck, Block
   and psychoticism. J. Abn. Psychol., 87, 664-668.
Claridge, G. S., and R. N. Herrington (1960). Sedation threshold,
   personality and the theory of neurosis. J. Ment. Sci., 106, 1568-
   1583.
Claridge, G. S., and E. Ross (1973). Sedative tolerance in twins.
   In G. S. Claridge, S. Canter, and W. I. Hume (Eds.), Personality
   Differences and Biological Variations. Pergamon Press, Oxford.
   pp. 115-131.
Claridge, G. S., J. R. Donald, and P. M. A. Birchall (1981). Drug
   tolerance and personality: some implications for Eysenck's theory.
   Pers. Ind. Diff., 2, 153-156.

Eysenck, H. J. (1947). Dimensions of Personality. Routledge & Kegan
    Paul, London.
Eysenck, H. J. (1957). Drugs and personality. I. Theory and methodo-
    logy. J. Ment. Sci., 103, 119-131.
Eysenck, H. J. (1967). The Biological Basis of Personality. Charles
    C. Thomas, Springfield, Ill.
Eysenck, H. J., and S. B. G. Eysenck (1975). Manual of the Eysenck
    Personality Questionnaire. Hodder and Stoughton, London.
Eysenck, H. J., and S. B. G. Eysenck (1976). Psychoticism as a Dimen-
    sion of Personality. Hodder and Stoughton, London.
Fink, M. (1958). Lateral gaze nystagmus as an index of the sedation
    threshold. EEG Clin. Neurophysiol., 10, 162-163.
Giberti, F., and R. Rossi (1962). Proposal of a psychopharmacological
    test (stimulation threshold) for differentiating neurotic from
    psychotic depressions. Psychopharmacologia, 3, 128-131.
Gray, J. A. (1970). The psychophysiological basis of introversion-
    extraversion. Behav. Res. Ther., 8, 249-266.
Gray, J. A., and G. G. Ball (1970). Frequency-specific relation
    between hippocampal theta rhythm, behaviour and amobarbital action.
    Science, 168, 1246-1248.
Kawi, A. A. (1958). The sedation threshold: its concept and use for
    comparative studies on drug-induced phenomena. Arch. Neurol.
    Psychiat., 80, 232-236.
Killam, E. K. (1962). Drug action on the brainstem reticular forma-
    tion. Pharmacol. Rev., 14, 175-223.
Perez-Reyes, M., and G. Cochrane (1967). Differences in sodium thio-
    pental susceptibility of depressed patients as evidenced by the
    galvanic skin reflex inhibition threshold. J. Psychiat. Res., 5,
    335-347.
Perez-Reyes, M., H. C. Shands, and G. Johnson (1962). Galvanic skin
    reflex inhibition threshold: a new psychophysiologic technique.
    Psychosom. Med., 24, 274-277.
Rodnight, E., and R. N.Gooch (1963). A new method for the determination
    of individual differences in susceptibility to a depressant drug.
    In H. J. Eysenck (Ed.), Experiments with Drugs. Pergamon Press,
    Oxford. pp. 131-168.
Shagass, C. (1954). The sedation threshold. A method for estimating
    tension in psychiatric patients. EEG Clin. Neurophysiol., 6,
    221-233.
Shagass, C., and A. L. Jones (1958). A neurophysiological test for
    psychiatric diagnosis: results in 750 patients. Amer. J. Psychiat.,
    114, 1002-1009.
Shagass, C., and A. B. Kerenyi (1958). The 'sleep' threshold. A simple
    form of the sedation threshold for clinical use. Canad. Psychiat.
    J.,1, 101-109.
Shagass, C., J. Naiman, and J. Mihalik (1956). An objective test which
    differentiates between neurotic and psychotic depression. Arch.
    Neurol. Psychiat., 75, 461-471.

PERSONALITY FACTORS IN SELF-MEDICATION BY SMOKING

D. M. Warburton, K. Wesnes and A. Revell

ABSTRACT

Self-medication refers to the therapeutic use of drugs that have been selected by the person himself and not prescribed by doctors or some other conventional medical source. Certain personality types are more likely to self-medicate than others; these people score highly on scales which measure desire from personal control. If people who self-medicate select psychoactive drugs that are appropriate for their mental health, three predictions are implied: 1. People will adopt a drug which matches their personality. 2. Reduction or elimination of use of that drug will result in an increase in the symptoms. 3. Drug use will increase in the situations to which the person is sensitive by virtue of their personality.

As an example of the self-medication, nicotine is used and these three claims examined. Evidence is cited that cigarette smoking is more likely to be adopted by individuals who score highly on extraversion and neuroticism although there are sex differences. Survey studies have shown that the amount of smoking and the strength of cigarette that is smoked are also related to the individual's personality and sex. Studies of smoking cessation are consistent with this data. Previous experimental studies have investigated the situation x personality x smoking interaction and shown that more nicotine is taken in when the subjects are susceptible to the demands of the situation. In particular, extraverts smoke more intensely towards the end of a boring test session, while neurotics smoke more intensely at the beginning of a test session. These data suggest that smoking is being used as self-medication by certain personality types.

KEYWORDS

Smoking; extraversion; neuroticism; self-medication; abstinence symptoms; anxiety; anger; depression.

The papers in this volume are concerned with differential psychopharmacology in the sense defined by Janke: "a subdiscipline of psychopharmacology which is concerned with the description, explanation and
prediction of individual differences in response to psychotropic drugs.
Individual differences may be found between subjects and within a
subject at various times." (Janke and others, 1979; p. 13). The other
contributors to this volume have taken a psychological response measure as their dependant variable and studied the interaction between
the independent variables of dose levels and individual differences
in a standard situation. We have made a different interpretation of
this definition by taking drug choice and dose level as our dependant
variables and studying the interaction between the independent variables of personality and situation on them. Thus we are trying to understand how individuals respond to psychotropic drugs when they are
allowed relatively free access to them and allowed to self-medicate.

In most circumstances drug availability is controlled by law and the
ordinary person only has access to them via a doctor's prescription.
The vast expansion of prescription drug use has been documented elsewhere (e.g. Warburton, 1978), and this explosion has resulted from
the acceptance by the ordinary person that drugs can be used to help
a person master, reduce, minimise or tolerate demands which tax or
excede his ability to cope. Thus drug taking is now accepted by the
average man as a rapid and certain coping strategy for the problems
of life. One of the most interesting aspects of psychotherapeutic
drug use is the fact that either people go to the doctor to obtain
drugs on prescription, or they self-medicate, but there are very few
people who do both (Parry and others, 1973). There is a clear sex
difference in these groups; women use prescription drugs more than
men, but men use alcohol and marijuana to a greater extent and so take
more psychoactive substances in total. In addition, self medication is
more common among young people and the use of medically-prescribed
drugs increases with age even though the levels of psychological dis-
tress are higher among young people (Parry and other, 1973).

In one set of our studies, we have investigated the hypothesis that
self-medication is characteristic of people who like to control their
own lives. This personality type can be assessed on the Internal-
External Control Scale of Rotter (1966) which measures the extent to
which people believe that success and failure are the product of their
own efforts and abilities (Internal Control) or stem from powers beyond their control including fate, chance and luck (External Control).
A great deal of evidence has accumulated to suggest that there are
differences in behaviour between people who perceive a causal relation
between events and their own action and those who do not. We have
found that people who self-treat score highly in the internal control
direction on the scale, and there was a negative correlation between
external control scores and attitudes to self treatment. This evidence
supports the notion that self-medicating people believe that they have
a greater understanding of their own bodies and that they can select
drugs to control their own emotional states and general health.

Drugs for self-medication can be obtained in a number of ways. They
can be non-prescription drugs obtained over the counter, prescription
drugs obtained from non-medical sources, or non-medical drugs that
are obtained legally or illegally. In our studies we have been more
interested in the much more common form of self-medication, the use
of non-medical drugs like caffeine, alcohol and nicotine. In a sepa-

rate paper (Warburton, 1979a), use of alcohol for self-medication has been examined and it was concluded that alcohol is used on occasions for mood elevation, anxiety reduction and as a hypnotic. In this paper we will be discussing the use of nicotine by smokers as self-medication to cope with the demands of life.

We conducted a survey of 468 young adults to determine their use of various coping strategies including smoking. Our results indicate three populations as defined by people's preferred coping strategy: (i) those who tend to turn to friends with their problems; (ii) those who tend to turn to parental or expert advice; (iii) those who tend to solve problems on their own, often with the use of drugs. There were some interesting sex differences in coping strategies which supported the findings of Parry and coworkers (1973). Women preferred to go to the doctor with their problems ($t = 3.96$; $p < 0.001$), while men reported that they liked to solve their problems on their own ($t = 5.22$; $p < 0.001$), and prefer to self-medicate to cope with problems ($t = 3.57$; $p < 0.001$).

It is interesting to note that solving problems with drugs correlated positively both with solving problems on one's own ($r = 0.274$; $p < 0.01$) and with the number of cigarettes smoked ($r = .341$; $p < 0.001$). Furthermore, those people who preferred to self-medicate did not take their problems to "expert advice agencies" such as doctors and counsellors, and not to discuss their problems with friends. Thus we have two "external" help strategies and one "internal" strategy. The more heavily someone smokes the more likely they are to be displaced towards the third strategy population.

Multicorrelational analysis showed that people who preferred to solve their own problems smoked more cigarettes per day ($r = 0.341$; $p < 0.001$); had smoked regularly for a longer period of time ($r = 0.288$; $p < 0.001$); started smoking at an earlier age ($r = 0.232$; $p < 0.05$); rated strength as an important factor in the choice of cigarette brand ($r = 0.28$; $p < 0.01$) and rated tar grouping as unimportant ($r = 0.276$; $p < 0.01$). The finding that people who solve problems by themselves rated strength of cigarette as an important factor in brand preference suggests that cigarettes are being used for pharmacological reasons. It suggests that these people are aware of the relative effects of different amounts of nicotine in different cigarettes and choose their cigarette to meet their needs. Thus it is our claim that people consciously or unconsciously discover drugs which are psychopharmacologically appropriate to help them with their problems. Of course, not all cigarette smoking can be considered as self-medication; there will be differences in use between individuals and even within the same individual on different occasions.

The claim of self-medication gives rise to three predictions about use of these drugs. Firstly, people will adopt a drug which matches their personality. Secondly, reduction or elimination of that drug will result in an increase in a set of psychological symptoms that can be predicted from the user's personality. Thirdly, drug use will increase in situations to which the person is sensitive by virtue of his personality. In this paper we will examine these predictions for smoking in the following three forms.
    (A) People who smoke will have certain personality
        characteristics (Personality of the Smoker)

(B) Reduction or cessation of smoking cigarettes will
    result in psychological symptoms which can be pre-
    dicted from the smoker's personality characteristics
    (Personality and Abstinence Symptoms)

(C) Cigarette use will increase in situations to which
    the smoker is sensitive by virtue of his personality
    (Personality and Situational Smoking).

(A) PERSONALITY OF THE SMOKER

The neurochemistry of behaviour is based on the assumption that many
aspects of human behaviour can be related to the function of specific
neurochemical systems in the brain, and individual differences in behaviour will be a consequence of quantitative variations in these
systems (Warburton, 1975, 1981). As a corollary of this assumption
that the effects of drugs on behaviour can be related to neurochemistry, and a specific assumption of differential psychopharmacology is
that differences in drug effects reflect different degrees of responsiveness of these neural systems (Janke and coworkers, 1979). We believe that qualitative and quantitative differences in drug taking
will result from neurochemical differences that will also underlie
behavioural differences, and so different patterns of self-medication
will be correlated with different behaviour patterns. In other words,
differences in cigarette smoking behaviour will be related to individual differences in behaviour.

One influential theory of individual differences in behaviour is based
on the dichotomy between extraverts and introverts. A personality
questionnaire such as the Eysenck Personality Inventory (Eysenck and
Eysenck, 1964) can be used to assess a person's degree of behavioural
extraversion on the basis of their life style attitudes. An extraverted person is characterised by a tendency to get bored easily and stop
concentrating. He is expansive, likes to have many friends, tends to
be optimistic, takes chances, acts on the spur of the moment and is
unreliable. In contrast, the introverted person tries to lead a quiet
and retiring life. He is introspective, reserved, keeps his feelings
under control and is distant except from intimate friends. He is reliable but pessimistic, so he does not like uncertainty, preferring
an orderly existence and planning ahead.

In the largest surveys of male smokers (Eysenck and others, 1960;
Eysenck, 1963) a very highly significant positive correlation was
found between cigarette smoking and extraversion. Heavy smokers were
the most extraverted, medium smokers were less extraverted, light
smokers were less extraverted still, and non-smokers were the least
extraverted. Ex-smokers scored in between light and medium on the
extraversion scale. Smaller studies on both sexes using other personality scales have confirmed this statistical relationship between
smoking and extraversion (Matarazzo and Saslow, 1960).

As well as the extraversion-introversion dimension, the Eysenck Personality Inventory has questions designed to assess behavioural neuroticism, which is an independent dimension of personality. The neurotic
person displays labile, emotional behaviour; he is anxious, irritable,
moody, restless, excitable, and changeable. In contrast, the stable
person is calm, and even tempered. There is less consistency in the
evidence for a relationship between smoking and neuroticism, and

Eysenck's studies of men gave no evidence for a significant correlation (Eysenck and others, 1960; Eysenck, 1963). Rae's (1975) survey of 253 female college students revealed no differences in neuroticism between non-smokers, ex-smokers, light smokers or medium smokers, but there were very few heavy smokers (over 15 per day) in the college. However, a number of studies have suggested a positive relationship. The interesting pattern that emerges from these surveys is that there is some relation between cigarette consumption and neuroticism at least for women (Dunnell and Cartwright, 1972; Meares and others, 1971; Waters, 1971).

In our own work a questionnaire was given to 259 male and female smokers to obtain information about the number of cigarettes smoked a day, the number of years that the individual had been smoking and the specific brands smoked. In addition, all the smokers were asked to complete the Eysenck Personality Inventory. For both sexes the distribution of number of cigarettes was bimodal with a separation around 15 cigarettes per day, which is consistent with the results of a survey by Schachter (1978). These results suggest that there are two populations of smokers, light smokers and heavy smokers, with a separation at 15 per day, and so the personality and smoking data were analysed separately according to sex and number of cigarettes smoked per day.

This analysis revealed that male, heavy smokers smoked more than female, heavy smokers, and male, light smokers smoked more than female, light smokers (F = 149, df = 3.255, p < 0.0001). Male, heavy smokers had been smoking longer than either of the other three groups (F = 3.7, df = 3.255, p < 0.05). The previous finding of Eysenck (1963) that heavy smokers are more extraverted than light smokers was confirmed but we also found that female smokers were more extraverted than male smokers (F = 3, df = 3.255, p < 0.05). No differences were found in the neuroticism scores of the four groups which again supports the work of Eysenck.

The personality and smoking information were then correlated within each of the four groups in order to determine any relationships which might exist between the various smoking and personality parameters. The correlations brought to light some interesting and unexpected associations. For each of the separate groups, a positive correlation was found between the number smoked per day and the degree of neuroticism, i.e. the more neurotic smokers in each group smoked more cigarettes per day, even though the mean neuroticism scores of light and heavy smokers did not differ. Thus neuroticism was not related to whether a smoker was either a heavy smoker or light smoker, but if a smoker was one of these types then the number that he or she smoked per day was related to the degree of the individual's neuroticism.

In contrast, no clear picture emerged when we considered the association between the number smoked a day and the degree of extraversion. We had found that light smokers were less extraverted than heavy smokers, and it might have been assumed that the level of extraversion scores would have correlated positively with the number of cigarettes smoked per day. However, the correlations between these two variables was zero for the female light and male heavy groups, and negative for the female heavy and male light smokers. The absence of any consistent pattern suggests that although the degree of extraversion was related to whether the individual was a light or a heavy smoker, if the individual was a light or heavy smoker then the number smoked per day was

not associated with the degree of extraversion, but only with neuroticism.

From this data one could speculate that constitutional factors, which
result in extraverted behaviour, determine whether a person becomes a
light or heavy smoker, whereas the factors that underlie neuroticism
are not associated with heavy or light smoking, but influence the
number smoked per day if an individual is a light or heavy smoker.

Another interesting relationship emerged when the correlations between
personality and the strength of cigarettes are considered. While extraversion scores were not correlated with the strength of cigarettes
smoked, neuroticism scores were positively correlated for women, un-
correlated for male light smokers and negatively correlated for male
heavy smokers. Thus the more neurotic females smoked higher delivery
cigarettes, but this was not true for males. For male, light smokers
the strength of their cigarettes did not correlate with their neuroticism scores, whereas male heavy smokers smoked weaker cigarettes if
they had high neuroticism scores. Of course, these correlations were
based on the machine-estimated yields of the cigarettes smoked and do
not tell us how much nicotine and tar were actually obtained. However,
we can safely conclude that the strength of cigarettes that are pur-
chased is related to the degrees of neuroticism of all groups except
male, light smokers. From this data it could be argued that the more
neurotic male, heavy smokers are more concerned about their health
and their cigarette consumption and so buy cigarettes of lower nicotine and tar yields than less neurotic male smokers. On the other
hand, the more neurotic female smokers smoke not only more, but also
smoke stronger cigarettes, which can be used as evidence that women
buy cigarettes in order to cope with their neuroticism.

One of the crucial studies of smoking and personality was done by
Cherry and Kiernan (1976, 1978). A cohort of 2,753 young people have
been followed for 25 years and at 16 years the subjects completed the
Maudsley Personality Inventory before most of them had begun to smoke.
At 20 years and at 25 years, they completed a smoking habits questionnaire and it was found that the cigarette smokers as a group were extraverted and neurotic as Eysenck (1963) and we would have expected.
Those teenagers who smoked regularly at before 16 years were more neurotic and more extraverted than smokers who did not. A statistical
analysis revealed that the two personality dimensions are independent
and additive in their effect on the likelihood of becoming a regular
smoker. Self-report of depth of inhalation varied among the personality groups, deep inhalers had a higher mean neuroticism score than
slight inhalers whose neuroticism scores were the same as non-smokers.
On the other hand, deep inhalers had the same mean extraversion score
as non-smokers while the slight inhalers were more extraverted than
non-smokers. Thus the deep inhaler can be characterised as more neurotic and less extraverted.

(B) PERSONALITY AND ABSTINENCE SYMPTOMS

Inferences about the therapeutic function of a drug can often be made
from the symptoms that occur when medication is terminated; for example, it is very obvious the function that insulin is serving for a
diabetic person when injections are discontinued. The withdrawal symptoms that follow cessation of smoking are not as clear cut as this

example, but evidence has accumulated of a pattern of symptoms that
are associated with abstinence from cigarettes (Shiffman, 1979;
Shiffman and Jarvik, 1976). These abstinence symptoms are often cited
as evidence of nicotine dependence, but this seems less likely in
view of the fact that about a quarter of smokers show no symptoms at
all when they stop smoking and withdraw from nicotine. This variability could easily be explained if a proportion of smokers were using
cigarettes as self-medication and abstinence symptoms resulted from
the removal of medication from this group.

One group of symptoms that are frequently found following smoking
cessation are changes in electrocortical arousal and "attention". It
has been observed that there is a shift in electrocortical arousal
from the higher frequencies, that are usually associated with alertness,
to slower activity (Knott and Venables, 1977). In comparison with his
non-deprived state, the deprived smoker reports that he feels less
alert, more fatigued and unable to concentrate as well as he did before (Shiffman and Jarvik, 1976). These subjective experiences are
associated with objective evidence of impaired vigilance performance
(Heimstra and others, 1967) although this impairment is not observed
in all subjects (Wesnes and Warburton, 1978). Thus it could be argued
that from this evidence that cigarettes help the smoker feel more
alert and function more efficiently. This sort of effect of cigarettes
would be most important for the extravert who is prone to boredom and
seeks stimulation of various kinds.

A second common set of abstinence symptoms are emotional states of
hostility and anxiety. The deprived smoker reports an increased irritability and hostility (Mausner, 1970; Thomas, 1973). Deprived smokers
reported much higher levels of aggression before smoking a cigarette
than after. Other studies have also shown hostility and aggressive
behaviour increase markedly during abstinence (Schechter and Rand,
1974). Anger is commonly reported as a triggering factor in relapse
among ex-smokers, and these relapses occurred in the absence of smoking-
related cues, e.g. "people around were smoking" (Shiffman, 1979a).
Clearly, the smoker is being deprived of some property of the cigarette which is sedative and in the questionnaire studies of Russell
and co-workers (1974) and our own studies with the same questionnaire
(Warburton and Wesnes, 1978), it has been found that many smokers
claim that they smoke when angry.

Stronger additional evidence for smoking for "sedative" effects appears
in the claims of many smokers that they smoke more when anxious
(Russell and others, 1974; Warburton and Wesnes, 1978). One of the
major symptoms of cigarette withdrawal is increased anxiety (Nesbitt,
1973; Shiffman and Jarvik, 1976) which is more likely to occur among
women, among whom there is the greatest proportion of neurotic smokers
(Guildford, 1966; Shiffman, 1979b). Anxiety is also given as one of
the major causes of relapse, especially among women (Shiffman, 1979b).

Recently, a large epidemiological study of British doctors was made
(Lee, 1979). As a group, doctors have reduced their smoking dramatically and as expected, there have been dramatic reductions in death
from the so called "smoker-related" diseases. However, the overall
death rates did not fall as dramatically as one would have predicted
from groups that were matched for socioeconomic status, and the reason
for this descrepancy was that mortality due to other causes had increased. In particular, stress-related deaths had increased relative

to the equivalent social classes; more doctors died from cirrhosis of
the liver, suicides and "accidents, poisonings, etc. which were ac-
corded open verdicts at the coroner's court". Lee concludes that "the
relative worsening in mortality from stress-related disease may have
been due partly to a possible adverse effect of giving up smoking, if
smoking had acted to reduce stress" (p. 1538).

An analysis of the situations which resulted in a return to smoking
was made by Marlatt (1979) and Shiffman (1979a). Retrospective reports
indicated that 80% of situations fell into three categories: coping
with anxiety and other negative emotional states (43%), social pressure (25%) and coping with social stress (12%). Few of Marlatt's smokers and those in Shiffman's study reported that physical withdrawal
symptoms triggered the relapse which tends to discount the nicotine
dependence hypothesis. In the Shiffman (1979a) study, two thirds of
the subjects were under stress at the time of relapse and anxiety was
particularly common among ex-smokers who relapsed at work, which suggests that work-related anxiety was a contributory factor. Neurotics
are more anxiety-prone and so it is not surprising that this group
·find it difficult to stop smoking or relapse if they do (Cherry and
Kiernan, 1978). These data on coping with stress fit neatly with two
studies which suggest that deprived smokers, as a group, are more
likely to respond with anxiety in situations in which they are stressed (Frankenhaeuser and others, 1971; Myrsten and co-workers, 1972).
Thus we have some suggestion that a situation is important in the occurrence of abstinence symptoms. The importance of situations and their
interaction with the individual will be emphasised in the next section.

(C) PERSONALITY AND SITUATIONAL SMOKING

In Section A evidence was reviewed which showed that smoking behaviour
was related to the trait dimensions of extraversion and neuroticism,
and it was proposed that use of cigarettes was a consequence of the
neurochemical characteristics which determined these traits. In Section B it was argued that the cigarette abstinence symptoms indicated
that cigarettes were being used as self-medication by some individuals.
Thus a simple trait model of smoking would predict that smoking behaviour is determined primarily by individual neurochemical differences and that smoking behaviour would be consistent over a wide variety of situations.

However, at the end of Section B some evidence was given that abstinence symptoms were more likely to occur in some situations than
others. These findings imply that the simple trait model for smoking
behaviour may be too limited because it ignores situational factors.
Situational factors in smoking have been studied by a number of researchers on the assumption that smoking behaviour is controlled by
environmental factors external to the organism. These studies have
counted the number of cigarettes in specific environmental and social
situations.

The problem with a simple situational analysis of smoking is that situational specification is ambiguous unless the situation is related
to the person. A person may be asked whether he smokes at work, but
work has many aspects which will have different meanings for different
people and even for the same person at different times. Working with
others may be interesting and challenging for one person or stressful

for another, and, for the same person, working with a superior will
be stressful but not with a colleague of equal status. For some individuals repetitive work will be tedious and boring, for others it
will be soothing and satisfying, while for most people it will be tedious on some occasions and soothing on others.

In this section we propose an interactive model of smoking which includes both personality and situational factors. This model assumes
that smoking behaviour results from the _interaction_ between the individual and the situations which he encounters. This model has features
in common with the interactionist views of behaviour that have been discussed by Endler and Magnussen (1976) and applied to smoking by
Schalling (1977). The model predicts that smoking behaviour can vary
across both individuals and situations; it can be both person-specific
and situation-specific, but the prime determinant is the individual-
situation interaction rather than either the individual alone or the
situation alone. This approach emphasises the importance of the environment as it is perceived by the individual, and it assumes that the
most influential situational factor is the meaning that the situation
has for the person.

(1)   Smoking Behaviour

When smoking a cigarette, subjects can vary the total number of puffs,
the strength of a puff, the duration of puff and the inter-puff interval, in order to change the nicotine intake from that expected on the
basis of a smoking machine. This titration enables the smoker to adjust his dose to his needs throughout a particular situation by his
mode of smoke generation and his mode of smoke manipulation. Smoke
generation will be a function of the puff number, the puff strength,
the puff duration and the interpuff interval, and can be estimated
from the amount of nicotine deposited on the filter (butt nicotine)
providing the filtration efficiency is known. In addition, smoke intake will be a function of smoke manipulation, the way in which the
smoker takes the smoke, blows it out or inhales it.

Adams (1978) studied smoke generation with cigarettes of different
nicotine levels and total particulate matter. He found that the type
of cigarette affected smoking behaviour; subjects adapted their smoke
generation in order to obtain what they wanted from the cigarette
whether this need be for nicotine, tar or gaseous products. For example, with low nicotine, low tar cigarettes, there was evidence of titration to obtain about 50% more than the machine-estimated smoke
yield.

Evidence of titration was also found by Ashton and Watson (1970) for
subjects smoking in a driving simulation task. They tested subjects
in an easy driving task, a stressful driving task and at rest. In all
situations they found that subjects puffed more frequently at the low
nicotine cigarettes (1.0 mg of nicotine on machine-estimated delivery)
than the high nicotine cigarettes (2.1 mg nicotine on machine-estimated delivery), so that they took into their mouths nearly the same
amount of nicotine from each brand. Interestingly, subjects obtained
more nicotine from the cigarettes during the more stressful test than
the easier test, (although the differences were not statistically
significant) which suggest that individual smokers titrate the delivery from the cigarette from situation to situation. We tested this
"titration for situation" hypothesis in a vigilance study.

(2) Vigilance Situation

Subjects observed the second hand of a clock and were asked to report whenever they saw the second hand stop. Previous work in our laboratory (Wesnes and Warburton, 1978) had shown that detection performance on this task declined markedly in subjects over an eighty minute session. Cigarettes were given to the subject at twenty, forty and sixty minutes, and so performance on the first 20 minutes was not under the influence of the drug, which gave a baseline score for each individual. The typical finding of the studies was that cigarettes containing nicotine improved the performance of the group, although there were wide individual differences in baseline scores and the magnitude of the cigarette effect.

In these studies the amount of nicotine each subject took into his mouth was estimated from the butt nicotine. These estimates do not tell us how much nicotine entered the blood stream because this amount will depend on the depth of inhalation but all our subjects said that they were deep inhalers and so we would expect a good positive correlation between butt nicotine and blood nicotine for our subjects. It was evident that there was titration of intake so that smokers obtained more nicotine in their mouth than one would expect from the machine estimates of delivery from the low nicotine cigarette and less than expected from the high nicotine brand. This titration pattern suggests that subjects are adjusting their intake to obtain their own optimum level of cigarette smoke (Warburton and Wesnes, 1978).

(3) Extraversion and Smoking Behaviour in a Vigilance Situation

The major prediction from the self-medication hypothesis is that smoking behaviour will vary according to the individual's needs in a particular situation. In vigilance tests, extraverts have lower levels of electrocortical arousal than introverts (Gale and others, 1971). From a review of the psychophysiological literature, Warburton (1979b) concluded that lower levels of electrocortical arousal were correlated with impaired information processing, and subjects had more lapses in attention as electrocortical arousal decreased. Vigilance decrements occur as a result of increased occurrence of these lapses in attention and so we would expect a greater vigilance decrement in extraverts. This prediction has been supported by tests of groups of introverts, extraverts and normals on attentional tasks; as a group, introverts performed best and extraverts performed worst (Davies and Hockey, 1966).

From this evidence it is obvious that in order to perform efficiently, extraverts need a drug which will maintain electrocortical arousal. Nicotine increases electrocortical arousal and produces improvements in attentional performance which are correlated with increased cortical arousal (Warburton and Wesnes, 1979). Thus cigarettes could be used to obtain nicotine to help the extraverts in a vigilance task.

When we examined smoking behaviour as a function of extraversion, there was a strong positive correlation between extraversion and smoke intake on the medium nicotine cigarette and small positive correlations with the low nicotine cigarette. These correlation coefficients give some support for the hypothesis that extraverts smoked the experimental cigarettes harder. The difference between the intake from the first cigarette of the session smoked at twenty minutes and the last cigarette taken at sixty minutes was calculated in order to test the prediction that extraverts smoked more at the end of a situation when they are bored, and have a greater need for nicotine to produce electrocortical arousal. There was evidence for this prediction: the association between extraversion and the smoking difference was significant for the intermediate delivery cigarette and the correlations for the other brands were in the same direction (Warburton and Wesnes, 1978).

In a previous study, Myrsten and others (1972) selected groups of subjects on the basis of a questionnaire which asked about the situations in which smokers felt a need to smoke. One group said that they smoked to calm themselves, "high arousal" smokers, while the second group smoked when bored, "low arousal" smokers. Low arousal smokers performed better in boring situations when they were allowed to smoke. In our study we found that the effect of smoking on subjects in the vigilance situation in comparison with the no smoking condition depended on their position on the constitutional extraversion-introversion continuum with the most dramatic effects on the performance of extraverts. Thus the subjects adjusted their dose of nicotine by smoking, extraverts smoked more intensely in the session, and especially at the end of a session when their electrocortical arousal would be lowest on the average. This data gives evidence for an extraversion by situation interaction in the control of self-medication by smoking behaviour.

(4) Neuroticism and Smoking Behaviour in a Vigilance Situation

Correlations were made between the neuroticism scores and the smoke intake from the test cigarettes. There was some evidence that the more neurotic subjects smoked more than the more stable subjects on the first cigarette. However, a more interesting association was found between neuroticism and the change in smoking pattern over the session; a positive correlation was found between neuroticism and the difference in intake between the first and last cigarette for both the low nicotine cigarette and the high nicotine cigarette, indicating that the more neurotic subjects smoke more intensely at the beginning of the session that at the end of the test. This result provides further evidence that smoking behaviour is the outcome of the interaction of the situation and the individual's constitution. Anxiety arises in situations of uncertainty when a person is subjected to an unpredictable pattern of stimuli or is faced with uncertainty about which response to choose, or both (Warburton, 1979c) and this effect will be greater in the more neurotic subjects in our test situation. Consequently, we can hypothesise that the more neurotic subjects found the test situation particularly stressful, and so they smoked more intensely because they have a need for some sedative chemical from the cigarette in order to cope with the experimental test. This result is consistent with the trend in the data of Ashton and Watson (1970) that stress increased smoking intensity.

In agreement with the notion of sedative smoking Matarazzo and Saslow's (1960) survey showed clearly that smokers had higher anxiety scores than non-smokers and a greater number of sings of psychological tension were found in heavy smokers than moderate and light smokers (Lawton and Phillips, 1956). In our survey of smokers (Warburton and Wesnes, 1978) we gave the Smoking Motives Questionnaire (Russell and co-workers, 1974) and it was clear that subjects who had high scores on neuroticism were <u>less</u> likely to be "stimulation" smokers, and were more clearly "sedative" smokers. Russell and others (1974) failed to find a sedative factor in their factorial analysis of smoking motives, but this factor had appeared in previous analyses (e.g. McKennell, 1970; Frith, 1971). If we examine the items on Russell and co-workers' (1974) questionnaire for his general population sample, his clinic sample and our student population, two of the most frequently answered items were smoking when worried and smoking when angry. The percentage of subjects saying "Yes" to these questions were 74% of the general, 93% of clinic and 88% of the student population. The hypothesis of sedative smoking by neurotic subjects was tested, subdividing our group into three classes on the basis of their replies to the two questions about "smoking when worried" and "smoking when angry" (Warburton and Wesnes, 1978). The subdivisions were a "high sedative" group, an "intermediate sedative" group and a "low sedative" group. When the neuroticism scores for these subjects in each group were compared, it was found that the high sedative and low sedative groups differed significantly, which is consistent with the prediction that subjects scoring high on neuroticism were more likely to smoke when worried or angry i.e. "under stress", than low neuroticism subjects.

Profiles of physicians showed that cigarette smokers had significantly higher levels of anxiety and anger than non-smokers, and that it was the physician's awareness of nervous tension which lead to increased use of cigarettes. Similarly, a survey of executives revealed that heavy smoking (more than 20 a day) was more common in patients that were judged by the examining doctor to be under excessive stress; interestingly one of the main reasons given by these patients for smoking was the tranquillizing effect of cigarettes (Pincherle and Williamson, 1971).

(5)   Smoking Behaviour During Examination Stress

In a recent study, 48 first year undergraduates filled in a detailed diary on their smoking habits during examination week, and then again 6 weeks later after the examination results had come out. This design enabled us to compare the student's smoking behaviour in a high stress and a low stress period of their lives.

The number of cigarettes smoked during and after the exams are summarised in Table 1. The data provides an excellent example of a group of people adjusting their cigarette intake according to their situation. Firstly if we look at the amount of smoking in the morning, the mean number smoked in the non-examination period is 2.2 cigarettes smoked, while the mean number during the examination period is 3.07 - an increase in the same group of almost 40%. A comparison by t-test between the scores for the two periods yielded a t of 2.2, indicating a difference which is significant beyond the 0.05 level. The mean number of cigarettes smoked during the morning before an afternoon examination was 3.95 - an increase of 80% over the average number for mornings during the non-examination period, and an increase of 29% over the mean morning consumption over the examination period as a whole. Testing the comparison between morning before an examination and the mean for post-examination mornings gave a t value of 4.45 - significant beyond the 0.0001 level.

TABLE 1   Number of Cigarettes Smoked During Examination Period

	Time period	Mean number of cigarettes smoked
EXAMINATION PERIOD	Evening before morning examination	6.6
	Morning before afternoon examination	3.95
	Evening before day off	7.78
	Mean for all mornings during period	3.07
	Mean for all afternoons during period	4.15
	Mean for all evenings during period	7.1
NON-EXAMINATION PERIOD	Mean for all mornings	2.2
	Mean for all afternoons	3.5
	Mean for all evenings	5.97

From the cigarette totals for the afternoons and evenings it was obvious that subjects smoked significantly more cigarettes at all times during the examination period than six weeks later. The mean number of cigarettes smoked during the afternoons of the non-examination period was 3.5, the mean for the exam period was 4.15 ($t = 1.63$; $p < 0.1$). The mean number smoked during the evening for the non-examination period was 5.97 and for the examination period the mean number was 7.1, an increase significant at the 0.005 level ($t = 2.82$). The individual data are highly consistent with this pattern; only two of the fifty subjects' data contradicted the trend for mornings, 8 for afternoons and 6 for evenings.

The mean number of cigarettes smoked on an evening before an examination (6.6), was lower than that for an evening before a day off during the examination period, which was 7.78, but both figures are still higher than the mean for evenings in the non-examination period which was 5.9 ($t = 1.58$; $p < 0.1$) for the evening before an examination compared to non-examination evenings ($t = 4.57$, $p < 0.0005$) for evening before day off compared to evenings in non-examination period. Perhaps this represented relaxation smoking after high stress.

Subjects gave a subjective indication of strength and depth of inhalation which followed exactly the same pattern as the data for number of cigarettes smoked i.e., highly significant increases in strength and depth of inhalation during the examinations with respect to the post-examination period. Once again the individual data are highly consistent. Depth and strength of inhalation for the evening before a morning examination was significantly higher than the mean for an evening prior to a free day (for strength $t = 4.88$, $p < 0.0001$; and for depth $t = 5.65$, $p < 0.0001$). The same pattern of greater inhalation during the morning before an afternoon examination compared with the mean for mornings of the non-examation period (for strength $t = 8.4$, $p < 0.00001$; for depth $t = 9.5$, $p < 0.00001$). Similarly, a

comparison of the evening before a free day within the examination
period with the mean for evenings in the non-examination period gave
significant differences for strength (t = 3.4, p< 0.001) and for depth
(t = 3.72, p< 0.001).

Comparing means for mornings in the examination and non-examination
periods, for strength we obtained a t of 2.3 (p < 0.05), whilst for
depth t = 3.08 (p< 0.005). The same comparison performed for afternoons gives for strength a t of 1.21 (non-significant trend) and for
depth a t of 2.82 (p< 0.005). The same comparison between evenings in
the examination and non-examination periods, for strength gives a t
of 2.98 (p< 0.005) and for depth a t of 2.95 (p< 0.005).

Thus the undergraduate students who took part in this study increased
the number of cigarettes they smoked quite dramatically when faced by
the period of examinations and the concomitant stress. They also felt
that they were inhaling more strongly and deeply than during the non-
examination period. It can be assumed that the two questionnaires were
independent, since the first one was completed and returned to us six
weeks before the second, and so the subjects did not have access to
the examination information when answering the second questionnaire.

These data demonstrate that smoking behaviour changes in stressful situations. Smokers use more cigarettes, they smoke them more intensely
and inhale the smoke more deeply. The more neurotic subjects (those
susceptible to stress) show the most dramatic effects. The question
arises whether the smoker's reliance on cigarettes to cope with stress
is justified or not. Accordingly we have analysed performance incre-
ments as a function of neuroticism, and found that there was a direct
association between the degree of neuroticism and the amount of performance improvement (Warburton and Wesnes, 1978). These results were
consistent with data obtained by Kucek (1975) in an experiment where
subjects were tested under conditions of information overload in
which they were required to track a target and do mental arithmetic.
A comparison of neurotic smokers allowed to smoke and neurotic subjects not smoking showed that smoking had a beneficial effect on the
performance of neurotic subjects allowed to smoke. Nicotine is the
most likely constituent of cigarettes for producing this improvement,
and another vigilance study tested nicotine tablets with doses similar to those estimated from butt analyses in the previous study. For
both females and males the improvement scores were directly correlated with neuroticism (Warburton and Wesnes, 1978).

This significant association with neuroticism gives strong evidence
for the hypothesis that nicotine is the ingredient of cigarettes which
is important in the effects of smoking on vigilance performance of
neurotics and it suggests that nicotine is having some sedative effect
which is beneficial especially for the more neurotic subjects in the
test situation. This finding was tested in another way by subdividing
the smoker subjects into a 'high' neuroticism group and a 'low' neuroticism group about the mean neuroticism score. The difference scores
for the subjects in each group were compared, and it was found that
there was a significantly greater effect of the nicotine on the high
neurotic group (Warburton and Wesnes, 1978). Clearly the smoker's
faith in the cigarette was not misplaced!

Our hypothesis to explain the finding with extraverts was phrased in terms of the beneficial action of nicotine on attentional pathways in the central nervous system, but the pattern of results with the neurotic favours the notion that nicotine is improving performance by reducing anxiety. At first sight this sedative action seems to be incompatible with the attention hypothesis, but there is a parsimonious way of resolving this apparent paradox.

Sarason (1972) has published a number of studies which suggest that the highly anxious individual is preoccupied with his inadequacies and his ability to cope with the problem and fear of failure. These preoccupations are bound to have a detrimental effect on attentiveness to external cues. In our situation the decreased attention will be re-flected in poorer vigilance performance initially until the subject is reassured by the simplicity of the task. In support of this notion there appears to be a relationship between the initial performance measured in terms of a probability of a hit and neuroticism (which indicates that lower hit rates are associated with higher degrees of neuroticism). If the neurotic is uncertain about his ability to re-spond appropriately, then these preoccupations will act as distracting stimuli that will interfere with the main task; there is considerable evidence to show that a high incidence of day-dreaming and phantasis-ing is correlated with poor vigilance performance (Warburton, 1979b).

An improvement of performance would be expected if these distracting preoccupations could be reduced. Warburton (1979b) has hypothesised that an increase in the activity of the cholinergic pathways ascend-ing to the cortex will result in improved information processing. The electrocortical arousal produced by nicotine provides evidence that these pathways are being activated by this drug. It follows from this finding that nicotine should reduce the effect of distracting stimuli on performance and the enhanced performance of subjects tested on the Stroop test after nicotine supports this idea (Wesnes and Warburton, 1978). It seems reasonable to conclude that nicotine will enable the distracting preoccupation with failure to be filtered out in a similar fashion and performance will improve. Subjects scoring highly on neuroticism will be more preoccupied with failure and so nicotine will restore their performance to the same level as more stable subjects by enhanced filtering of these distracting stimuli.

   (D) CONCLUDING COMMENTS

The data in the preceding sections give strong evidence that some ci-garette smoking can be regarded as self-medication, especially for certain groups. It seems that, depending on the situation, smokers will adjust their smoking behaviour in terms of number of cigarettes smoked, intensity of smoking and depth of inhalation. Deprivation of cigarettes results in marked abstinence symptoms which also depend on the situation, and so relapse occurs in these contexts.

In the previous sections we have discussed the "extravert" or "stimu-lations" smoker and the "neurotic" or "sedative" smoker as if they were homogenous groups who self-medicated in the same fashion. How-ever, there are probably differences in smoking behaviour as a func-tion of the intensity of the individual-situation interaction, its duration and more probably its density (the product of intensity and duration). Thus an extravert will smoke less in brief, slightly boring tasks than a prolonged tedious situation, but conceivably the same smoking behaviour could occur during a brief, very boring experience and a long, but moderately interesting task. In other cases smoking may not even be initiated until the intensity, duration or density of the interaction reaches a critical level. Clearly starting a cigarette and the pattern of smoking behaviour depends on the individual-situation interaction. An important extension of these concepts can be made on the basis of the observation that some smokers smoke in anticipation of a future need while they are still coping because either the situation has not occurred or the critical stress level has not been reached. Here the smoking behaviour is very clearly a response to the individual's interpretation of the situation, i.e. the person-situation interaction, rather than the objective characteristics of the situation. The person has learned that self-medication by smoking will avoid the undesired consequences of the situation and so the anticipatory smoking can be seen as a rational coping strategy on the basis of his past experience.

ACKNOWLEDGEMENTS

We are grateful to Carreras-Rothmans Ltd., The Medical Research Council and the Tobacco Research Council for financial support of the research discussed in this paper.

REFERENCES

Adams, P. I. (1978). The influence of cigarette smoke yields on smoking habits. In R. E. Thornton (Ed.), Smoking Behaviour: Physiological and Psychological Influences. Churchill Livingstone, Edinburgh.

Ashton, H., and D. W. Watson (1970). Puffing frequency and nicotine intake in cigarette smokers. Brit. Med. J., 3, 679-681.

Cherry, N., and K. Kiernan (1976). Personality scores and smoking behaviour. Brit. J. Prev. Soc. Med., 30, 123-131.

Cherry, N., and K. Kiernan (1978). A longitudinal study of smoking and personality. In R. E. Thornton (Ed.), Smoking Behaviour: Physiological and Psychological Influences. Churchill Livingstone, Edinburgh.

Davies, D. R., and G. R. J. Hockey (1966). The effect of noise and doubling the signal frequency on individual differences in visual vigilance performance. Brit. J. Psychol., 57, 381-389.

Dunnell, K., and A. Cartwright (1972). Medicine Takers, Prescribers and Hoarders. Routledge & Kegan Paul, London.

Endler, N. A., and D. Magnussen (1976). Interactional Psychology and Personality. Hemisphere Publ. Corp., Washington D.C.

Eysenck, H. J. (1963). Personality and cigarette smoking. Life Sci., 3, 777-792.

Eysenck, H. J., and S. B. G. Eysenck (1964). Manual of the Eysenck Personality Inventory. University of London Press, London.

Eysenck, H. J., M. Tarrant, M. Woolf, and L. England (1960). Smoking and personality. Brit. Med. J., 2, 1456-1460.

Frankenhaeuser, M., A. L. Myrsten, B. Post, and G. Johansson (1971). Behavioural and physiological effects of cigarette smoking in a monotonous situation. Psychopharmacologia, 22, 1-7.

Frith, C. D. (1971). Smoking behaviour and its relation to the smoker' immediate experience. Brit. J. Soc. Clin. Psychol., 10, 73-78.

Gale, A., M. Coles, P. Kline, and V. Penfold (1971). Extraversion-introversion and the E.E.G.: basal and response measures during habituation of the orienting response. Brit. J. Psychol., 62, 533-542.

Guilford, J. S. (1966). Factors related to successful abstinence from smoking. American Institutes for Research, Pittsburgh.

Heimstra, N. W., N. R. Bancroft, and A. R. Dekock (1967). Effects of smoking on sustained performance in a simulated driving test. Ann. N.Y. Acad. Sci., 142, 295-306.

Janke, W., G. Debus, and N. Longo (1979). Differential psychopharmacology of tranquilizing and sedating drugs. Mod. Probl. Pharmaco-Psychiat., 14, 13-98.

Knott, V., P. Venables (1977). EEG alpha correlates of non-smokers, smokers, smoking and smoking deprivation. Psychophysiology, 14, 150-156.

Kucek, P. (1975). Effect of smoking on performance under load. Studia Psychologica, 17, 204-212.

Lawton, M. P., P. W. Phillips (1956). The relationship between excessive cigarette smoking and psychological tension. Am. J. Med. Sci., 232, 397-402.

Lee, P. N. (1979). Has the mortality of male doctors improved with the reductions in their cigarette smoking? Brit. Med. J., 2, 1538-1540.

Marlatt, G. A. (1979). A cognitive-behavioural model of the relapse process. In N. A. Krasnegor (Ed.), Behavioral Analysis and Treatment of Substance Abuse. National Institute on Drug Abuse, Washington D.C.

Matarazzo, J. D., and G. Saslow (1960). Psychological and related characteristics of smokers and non-smokers. Psychol. Bull., 57, 493-513.

Mausner, J. S. (1970). Cigarette smoking among patients with respiratory disease. Am. Rev. Respir. Dis., 102, 704.

McKennell, A. C. (1970). Smoking motivation factors. Brit. J. Soc. Clin. Psychol., 9, 8-22.

Meares, R., J. Grimwade, M. Bickley, and C. Wood (1971). Smoking and neuroticism. Lancet, 2, 770.

Myrsten, A.-L., B. Post, M. Frankenhaeuser, and G. Johansson (1972). Changes in behavioural and physiological activation induced by cigarette smoking in habitual smokers. Psychopharmacologia, 27, 305-322.

Nesbitt, P. D. (1973). Smoking, physiological arousal, and emotional response. J. Pers. Soc. Psychol., 25, 137-145.

Parry, H. J., M. B. Balter, G. D. Mellinger, P. H. Gisin, and D. I. Manheimer (1973). National patterns of psychotherapeutic drug use. Arch. Gen. Psychiat., 28, 769-784.

Pincherle, G., and J. Williamson (1972). Smoking and neuroticism. Lancet, 2, 981.

Rae, G. (1975). Extraversion, neuroticism, and cigarette smoking. Brit. J. Soc. Clin. Psychol., 14, 429-430.

Rotter, J. B. (1966). Generalized expectancies for internal versus external control of reinforcement. Psychol. Monogr., 80, Whole Number 609.

Russell, M. A. H., J. Peto, and U. A. Patel (1974). The classification of smoking by factorial structure of motives. J. Roy. Stat. Soc., A 137, 313-333.

Sarason, I. G. (1972). Anxiety and self-preoccupation. In I. G. Sarason, and C. Spielberger (Eds.), Stress and Anxiety. Wiley, New York. pp. 27-44.

Schachter, S. (1978). Pharmacological and psychological determinants of smoking. In R. E. Thornton (Ed.), Smoking Behaviour: Physiological and Psychological Influences. Churchill Livingstone, Edinburgh.

Schalling, D. (1977). The trait-situation interaction and the physiological correlates of behavior. In D. Magnussen, and N. S. Endler (Eds.), Personality at the Crossroads: Current Issues in Interactional Psychology. Lawrence Erlbaum Assoc. (John Wiley), Hillsdale, N.J.

Schechter, M. D., and M. J. Rand (1974). Effect of acute deprivation of smoking on aggression and hostility. Psychopharmacologia, 35, 19.

Shiffman, S. M. (1979a). The tobacco-withdrawal syndrome. In N. A. Krasnegor (Ed.), Cigarette Smoking as a Dependence Process. National Institute on Drug Abuse Monograph, Washington D.C.

Shiffman, S. M. (1979b). Analysis of relapse episodes following smoking cessation. Paper presented at the Fourth World Conference on Smoking and Health.

Shiffman, S. M., and M. E. Jarvik (1976). Smoking withdrawal symptoms in two weeks of abstinence. Psychopharmacology, 50, 35-39.

Thomas, C. B. (1973). The relationship of smoking and habits of nervous tension. In W. L. Dunn (Ed.), Smoking Behaviour: Motives and Incentives. Winston and Sons, Washington D.C.

Warburton, D. M. (1975). Brain, Drugs and Behaviour. Wiley, London.

Warburton, D. M. (1978). Internal pollution. J. Biosoc. Sci., 10, 309-319.

Warburton, D. M. (1979a). Self-medication. In D. J. Oborne, M. M. Gruneberg, and J. R. Eiser (Eds.), Research in Psychology and Medicine, Vol. 2. Academic Press, London.

Warburton, D. M. (1979b). Neurochemical basis of consciousness. In K. Brown, and S. J. Cooper (Eds.), Chemical Influences on Behaviour. Acadmic Press, London.

Warburton, D. M. (1979c). Physiological aspects of anxiety and schizophrenia. In V. J. Hamilton, and D. M. Warburton (Eds.), Stress and Cognition. Wiley, London.

Warburton, D. M. (1981). Neurochemical bases of behaviour. Brit. Med. Bull., 37, 121-125.

Warburton, D. M., and K. Wesnes (1978). Individual differences in smoking and attentional performance. In R. E. Thornton (Ed.), Smoking Behaviour: Physiological and Psychological Influences. Churchill Livingstone, Edinburgh.

Warburton, D. M., and K. Wesnes (1979). The role of electrocortical arousal in the smoking habit. In A. Rémond, and C. Izard (Eds.), The effects of nicotine. Elsevier, Amsterdam.

Waters, W. E. (1971). Smoking and neuroticism. Brit. J. Prev.Soc. Med., 25, 162-164.

Wesnes, K., and D. M. Warburton (1978). The effects of cigarette smoking and nicotine tablets upon human attention. In R. E. Thornton (Ed.), Smoking Behaviour: Physiological and Psychological Influences. Churchill Livingstone, Edinburgh.

PHARMACOPSYCHOLOGICAL EXPERIMENTS WITH HEXOBARBITONE

Ewald-Heinz Strauß

ABSTRACT

This investigation examined the general validity of Lienert's 'regression of intelligence' hypothesis. Furthermore, we tested the influence of personality traits (extraversion vs. introversion, and high vs. low neuroticism) as moderating variables of drug effects. One hundred subjects in a double-blind design (0.4 g hexobarbitone vs. placebo) were given five achievement tests and three questionnaires in a balanced order. Evidence which could be used to support the regression hypothesis was not found. In the achievement tests, only a few significant differences were found between the extreme groups. The dimension of neuroticism was a better determinant of the drug effect experienced by the subjects than was the dimension of extraversion-introversion. The data were discussed critically in connection with Eysenck's drug postulate and with the concept of activation.
1. The pharmacology of the drug;
2. The influence of hexobarbitone on intellectual performance capability
   - a contribution to the testing of the hypothesis of regression of intelligence;
3. Personality traits as moderating variables of the drug effect.

KEYWORDS

Regression hypothesis of intelligence; drug postulate; personality traits; drug effects and personality traits; neuroticism; extraversion/introversion; drug effects and level of activation.

1. INTRODUCTION

Hexobarbitone (Evipan) is the N-methyl-cyclohexenylmethyl-barbitone. The drug is manufactured as sodium salt, and is classified as a sedative. The average hypnotic dose ranges from .25 to .50 g and the letal dose is 11 g. Hexobarbitone is quickly absorbed (in about 30 minutes) and is metabolized in the liver. Half of the dose has left the plasma after 5 hours and after 24 hours, 95% of the given dose has been eliminated.

The explanation for the effect of the barbiturate is disputed. Various possible causes have been considered, one of them being the impairment of metabolic processes by inhibition of phosphorylation. The individual regions of the central nervous system react with differing degrees of sensitivity to barbiturate concentrations. As suggested by Hauschild (1956), the phylogenetically youngest zones are paralysed while other, older regions (e.g. medulla oblongata) have scarcely been touched. The effect of the drug on the cortex and the thalamus is reversible in low dosage. It leads to drowsiness and eventual inhibition of convulsions. Breathing and circulation remain unaffected. When the dosage is increased paralysis takes place in the following order: cerebrum, spinal cord, medulla oblongata .

Each subject received a dose of .40 g hexobarbitone, i.e. we restricted ourselves to the average dosage of the hypnotic drug. Subsequently most of the subjects experienced impairment (symptoms: tiredness, dizziness, feeling "as if you had drunk too much alcohol"). The applications of the drug followed the double-blind method. The reasons for using the drug are as follows:
(1) LSD, a very powerful drug is banned in the GDR and was therefore not available for our experiments. In addition there are ethical questions regarding experiments which use LSD, questions which have been raised since 1964 (the year of Lienert's publication).
(2) The effect of barbiturates on cortical functions is reversible, whereas tranquilizers and other neuropsychopharmacological drugs, which were more often used at that time, mainly affect other regions of the CNS.
(3) Hexobarbitone is the least toxic of all the barbiturates (principle of "nil nocere").

The regression hypothesis of intelligence as put forward by Lienert (1964) consists of two main statements:
(1) Pharmacological impairment results in a quantitative decrease of intellectual functions.
(2) Similarly, a qualitative change in the structural frame of intelligence will be noticed in the sense of regression to an ontogenetically earlier stage of development of intelligence.
    If we assume the validity of the regression hypothesis we should expect, with our conditions, to obtain the following results: 1. Increase of the mean intercorrelations of tests, 2. Increase of the loadings on the first factor and thus a decrease of the loadings on the specific factors, 3. Increase of the mean communalities, and 4. Decrease rather than increase of the number of factors.

The object of our investigation was to find out whether the hypothesis of regression is of general validity (aspect of general pharmacopsychology) and to which extent the effect of a psychotropic drug (hexobarbitone) would depend on the specific characteristics of the subject's personality (aspect of differential pharmacopsychology).

2. METHOD

Sixty minutes after having received .40 g hexobarbitone (or placebo) 100 students were given five achievement tests: the achievement test system ("Leistungs-Prüfsystem", LPS, Horn) - German version of Thurstone's primary mental ability test, the Cattell-figure test (scale 3), d2-concentration-test ("d2-Test", Brickenkamp), the concentration-achievement-test ("Konzentrations-Leistungstest", KLT, Düker and Lienert), and a stimulus-response experiment for measuring perceptual speed. These achievement tests were used in combination with three questionnaires: the MPI (Eysenck), the ENR (Brengelmann), and a scale for the assessment of subjective drug effects (Janke). The whole battery of tests had to be carried out within 180 minutes. With regard to the main conditions, the experimental set-up was balanced. The data obtained were analysed by correlation and factor analysis, transformation analysis, calculation of similarities between the two different matrices, analysis of constitution, and non-parametric methods.

3. RESULTS

3.1 Changes of Factorial Structure

Even the use of hexobarbitone produces a distinct change (in comparison to the placebo group) in the factorial structure (index of similarity S = .844). As expected, this change was less pronounced than the change brought about by LSD in Lienert's experiment. One interesting fact, however, is that though there were distinct structural changes, we observed only a few significant differences in the test results. Pharmacological influence was most significant with respect to impairment of the reasoning factor. Further significant changes were noted in those specific variables which measure the quality of achievement: the rate of errors in the concentration-test (KLT) as well as the number of mistakes in the LPS (Horn) and in the d2-test (Brickenkamp). The considerable deviation in the factorial structure (see above) observed in several subtests of our battery was confirmed by corresponding similarity coefficients. However, there was no significant change in general mental ability (S = .95).

Factor

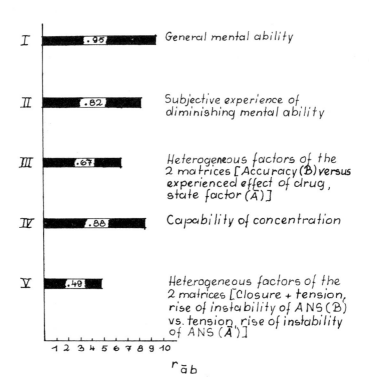

Fig. 1.   Similarities of the 5 factors of the battery
           of tests used (comparison of the matrices after
           the administration of placebo and hexobarbitone,
           calculations of similarities as done by Fischer
           and Roppert, 1964).

Figure 1 presents the similarities of the two matrices (hexobarbitone
versus placebo) of the other four factors we found. Only the factors
II (subjective experience of diminishing mental capability) and IV
(capability of concentration) still showed satisfying similarities
between the two factor matrices in question.

In answering our initial question, we may state that in our experiment
the essential data supporting the regression hypothesis could not be
found. It must be emphasized that we did not find evidence of a simultaneous overlap (Kalveram), which is a well-known source of error.

3.2 Differential Drug Effects

In accord with the subject of this book some of the results of the
experiment should now be described from a differential aspect.

3.2.1 The relation between test achievement and the neuroticism factor.
From a total of 100 subjects we selected 15 subjects scoring low in
neuroticism (n-group). We used the standardised ratings of the MPI or
the Brengelmann questionnaire (T-scale, M = 50 ± 10 z). The sample was
balanced in accordance with most important criteria of our experiment.
For the parallel group we used 20 subjects scoring high in neuroticism
(N-group). The same criteria were used for their selection.

The findings were: Only 2 of the 15 results of the achievement data
examined could be statistically verified (Kullback test):
(1) Group N/n: Test variable word-fluency in the LPS (Horn):
    2↑-Test: 19.246, df = 5, p < 1 %.
    The result indicates that subjects scoring low in neuroticism are
    significantly worse at handling exercises which demand word-fluency.
(2) Group N/n: Test variable number of errors in the d2-test:
    Chi² = 4.536, df = 1, p < 5 %.
    The result shows that subjects scoring low in neuroticism improve
    significantly less often when working under the effect of hexobar-
    bitone than those subjects scoring high in neuroticism. They are,
    therefore, liable to make fewer mistakes in short-term concentra-
    tion tests.

Discussion: We are not aware of any special investigations with the
help of drugs into the word-fluency of corresponding groups of subjects.
Janke's table (1965) for the effect of tranquilizers, neuroleptics, and
sedatives in very small dosages does not seem applicable to the conditions of our experiment. The administration of 400 mg hexobarbitone is
probably a more serious matter in comparison with the very low dosages
of the afore-mentioned drugs (fluphenazine 1 mg, promazine 25-75 mg)
in Janke's experiment. We should like to see a similar table incor-
porating the more common drugs and dosages as well as personality and
achievement variables. Generalisations about the effects of similar,
but not specifically tested drugs, have a high degree of uncertainty,
however, even with regard to changes in subjective and objective
achievement parameters (Strauß, 1979). The inclusion of psychophysiological parameters, however, seems to be useful for an exact characteri-
sation of work loading.

As for our second result (subjects scoring high in neuroticism make
fewer mistakes in a short-term test of concentration (d2-test of
Brickenkamp) than those scoring low in neuroticism (n-group)) we would,
like Janke (1964), have expected a worsening of achievement. He found
definitely worse results for unstable subjects after the administration
of .4 g heptabarbital (Medomin) in the error quotient of the KLT (long-
term concentration test of Düker and Lienert). Our short-term concentration test demanded relatively low psychical strain, however, and
there was no additional emotional loading with noise. Subjects scoring
high in neuroticism showed, therefore, a tendency towards emotional
stabilisation and a slightly increased readiness to perform. The
n-group, on the other hand, tended towards emotional lability, a paradoxical state of arousal which found expression in a higher error
quota in the d2-test.

Janke's discovery seems to be confirmed in as far as the neuroticism
variable is manifest predominately in emotional reactions (and motor
achievements). We could only verify few data statistically in the
achievement tests we conducted.

3.2.2 The influence of extraversion/introversion on achievement data.
We followed a similar procedure to that described in section 3.2.1
and chose, on the basis of the ENR-Brengelmann questionnaire and the
MPI, 20 subjects scoring high in extraversion (E-group) and 20 subjects
scoring low in extraversion (I-group) from our total of 100 subjects.
The groups were well balanced.

Results: Only 2 results out of the 15 achievement variables that we
looked at from our battery (section 2) proved to be significant.
(1) Group E/I: Number of errors (display)
      χ^2-Test: χ^2 = 19.246, df = 5, p < 1 %.
      The result means that extraverts show a considerably bigger drop
      in achievement than introverts for the same short-term demands on
      perception (perceptual speed, display). This fall off in achieve-
      ment is manifest in the much higher number of mistakes made.
      (The subjects were asked to judge the number of times a given
      figure (e.g. 7.189) appeared in front of them - between 3 and
      12 frames were lit up at any one time. They were seated 3.5 m
      away from the display. The subjects noted the number of frames
      containing the figure in question and each subject stopped the
      electric clock next to him.)
(2) Group E/I: Error quotient in the KLT (Düker and Lienert)
      χ^2-score = 9.957, df = 4, p < 5 %.
      The result shows that introverts are significantly more impaired
      than extraverts by the use of hexobarbitone as regards high
      achievement in long-term demands on their capacity for concentra-
      tion. If we consider the absolute scores of I and E subjects, we
      observe interesting relationships (see section 3.2.4.2 for a com-
      parison with the subjects' subjective assessment of impairment).

Discussion: We are not aware of similar experiments with a display
relating to the first result. Since Eysenck (1957, 1963) did not use
selected extreme groups for his drug postulate we looked forward to
our result with great interest. Our result seems to fit the drug
postulate very well. Since the extraverts produced significantly more
mistakes, it was possible to conclude that they were nearer to the
sedation threshold and made, therefore, more mistakes. Although our
results agreed with those of Eysenck's drug postulate, we could not
see further direct evidence for it. Our reasons are as follows:

- The conditions for the experiments were not systematically varied
  as regards the degree of additional emotional loading either by
  Eysenck or by us. We lack the equivalent of the table by Janke
  (see section 3.2.1) for the relationship extraversion-introversion.
  The analysis of systematic variations in conditions (changes in
  dosage, additional emotional loading, etc.) could produce interesting
  evidence as to the validity and limits of the drug postulate.

- We lack systematic examinations of this problem, but our everyday
  experience does not indicate that "typically" extraverted and predominately less "neurotic" subjects (i.e. stable in A.N.S.) are
  more impaired by the administration of a sedative drug than introverted subjects. Our result could be an indication of this relationship but it needs closer examination with larger groups and
  variations in conditions with this aim in mind.

- According to Legewie (1968, p. 62) the relationship between the
  sedation threshold and N is more certain than the relationship with

extraversion. For this the examination of extreme groups would be
less favourable than that of subjects scoring high in neuroticism.
The procedural difficulties in determining the sedation threshold
are certainly a further factor in explaining the divergent results
which Legewie found. A solution to this problem should be possible
with the help of partial correlations which allow E and N to be
controlled simultaneously.
Finally, our result should be related to the activation concept.
We relied on Legewie's work (1968, p. 66 ff). He devised a table
showing the effect of drugs in relation to the level of activation
and type of achievement (Yerkes-Dodson's law). If we assume that
in contrast to the very strenuous KLT, the demands of the display
only provide an average degree of complexity, then subjects with a
high level of activation (introverted according to Eysenck) should
benefit from a sedative or hypnotic drug with regard to their capacity for achievement. Subjects scoring high in extraversion, on the
other hand, bordering on the sedation threshold and with a lower
level of activation, feel impaired by such drugs. Our result is
compatible with this concept.

Let us now relate our second result (concerning the error quotient of
the KLT of Düker and Lienert) to the activation concept. If we accept
the idea that the lengthy KLT provides a high degree of complexity,
extraverts (with a tendency to a low level of activation) should benefit somewhat from sedatives, whereas subjects with a high level of
activation (inclined to introversion) benefit considerably. In fact,
we found the reverse to be the case. The introverts' achievements
were significantly worse in comparison to the extraverts. For long-
term demands on capacity for concentration - in relative contrast to
short-term achievement in alertness tested by the display - the sup-
position, which we described in section 3.2.4.2, for the comparison of
subjective and objective achievement data, would seem to work.

3.2.3 Regarding possible differences between the sexes in their
       capacity for intellectual achievement.
In order to answer this question we chose 21 male and 21 female subjects from a total of 100 subjects. These subjects had all worked in
mixed groups and therefore under the same conditions.

The results were as follows: Only total achievement on the LPS (Horn)
produced significant differences between male and female subjects
($2\uparrow = 15.844$, df = 8, p < 5 %). Achievements of male subjects were
more often found at extreme points. Male subjects were, therefore,
more often considerably impaired but they also showed an improvement
in achievement more often after the administration of the drug than
female subjects. Real differences in achievement, however, did not
occur. We found out, on the other hand, that there was a clear difference as regards their experience of the drug effect. Janke (1964) had
similar results for stable and unstable subjects amongst others. In
the following section we pursue this question.

3.2.4 Analysis of the results of the questionnaire to determine the
       subjects' situational condition after the administration of
       drug.
A synopsis of the results of the experiments with the questionnaire
(Janke, 1964) given to 100 subjects after administration of placebo

and drug will be given in this section. We will then take up the question
of possible differences between the subgroups (N, E, I) we described
previously. Above all, following Janke's investigations (1964), we might
expect that the differential effect of the drug relates predominately
to emotional events. Janke's questionnaire (now mostly superseded by
the so-called list of adjectives (EWL by Janke and Debus, 1978) has been
verified by pharmacopsychological experiments for the assessment of
emotional effects. The subjects were asked to rate themselves in regard
to each of 8 categories shown in diagrams 2 - 4 from 5 distinct grades.
Category 3 is given as an example. The 5 questions are:

    5   Is your capacity for concentration very good?
    4   Is your capacity for concentration good?
    3   Is your capacity for concentration average?
    2   Is your capacity for concentration slightly impaired?
    1   Is your capacity for concentration severely impaired?

3.2.4.1 The results of the analysis of Janke's questionnaire for the
         whole group.
This questionnaire was administered to 100 students and Abitur year
pupils of both sexes whose ages ranged from 18 to 33. The questionnaire
was completed one hour after subjects had taken the placebo or the
drug hexobarbitone (double-blind method) both at the beginning of the
battery of tests as well at the end of the experiment four hours later.
Each subject, therefore, answered the questionnaire four times.

For the category "psychic achievement capacity", 90 to 100 of the subjects rated their psychic capacity as average after the administration
of the placebo and did not fall back on possible excuses as is more
frequently the case in an achievement test. After 4 hours working through
the battery the degree of tiredness approached that reached after the
administration of the drug. The differences in this category are, however, still highly significant (placebo vs. drug group, p <.1 %).

Figure 2 depicts the mean ratings of the questionnaire (Janke) with
regard to the self-ratings of 100 subjects in the afore-mentioned
8 categories. As expected, it shows a clear fall in means in all categories after the placebo at the end of the experiment or under sedation after one hour and four hours. An exception was found in category 8 (mood). The biggest differences were found between the initial
and final evaluation one hour and four hours after the intake of the
placebo. The lowest evaluations of all were seen after four hours,
at the end of the battery of tests, to which therefore both physiological tiredness and pharmacological impairment contributed.

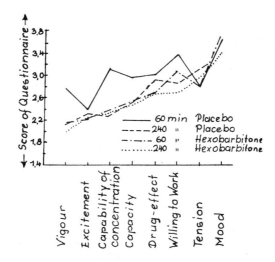

Fig. 2.   Mean ratings of Janke's questionnaire
          (Self-ratings of 100 subjects; comparison
          placebo vs. 0.4 g hexobarbitone, 60 and
          240 min p.a.)

Table 1 gives an overall view of the post-hoc statistics (2↑-Test,
Kullback) of the effects experienced by all 100 subjects.
The first column shows the results of group comparisons one hour after
the administration of the placebo or the drug at the start of the
battery of tests. The second column presents the results of the group
comparison 4 hours after dosage.

TABLE 1   Synopsis of the Post-hoc Statistics of
          Janke's Questionnaire (by 2↑-Test, Kullback)

Categories of questionnaire	1 Placebo/drug 60 min p.a. n = 100	2 Placebo/drug 240 min p.a. n = 100
1 Vigour	+ + +	(+)
2 Excitement	+ +	n.s.
3 Capacity for concentration	+ + +	n.s.
4 (psychic) capacity	+ + +	+ + +
5 Effect of drug (activating vs. sedating)	+ + +	+ +
6 Readiness to work	+	+ +
7 Tension	(+)	+
8 Mood	n.s.	n.s.

+++ = p < .1%;   ++ = p < 1%;   + = p < 5%;   (+) = p < 10%;

n.s.= not significant.

The statistical evaluation was carried out here as in the following
tables by Kullback's 2↑-Test. This method (similar to the chi² method)
proved very useful for our purposes.
After one hour we find in most categories highly significant to significant differences in (subjective) ratings after the administration of
placebo and hexobarbitone. In categories 2 (excitement) and 3 (capacity for concentration) the results show no further significant differences 4 hours after the administration of placebo or drug. A possible
explanation is that "physiological" tiredness from high work loads
cannot be increased further by the drug in the dosage used. It is also
possible that the diminishing effect of the drug is almost compensated
for by the so-called "reactive increase in tension" (Düker, 1963). We
consider the latter explanation to be more probable since Steinberg
(1961), for example, found that in competetive situations the effect
of sedatives can be fully compensated for by motivational or social
factors. What remains unanswered is why this trend could not be found
in other categories.

3.2.4.2 Questionnaire analysis for groups scoring high (E) and low
         (I/e) in extraversion.
In order to get a precise analysis of the relationships, we formed
4 extreme groups (each with 20 or 15 subjects) from a total of 100
subjects classified with high (E) or low extraversion (I/e) scores
and high (N) or low (n) scores in neuroticism. The tests used, as
already mentioned, were the MPI (Eysenck) and Brengelmann's questionnaire. In order to compare the results we made a linear transformation
to a uniform T-scale (T = 50 ± 10 z). Twenty subjects with 36 or more
E-points in the MPI or 24 or more E-points in the Brengelmann test
were classified as extraverts. Twenty subjects with 10 or fewer E-
points in the MPI or 13 or fewer points in the Brengelmann test were
called introverts.

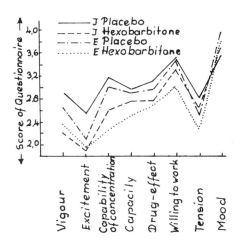

Fig. 3.   Mean ratings of Janke's questionnaire (self-
          ratings related to 8 categories of 20 extra-
          verts and introverts, resp. comparison placebo
          vs. 0.4 g hexobarbitone, 60 min p.a.)

Diagram 3 shows the mean ratings of Janke's questionnaire of 20 extraverts (E) and introverts (I) one hour after the administration of a placebo or drug. The corresponding values for the end of the experiment have been omitted here.

With the exception of category 8 (mood) the means of the other 7 categories were for the introverts somewhat higher than those of the extraverts, both after the administration of drug and placebo at the beginning and at the end of the battery of tests. At first glance, against expectations, apparently very large differences for the extra- and introverts after the administration of the drug could not be statistically verified on account of remarkable variance.   The statistical verification of other differences, however, was better than expected.

Table 2 gives a survey of the results of the significance testing of each 20 extra- and introverts (see diagram 3). In the third column are the results of the comparison of the differences in effect between extra- and introverts. What we did find interesting and in accord with Eysenck's drug postulate was the discovery that extraverts unlike introverts did not feel significantly impaired as far as the category vigour vs. tiredness was concerned.

TABLE 2   Survey of the Post-hoc Statistics of
Janke's Questionnaire (by $2\hat{\,}$-Test, Kullback)
Related to 20 Subjects Scoring High (E) vs.
Low (I) in Extraversion, see Fig. 3 and Table 1

Categories of questionnaire	Extraverts(E) placebo/drug 60 min p.a. n = 20	Introverts(I) placebo/drug 60 min p.a. n = 20	Difference between the self-ratings of E vs. I D_E/D_I
1 Vigour	n.s.	+	n.s.
2 Excitement	+	+ +	n.s.
3 Capacity for concentration	+	(+)	n.s.
4 (psychic) capacity	n.s.	n.s.	n.s.
5 Effect of drug (activating vs. sedating)	+ +	+	n.s.
6 Readiness to work	n.s.	n.s.	n.s.
7 Tension	(+)	n.s.	+
8 Mood	n.s.	n.s.	n.s.

++ = p < 1%;   + = p < 5%;   (+) = p < 10%; n.s. = not significant.

Alongside the very significant sedating effect in introverts (category 2) after the administration of sedatives, there is in column 3 only one significant result. This shows that there are significant differences between E and I concerning self-rating for the category tension. Extraverts tend then to score 2 (calm) and introverts tend to score 3 (neither tense nor calm). We will now undertake a comparison with achievement data using as an example the error quotient in the KLT (Düker and Lienert). It has proved to be a good indicator of capacity for concentration in many experiments done by Düker and his co-workers. The differences after the administration of the drug

as compared with the placebo prove to be statistically significant in
the error quotient of the KLT (p < 5 %) for extraverts and introverts,
in the sense that subjects scoring low in extraversion were more impaired. Within the group of introverts, the results showed an increase
in the error quotient of the KLT from 12.24 to 35.97 (p < .1 %). The
increase of the error quotient for the 20 extraverts from 18.62 to
23.32 could not be statistically verified. On the other hand, the extraverts (Table 2) felt in the category capacity for concentration
significantly impaired after the administration of the drug whereas
the introverts felt only symptomatically impaired. The following can
serve as a summary:

Error quotient (KLT) placebo drug (n = 20)   Category capacity for
                                             concentration

Difference I/E I 12.24   35.97 (p < .1 %)   self-rating p < 10 % (+)

  p < 5 % +   E 18.62   23.32 n.s.   self-rating p < 5 %   +

Consequently, extraverts may indeed feel more impaired than introverts
but objectively they make fewer mistakes. The reverse relationship is
true for the introverts. A correlation between the values of the error
quotients and the self-ratings of introverts revealed no significant
relationship. Achievement and self-rating differ therefore considerably.
One could follow Eysenck and accept that introverts with their precise
style of work and high level of arousal are very sensitive to the
disruption of their objective capacity for concentration. On the other
hand, an additional sedative has a less serious effect on the achievement of the extraverts with their strong inhibition potentials and who
from the beginning had a more easy-going approach to their work. But
perhaps here, too, there are other explanations, for example, the law
of initial value (Wilder) can be considered.

3.2.4.3 Questionnaire analysis for groups scoring high (N) and low
         (n) in neuroticism.
Finally there are still the results of subjects scoring high and low
in neuroticism to be described.

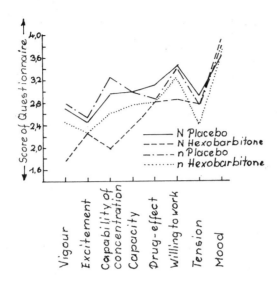

Fig. 4.   Mean ratings of Janke's questionnaire (self-
          rating related to 8 categories of 20 subjects
          scoring high (N) and 15 subjects scoring low
          (n) in neuroticism; comparison placebo vs.
          .4 g hexobarbitone, 60 min p.a.)

Figure 4 shows the mean ratings of Janke's questionnaire by 20 subjects
scoring high and 15 subjects scoring low in neuroticism one hour after
administration (p.a.) of a placebo or drug. The 20 subjects scoring
high in neuroticism (N) produce 28 and more points in the MPI and 27
and more points in the Brengelmann-test. People scoring low in neuroticism (n) achieve only 5 or fewer points in the MPI or 8 or fewer
points in the Brengelmann-test.

The particularly low scores of subjects with a high degree of neuroticism one hour after the administration of the drug is immediately
noticeable. Only in the category mood they do achieve higher scores
than under placebo. Perhaps this can be seen as an expression of
"emotional instability". Table 3 strengthens our impressions.

TABLE 3   Survey of the Post-hoc Statistics of
Janke's Questionnaire (by $2\uparrow$-Test, Kullback)
Related to 20 Subjects Scoring High (N) and
15 Subjects Scoring Low (n) in Neuroticism,
see Fig. 4 and Table 1

Categories of questionnaire	Ss scoring high in neuroticism (N) placebo/drug 60 min p.a. n = 20	Ss scoring low in neuroticism (n) placebo/drug 60 min p.a. n = 15	Differences between the self-ratings of N vs. n D_N/D_n
1 Vigour	+ + +	n.s.	n.s.
2 Excitement	+	+	(+)
3 Capacity for concentration	+ + +	(+)	n.s.
4 (psychic) capacity	+ + +	n.s.	+
5 Effect of drug (activating vs. sedating)	+ + +	n.s.	n.s.
6 Readiness to work	(+)	n.s.	n.s.
7 Tension	n.s.	+ +	n.s.
8 Mood	n.s.	n.s.	n.s.

+++ = $p < .1\%$;   ++ = $p < 1\%$;   + = $p < 5\%$;   (+) = $p < 10\%$;

n.s. = not significant

Here, too, the self-ratings within the two groups (N, n) were tested one hour after the administration of the placebo and .4 g hexobarbitone. In the third column are the results of the comparison of the differences in effect between drug and placebo in the two groups in question. In 4 out of 8 categories, the N-subjects experienced highly significant impairment. One result could only be confirmed at the 5 % level of significance. Quite obviously, such changes in the general level of activation affect the regulation of the A.N.S. (and in a narrower sense the dimension of neuroticism) in a very distinct way. Legewie (1968, p. 68 ff.) also mentioned this aspect in the field of achievement tests. We can accept that subjects with high I- and N-scores (as is considered typical for "true" neurotics) should have shown even clearer differences. We could not pursue this question, as only 3 out of 100 subjects showed this combination of I- and N-scores. The n- subjects proved to be much less susceptible to stress situations. Only in 3 categories did we calculate significant or symptomatic differences in comparison with the placebo experiment. Real differences between the groups of subjects in question exist only in the category 4 (psychic capacity).

The error quotient in the KLT rose by 10.91 to 16.73 for the N-subjects and from 11.32 to 17.28 for the n-subjects: The N-subjects felt themselves most significantly impaired by the sedative. In the achievement test. However, there is only a slight indication of this. Subjects scoring low in neuroticism were only symptomatically influenced; a more definite influence on their achievement could not be found.

3.2.4.4 An analysis of the questionnaire on the situational
         disposition (Janke) of the two sexes

We examined this question as to whether the two sexes may have completed the questionnaire differently in the sample of 21 subjects
described in section 3.2.3. In comparison with the aspect of achievement mentioned there, we found clearer differences in the answers   to
the questionnaire. These are given in Table 4.

TABLE 4 Differences between the Sexes in their Answers
         to the Questionnaire (Janke), $2 \uparrow$ -Test,
         n = each 21

Variable within the battery	$2 \uparrow$ -score	df	p	Interpretation
3 Capacity for concentration	8.799	3	<.05	female subjects feel significantly more impaired
5 (psychic) capacity	14.676	3	<.05	ditto
6 Effect of drug	8.368	4	<.10	female subjects symptomatically activated less often
43 Mood	10.830	5	<.10	female subjects symptomatically tend more to both poles, male subjects more to the positive pole
44 (psychic) capacity	14.114	4	<.01	female subjects very significantly more impaired
46 Readiness to work	10.174	4	<.05	female subjects rated themselves significantly less involved in work

Table 4 gives the significant data from the questionnaire for the
beginning (variables 3, 5, 6) and the end of the battery of tests
(variables 43, 44, 46). The calculations are taken from the differences between the two types of test conditions (placebo, drug).

Discussion: As far as we know there have been, up to now, few specific
results on the effect of drugs on the sexes in the context dealt with
here. Janke (1964) himself did not go into this problem, despite the
very comprehensive nature of his investigation. Even Munkelt's
description (1965) of various interrelationships between meprobamate,
alcohol, stability, and sex are difficult to interpret. Our main
question was not, however, directed towards a solution to this problem and this may restrict the significance of our findings to a
certain extent. Before evaluating the significant data from Table 4

we must warn against the inclusion of interfering components, above
all stability-instability. Therefore, it should be noted that the two
groups of female and male subjects did not differ significantly as
regards the possible pharmacologically determined changes for extraversion and neuroticism (2↑-test). Even the work conditions matched
completely since pairs of subjects came from the same subgroup.

Under our conditions the female subjects experienced a clear impairment of their disposition in 5 out of the 6 parameters (Table 4) at
the beginning of the experiment (60 min after the administration of
hexobarbitone) and towards the end of the experiment (240 min after
receiving hexobarbitone).
A pharmacologist would, in the end, attribute these facts to the body
weight of the female subjects being on average lighter than that of
the males. We would counter with the following points:
(1) If the above mentioned factor had played an important role, the
    fact that the results of the female participants in the objective
    achievement tests were as good as those of the male subjects would
    have been even more pronounced.
(2) The assessment of the variable 43 (mood) verifies that female sub-
    jects tend both more to the positive and to the negative poles.
    Obviously, therefore, "psychic information processing" (c.f.,
    Janke 1964) rather than pure drug effect is the predominate factor.
    This assumption has been made possible by Janke's experiments
    (1964) despite the acknowledged relationship between dosage and
    body weight. Lienert (1964) too, in his experiment, moved from
    the principle of drug administration per kg body weight, having
    established that unstable subjects (re. A.N.S.) with greater
    body weight needed a somewhat smaller dosage of LSD than had been
    originally calculated.

Nevertheless we agree that the weight factor must be eliminated, for
example, through partial correlations in experiments on this problem
in particular.
One by-product of our investigation that we can accept then is that
female subjects do feel more impaired by hexobarbitone than their
male counterparts. They appeared more unstable, but in achievement
tests they had the same results.

        4. SOME CONCLUSIONS

It is our opinion that investigations on the differentiation of intelligence and the reverse approach, i.e. its regression, by means
of factor analysis seem to have reached a limit. Future research should
avoid complex tests and instead favour experimental designs which give
a better insight into human information processing. This is because
many details and the process of achieving the final result is still
an open question. The relative invariance of achievement results allows
conclusions to be made as to the practice of testing; that is to say,
essential distortions of the results are not to be expected under conditions similar to those used in our experiment (e.g. normal subjects,
single administration of drug, high-work load condition, etc.). In
the first instance, however, we may expect that impairment of long
and short-term concentration and reasoning will occur.

It is worth noting from a differential aspect that only in a few
achievement tests were there any significant differences between the

extreme groups that we examined (E, I, N, n). As regards the personality variables extraversion-introversion, our results only partially
concurred with the hypothetical drug postulate of Eysenck, a postulate
not previously tested using extreme groups of extraverts and introverts. The dimension of neuroticism seems to be more useful than the
dimension of extra-introversion at least in accounting for the situational impairment experienced by the subjects.

We came to the conclusion that a limitation of the drug postulate from
the results using the extraversion-introversion dimension seems not to
be sufficient. There is no doubt about the heuristic importance of
Eysenck's postulate. The use of only two dimensions, however, seems
too limited. Situational influences and a gradation of difficulties
as expressed in different levels of achievement are not given due
consideration in this model.

In agreement with Janke and co-workers (1979) we think that if two
groups of introverts and extraverts are formed, one should not only
use questionnaires but also experimental data. Besides, the variable
of neuroticism (stable vs. instable subjects) should always be considered simultaneously. Situational aspects (high work load conditions,
experienced difficulty, ect.) should also be utilized in conjunction
with the activation concept (activation meant as "state"). On the
basis of Legewie's proposals regarding experiments (1968), the inclusion of these factors would probably provide use with more valid
results.

REFERENCES

Brengelmann, J. C., and L. Brengelmann (1960). Deutsche Validierung
    von Fragebogen der Extraversion, neurotischen Tendenz und Rigidi-
    tät. Z. exp. angew. Psychol., 7, 291-331.
Brickenkamp, R. (1962). Test d2, Aufmerksamkeits-Belastungstest.
    Hogrefe, Göttingen.
Cattell, R.B., and A. K. S. Cattell (1959). IPAT Culture Fair Intelli-
    gence Test. Illinois.
Dittrich, A. (1974). Probleme der pharmakopsychologischen Forschung.
    In W. J. Schraml, and U. Baumann (Eds.), Klinische Psychologie II.
    Huber, Bern, pp. 523-558.
Düker, H. (1963). Über reaktive Anspannungssteigerung. Z. exp. angew.
    Psychol., 10, 46-72.
Düker, H., and G. A. Lienert (1959). KLT Konzentrations-Leistungs-Test.
    Hogrefe, Göttingen.
Eysenck, H. J. (1957). Drugs and personality I. Theory and methodology.
    J. Ment. Sci., 103, 110-131.
Eysenck, H. J. (1959). Das"Maudsley Personality Inventory" als Bestim-
    mer der neurotischen Tendenz und Extraversion. Z. exp. angew. Psychol.,
    6, 167-190.
Eysenck, H. J. (Ed.) (1963). Experiments with Drugs. Pergamon Press,
    Oxford.
Fischer, G., and J. Roppert (1964). Ein Verfahren der Transformations-
    analyse faktorenanalytischer Ergebnisse. Schriftenreihe des Insti-
    tuts für Höhere Studien und Wissenschaftliche Forschung, Band 1.
    Wien.
Hauschild, F. (1956). Pharmakologie und Grundlagen der Toxikologie.
    VEB, Leipzig. pp. 729-741.

Horn, W. (1962). Das Leistungsprüfsystem (LPS). Hogrefe, Göttingen.

Janke, W. (1964). Experimentelle Untersuchungen zur Abhängigkeit der Wirkung psychotroper Substanzen von Persönlichkeitsmerkmalen. Akad. Verlag, Frankfurt/M.

Janke, W. (1965). Über einige methodische Probleme bei pharmakopsychologischen Untersuchungen mit Tranquilantien, Neuroleptika und Sedativa. Arch. ges. Psychol., 117, 306-318.

Janke, W., and G. Debus (1978). Die Eigenschaftswörterliste (EWL). Hogrefe, Göttingen.

Janke, W., G. Debus, and N. Longo (1979). Differential psychopharmacology of tranquilizing and sedating drugs. In Th.A. Ban et al. (Eds.), Modern Problems of Pharmacopsychiatry, Vol. 14. Karger, Basel. pp. 13-98.

Kalveram, K. Th. (1965). Die Veränderung der Faktorenstruktur durch "simultane Überlagerung". Arch. ges. Psychol., 117, 296-305.

Legewie, H. (1968). Persönlichkeitstheorie und Psychopharmaka. Hain Meisenheim.

Lienert, G. A. (1964). Belastung und Regression. Versuch einer Theorie der systematischen Beeinträchtigung der intellektuellen Leistungsfähigkeit. Hain, Meisenheim.

Munkelt, P. (1965). Persönlichkeitsmerkmale (psychische Stabilität und Geschlecht) als Bedingungsfaktoren der psychotropen Arzneimittelwirkung. Psychol. Beitr., 8, 98-183.

Steinberg, H. (1961). Methods and problems of drug-induced changes in emotions and personality. Rev. Psychol. Appl., 11, 361-372.

Strauß, E.-H. (1970). Pharmakabedingte Veränderungen im Ergebnis von Persönlichkeitstests. In H.-D. Rösler, H.-D. Schmidt, and H. Szewczyk (Eds.), Persönlichkeitsdiagnostik. VEB Deutscher Verlag der Wissenschaften, Berlin. pp. 264-277.

Strauß, E.-H. (1972). Zur Frage der Veränderung der Intelligenzstruktur. In H. Rennert, K. H. Liebner, and H.-D. Rösler (Eds.), Zu aktuellen Problemen der Medizinischen Psychologie. Wiss. Beiträge der Martin-Luther-Univ., Halle/Wittenberg. pp. 230-236.

Strauß, E.-H. (1979). Beiträge zur Regressionshypothese der Intelligenz und zur differentiellen Pharmakopsychologie. Dissertation (B) Humboldt-Universität, Berlin. (unpublished)

Wilder, J. (1931). Das "Ausgangswert-Gesetz" - ein unbeachtetes biologisches Gesetz; seine Bedeutung für Forschung Praxis. Klin. Wochenschrift, 10, 1889-1893.

DIFFERENTIAL EFFECTS OF A TRANQUILIZING DRUG AND PERSONALITY TRAITS

Uta Heinze, Ingrid Kästner and H. Kulka

ABSTRACT

The experiments showed that depending on the test and on medication, the personality traits lability, excitability, and nervousness influence behavioral performance. With the determination apparatus, the performance of the subjects with the traits stable, unexcitable, and not nervous improved when tranquilizer and placebo were administered, compared with normal, whereas the unstable, excitable, and nervous subjects showed a decline in performance after a dose of tranquilizer. Depending on the tests selected and on medication, the selected personality traits proved to be significant factors affecting performance.

KEYWORDS

Personality traits; Reaktive Anspannungssteigerung; emotional lability.

INTRODUCTION

In this investigation we attempted to answer questions arising from the relations between behavioral performance and personality traits. Since behavior is dependent both on objective factors, for instance the type of demand and the structure of the task set, and on subjective ones, such as psychological characteristics, we tried to account for this in selecting subjects and through an appropriate course of investigation.

Task differences could be realized through the tests used; the structure of demands was varied by means of diazepam and placebo. We used the Freiburger Persönlichkeitsinventar (Freiburg personality inventory) of Fahrenberg (Fahrenberg and Selg, 1970), to determine the degree of emotional lability, excitability, and nervousness of the subjects, who were then divided into groups.

The investigation was in the nature of a pilot study. The aim was to answer the following questions:

- What influence do the selected personality traits have on performance
  under the conditions of the experiment?
- Is there a connection between these personality traits and performance
  under the varied conditions brought about by the application of
  tranquilizer and placebo?

COURSE OF THE INVESTIGATION AND DESCRIPTION OF METHODS

The investigations were carried out on 33 healthy female students at
a medical college. Each subject was examined on four separate days.
The tests were divided into a practice-phase, a neutral experiment,
and a main experiment. In the practice-phase, the subjects were made
familiar with the testing situation and were administered a series of
tests in a definite order. The neutral and main experiments included
the same tests which were conducted in the same order, the only difference being that in the main experiments the subjects received
either a medium-sized dose of diazepam (10 mg) or placebo. The order
in which tranquilizer and placebo were administered was governed by
methodical considerations: 17 received tranquilizer first and 16 placebo. The instructions as to the effects of the drug were in both
cases the same, and were intended to produce an expectation of a sedative effect.
Each group of 3 or 4 subjects carried out all the experiments with the
same experimenter, and each subject began the experiments at the same
time on each day.
The application of tranquilizer and placebo was carried out in a single
blind procedure.

The following tests were carried out:
- Course of Stress test (Department of Psychology, Humboldt University
  Berlin)
- Concentration test (Konzentrations-Leistungstest; Düker and Lienert,
  1965)
- Determination apparatus (Determinationsgerät) with 200 trials at
  stimulus intervals of 1 sec for measuring complex reaction times
- Determination apparatus with 200 trials at stimulus intervals of
  0.8 sec
- Course of Stress test.

The Course of Stress test is a six-point rating scale which makes it
possible for the subject to make a self-estimation of psychic strain,
personal performance, motivation, and fatigue.
In Düker's concentration test, the subject calculates for 20 min according to certain rules. With this test it is possible to measure
concentration in terms of understanding, calculating, perceiving and
visualizing. The total number of tasks carried out and the number of
mistakes were recorded.
The determination apparatus (ZAK) demands from the subject reactions
to colour, light, and sounds. The intervals between stimuli are given
in advance by the experimenter. The number of correct and delayed but
correct reactions were assessed and given a value in points. The number of mistakes was also recorded.

The subjects were divided into groups according to their degree of
emotional lability, excitability, and nervousness measured by the
FPI. In the statistical evaluation, groups were compared which differed

in only one respect, for instance unstable/stable. The two groups which differed in all three respects (unstable/excitable/nervous - stable/ unexcitable/not nervous) were also compared.
For the statistical calculations, we used the Friedman test, the multiple average value comparison for the Friedman totals, the Wilcoxon comparison of pairs, and the U-test of Mann and Whitney.

RESULTS AND INTERPRETATION

The results of the tests with the determination apparatus showed similar tendencies, despite different stimulus intervals (see Fig. 1).

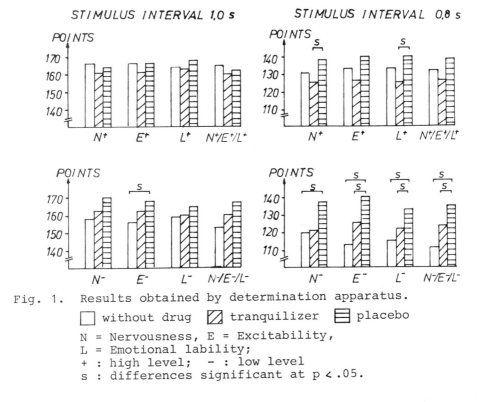

Fig. 1.   Results obtained by determination apparatus.

☐ without drug   ▨ tranquilizer   ▤ placebo

N = Nervousness, E = Excitability,
L = Emotional lability;
+ : high level;   - : low level
s : differences significant at p < .05.

On the other hand, the performance of the groups under the different conditions could be clearly distinguished. While the performance of the subjects in group 1 (unstable, excitable, nervous) deteriorated when the tranquilizer was administered and improved with placebo, the performance of subjects in group 2 was consistently better under the influence of the drug than that achieved under normal conditions. The subjects all experienced the effect of the tranquilizer subjectively; those in group 1 could not compensate for their impaired performance on this type of task, so that their performance became worse. When placebo was administered there was no impairment, neither objectively nor subjectively. The performance corresponded to those under normal conditions (group 1 with intervals between stimuli of 1 sec) or rose (group 2 with stimulus intervals of 0.8 and 1 sec).

We believe that the reason for the increase in performance is the
"Reaktive Anspannungssteigerung" (reactive rise in tension; Düker,
1963). Since the stress for the subject was greater with an interval
between stimuli of 0.8 sec, the rise in tension was more clearly seen
with this stimulus interval. The rise in performance of the subjects
of the second group could also be attributed to the reactive rise in
tension. Since when placebo was administered a deadening effect failed to appear, the improvement in performance between normal and placebo conditions was significantly greater than between normal and
tranquilizer conditions.
Since the motivation of all subjects in relation to the test was positive, it seems justified to attribute the changes in performance
above all to the reactive rise in tension which is variously dependent
on the selected personality traits; that is instability, excitability,
and nervousness.

Düker's concentration test measures other psychic components and yielded in our experiments other results, too. All subjects showed the same
tendencies, both in the total number of tasks carried out and in
the number of mistakes (see Fig. 2).

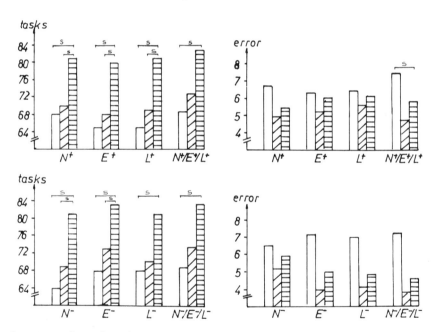

Fig. 2. Results in the concentration test (KLT; Düker and
         Lienert, 1965).

         ☐ without drug ▨ tranquilizer ☰ placebo

         N = Nervousness, E = Excitability,
         L = Emotional lability;
         + : high level;   - : low level
         s : differences significant at p< .05.

When placebo was administered, the total number of tasks carried out
rose steadily and the number of mistakes fell, but not so strongly
as with tranquilizer. The differences in the number of mistakes, in

comparison with that under neutral conditions, were purely accidental. In the total number of tasks carried out, significant improvements appeared in neutral-placebo and tranquilizer-placebo comparisons. The characteristics measured by the concentration test were obviously not as easily disrupted as the performance required with the determination apparatus. A further reason for this result could also be seen in the fact that in the concentration test, the subjects could work at their own speed; the pressure of time arising from the fixed stimulus intervals at the determination apparatus was not there.

When we compared the average values of the tasks carried out, we found that the results of subjects with the characteristics unexcitable and stable are superior to those of the excitable and unstable subjects, but not to a statistically significant extent (see Fig. 3).

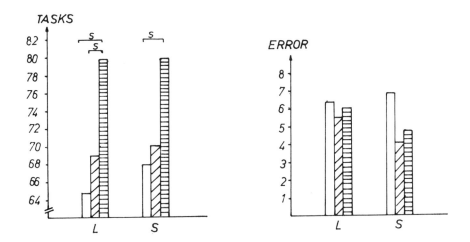

Fig. 3.   Comparison of results in the concentration test (KLT; Düker and Lienert, 1965).

☐ without drug   ▨ tranquilizer   ⊟ placebo

L = Emotionally labile subjects;
S = Emotionally stable subjects;
s : differences significant at p<.05.

The different task structures could also be the reason for the discrepancies between the concentration test results and those at the determination apparatus (see Fig. 4).
Perhaps, the subjects of group 1 adapted themselves, although with great exertion, to a set tempo which did not necessarily correspond with their individual tempo. The subjects of group 2 may not have allowed themselves to be as strongly influenced by the test situation or may not have significantly altered their individual tempo.

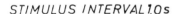

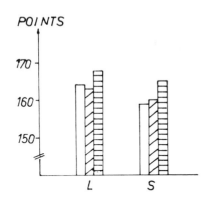
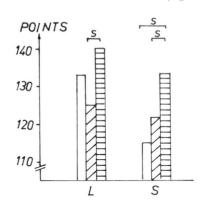

Fig. 4.   Comparison of results obtained by determination
          apparatus.

          ☐ without drug   ▨ tranquilizer   ⊟ placebo

          L = Emotionally labile subjects;
          S = Emotionally stable subjects;
          s : differences significant at p < .05.

The results of the subjective estimation of psychic strain, personal
performance, motivation, and fatigue by the subjects support our interpretation of the test results. The test situation was experienced
by group 1 as a greater strain and as demanding greater effort to
fulfil the tasks when tranquilizer is administered. The fact that
performance under these conditions varies is in all probability due
to different degrees of strength in personality traits.

REFERENCES

Düker, H. (1963). Über reaktive Anspannungssteigerung. Z. exp. angew.
    Psychol., 10, 46-72.
Düker, H., and G. A. Lienert (1965). Konzentrations-Leistungstest
    (KLT). Hogrefe, Göttingen.
Fahrenberg, J., and H. Selg (1970). Freiburger Persönlichkeitsinventar
    (FPI). Hogrefe, Göttingen.
Janke, W., and K. D. Stoll (1965). Untersuchung zur Wirkung eines
    Tranquilizers auf emotional labile Personen unter verschiedenen
    Bedingungen. Arzneim.-Forsch. (Drug Res.), 15, 366-474.
Janke, W., G. Debus, and N. Longo (1979). Differential psychopharma-
    cology of tranquilizing and sedating drugs. In Th. A. Ban et al.
    (Eds.), Modern Problems of Pharmacopsychiatry, Vol. 14, Karger,
    Basel. pp. 13-98.

MULTIPLE PREDICTION OF REACTIONS TO A PSYCHOTROPIC DRUG (PROMETHAZINE) BY PERSONALITY TRAITS

Wolfram Boucsein

ABSTRACT

Research concerning the influence of personality variables on drug response in normal subjects usually is limited to broad personality traits such as extraversion/introversion and neuroticism.

As a first approach in describing the predictive value of different kinds of traits including narrow traits, attitudes towards drugs, and experience with drugs, have been used in a multiple correlation procedure to predict objective and subjective responses to 25 mg promethazine in healthy male students either under white noise stress or under a control condition.

Drug-induced performance changes could easier be predicted by broad personality characteristics, whereas narrow traits, including attitudes towards drugs and drug consumption served best to predict changes in subjective activity.

The superiority of broad traits in predicting drug influence upon performance may be due to neurophysiological correlates of these personality characteristics.

KEYWORDS

Multiple prediction of drug response; multiple correlation; personality traits.

1. INTRODUCTION

In their extensive review of the literature dealing with differential effects of tranquillizing and sedating drugs, Janke, Debus and Longo (1979) stated that almost all investigations carried out with normal subjects to evaluate the relationships between personality traits and drug responses made use of broad personality characteristics, like emotionality (or neuroticism, emotional lability), extraversion/introversion, and a pattern of traits which might be called action-orientation. Measures of attitudes, interests and needs have not yet been used.

It is highly possible that broad traits are such good predictors of
drug action because they are more related to physiological constructs
than specific traits are.

In spite of this, since a response to a drug condition is a rather
specific characteristic of the individual, it is possible that narrow
traits might turn out to be as suitable predictors as broad traits are.
In addition, like pharmacotherapeutical findings showed, there is some
evidence that attitudes towards and experiences with drugs may have
predictive value for the actual drug response (Janke and others, 1979).

In the present experiment, multiple correlations including relatively broad and general traits such as neuroticism and extraversion/intro-
version, specific traits, attitudes towards drug intake, and experience
with drugs were performed as a first approach to compare the quality of
different kinds of traits for the prediction of response to a depressan
drug, promethazine, a highly sedating antihistaminic.

Multiple correlation technique was used for evaluating the predictive
value of the different trait measures. Although this may only be a
rough method, and any results obtained by it may not be replicable in
detail, it was chosen for it has the enormous economic advantage to
investigate the influence of more than 2 or 3 traits at the same time.
Anova-designs with many organismic factors, even with only 2 groups on
each factor, are so demanding for such large samples that their real-
ization is nearly impossible.

2. METHOD

2.1 Design of the Experiment

Forty-four healthy male students volunteered for the experiment, a
4 x 2 mixed design, which consisted of 7 sessions. Two drugs, one placebo and a non-medication condition, were proceeded by a session to
obtain personality variables which were again recorded on the 7th day,
and a practice session to avoid too large practice gains from the firs
to the second session. Half of the subjects were treated with a white
noise of 90 dbA through earphones; the other half had earphones but no
noise.

The following drugs were administered orally utilising a doubleblind
technique: 25 mg promethazine, 25 mg propiram fumarate, and a placebo,
all in identical capsules. To maintain the doubleblindness even with
the non-medication condition, drugs were administered by someone other
than the experimenter. Half of the subjects took part in the morning,
half in the afternoon and a oneday washout followed each drug session.

Each 5 hour experimental session consisted of 3 identical cycles; the
first to obtain initial values, the following 2 to obtain reactions
to drugs administered at the end of cycle 1. Within each cycle, a set
of subjective and performance measures were obtained.

Eight subjects took part in each session, separated by screens. The
places were permutated throughout the days. Subjects received standard
food at the beginning of each experiment and between the test cycles.

To evaluate subjective reactions to the drugs, an adjective checklist
(EWL by Janke and Debus, 1978) was used. Additionally, a symptom list

and a series of subjective rating-scales derived from the subscales of
the EWL was used, the results of which are not reported in the present
paper.

Performance measures included in the study were: choice reaction time,
tapping, tremor and 2 tests of cognitive performance, in which numbers
had to be found in matrices. In addition, tachistoscopic recognition
and word-fluency were recorded but not included in the present evaluation.

On the day before the practice session, a set of personality variables
had been obtained for the sake of prediction: extraversion and neuroticism, as measured by the ENNR (Brengelmann and Brengelmann, 1960),
phobic tendencies as measured by the FSS II (Geer, 1965), the EWL
(Janke and Debus, 1978), but with the instruction to answer according
to the habitual, long-lasting states, a questionnaire for mental activity and sensation seeking (Janke, 1963), a questionnaire to obtain
attitudes towards drugs, and one to find out the amount of drugs used
by the subjects, both from Janke and Schmidt (1967).

2.2   Evaluation of Data for Multiple Prediction

Results concerning drug effects were reported in another paper (Boucsein
and Janke, 1974). For multiple prediction, only reactions to the marketed
drug, promethazine, were selected. Because of the clearer drug effects,
reactions to the drug within cycle 3 (between 130 and 215 min p. appl.)
were predicted. Double differences, drug-placebo for cycle 3 - cycle 1,
were computed as criterion measures for the individual reactions to
promethazine.

As the technique of multiple correlations allows only one criterion
measure to be predicted by several predictors at the same time, the
number of variables used for the evaluation of drug effects had to be
reduced for the sake of multiple prediction. Therefore, only those
variables in which significant reactions in either the noise - or the
control group were obtained were taken into account as criterion measures.
Two kinds of criterion data were evaluated for multiple prediction:
first, speed of performance and second, subjective activity, were formed
as global measures by adding standard t-scores from variables correlating
highly in cycle 1 on the first day. In addition, this served as a method
to improve the reliability of criterion measures. Speed of performance
was computed from choice reaction time and speed of cognitive performance; subjective activity was composed by the activity and concentration
categories of the EWL.

3. RESULTS

For the noise group, for the control group, and for both criterion
measures, multiple regression was computed with the 13 predictor variables mentioned in Table 1. In this table, all predictors are shown
with their single correlation to the appropriate criterion measure, and
with their ß-weights for multiple regression.

TABLE 1 Multiple Prediction of Drug Effect in Both Criterion Measures Under Both Experimental Conditions with Unselected Predictors

Criterion:	Speed of performance				Subjective activity			
	Noise group		Control group		Noise group		Control group	
Predictors:	simple r	β-weight	simple r	β-weight	simple r	β-weight	simple r	β-weight
Neuroticism	-.16	-.53	.42	.34	-.20	-.23	.18	-.05
Extraversion	.54	.73	.24	.45	.14	.02	-.15	.31
Anxiety	.39	.60	-.02	.60	.17	-.05	-.18	-.27
Phobic tendencies	.00	.10	.17	.19	.17	.12	.39	.48
Mental activity	.28	.32	-.08	-.11	-.26	-.40	.27	.74
Deactivation	.14	-.05	-.10	-.11	.33	.09	-.42	.82
Sensation seeking	.28	-.09	-.29	-.38	.28	.34	-.22	-.39
Well-being	.25	-.74	.01	-.38	.07	-.08	-.22	-.83
Attitudes towards sleeping pills	-.49	-.27	.23	.36	-.30	-.38	.33	.71
Attitudes towards nicotine	-.15	.28	.42	.23	.30	.38	.11	-.34
Attitudes towards alcohol	-.09	-.35	.18	-.52	.33	-.14	.26	.14
Nicotine consumption	-.06	-.12	.20	.01	.17	.04	-.01	-.13
Alcohol consumption	.03	-.16	-.04	.09	.27	.22	-.10	-.24
multiple R		.83		.69		.73		.75

As Table 1 indicates, suppressor variables, i.e. variables with negative
ß-weights (Lord and Novick, 1968) are included in each of the 4 sets
of predictors. The inclusion of variables with suppression effects in
a multiple prediction raises two problems: first they don't seem to be
as good in cross-validation as other predictors (Lord and Novick, 1968),
and second, in the case of more than 2 or 3 predictors, a psychological
interpretation of suppression effects is nearly impossible. Therefore
all suppressor-variables were eliminated from each set of predictors
in the next step. With the remaining predictors, a step-by-step multiple
regression analysis was performed, until the multiple correlation that
was corrected concerning shrinking reached a maximum. Within each step
the predictor variable with the highest F-score for inclusion was selected. It is obvious that this procedure leads to different sets of
predictors for each of the 4 predictions.

Table 2 shows for each criterion measure under noise- or control condition the set of predictors which led to the highest multiple correlation.
Additionally a correction for shrinking was performed to make multiple
correlations based on different numbers of predictors comparable.

As Table 2 shows the best multiple predictions of drug effects could
be performed in 3 cases with 3 and in one case with 5 predictors. Only
10 out of the 13 predictors included in the initial calculation (Table 1)
were used. Though obviously the uncorrected multiple correlations in
Table 1 were higher than those in Table 2, because of a greater number
of predictors which have been taken into account, the appropriate corrected coefficients could not be computed except in one case because
they were undefined.

In each of the 4 predictions, there has been an important gain of
multiple prediction as compared to the greatest single correlation
including the correlations with predictors which had not been taken
into multiple prediction because of their suppressor function.

TABLE 2 Multiple Prediction of Drug Effect in Both Criterion Measures Under Both Experimental Conditions with the Set of Best Predictors

Predictors:	Speed of performance				Subjective activity			
	Noise group		Control group		Noise group		Control group	
	simple r	β-weight	simple r	β-weight	simple r	β-weight	simple r	β-weight
Neuroticism			.42	.40				
Extraversion	.54	.48	.24	.20				
Anxiety	.39	.29						
Phobic tendencies					.17	.20	.39	.46
Mental activity	.28	.33					.27	.43
Deactivation					.33	.37		
Sensation seeking					.28	.29		
Attitudes towards nicotine			.42	.28	.30	.32		
Attitudes towards sleeping pills							.33	.33
Alcohol consumption					.27	.25		
multiple R	.68		.58		.64		.64	
multiple R corrected	.63		.51		.51		.58	

4. DISCUSSION

Results obtained by stepwise multiple regression analysis must be interpreted cautiously because the inclusion of a single predictor may partially be influenced.

Therefore, including a specific personality variable into a multiple prediction of reactions to the drug in question does not necessarily prove this variable to be a good predictor in a different set of personality variables or even in a different situational context. This can already be seen in the actual prediction where there is little concordance between predictors for drug responses under noise and control conditions, as the results in Table 2 show.

Nevertheless, a noticeable difference between the classes of variables used for prediction of the performance and the subjective criterion appears in Table 2. Relatively broad traits such as neuroticism and extraversion were only used for the prediction of performance changes but not for changes in subjective activity due to promethazine action. Relatively narrow traits such as phobic tendencies, mental activity, deactivation, and sensation seeking are mainly used in the prediction of drug action on subjective activity, although anxiety and mental activity served as predictors of drug-induced performance under noise conditions, too.

The third class of predictors, namely attitudes towards and the consumption of drugs, also served more as predictors for subjective changes than for changes in performance measures.

The drug-action-modifying features of neuroticism and extraversion are well established in the performance area as well as in the area of subjective reactions to drugs (Janke and others, 1979).

In contrast the effects of narrow traits have not been investigated thoroughly up to now. The present investigation supports a hypothesis that should be tested in further research in differential psychopharmacology: broad traits may be better predictors for drug induced changes of performance probably because of their neurophysiological correlates (Eysenck, 1967) whereas narrow traits and attitudes towards drugs may be better predictors for subjective changes due to drugs. For the time being this can only be stated for one sedating drug, promethazine.

Although the results may not be replicable in detail, the multiple prediction approach in differential psychopharmacology seems to be fairly promising, especially in the investigation of narrow traits and for special attitudes and other personality variables closely related to the habit of drug use.

However, the theoretical background for the inclusion of drug action modifying variables of this kind should be established as well.

REFERENCES

Boucsein, W. (1971). Experimentelle Untersuchungen zum Problem inter-
    individueller Reaktionsdifferenzen auf Psychopharmaka. Gießen,
    unpublished dissertation.
Boucsein, W., and W. Janke (1974). Experimentalpsychologische Unter-
    suchungen zur Wirkung von Propiramfumarat und Promethazin unter
    Normal- und Streßbedingungen. Arzneim.-Forsch. (Drug Res.), 24,
    675-693.
Brengelmann, J. C., and L. Brengelmann (1960). Deutsche Validierung
    von Fragebogen der Extraversion, neurotischen Tendenz und Rigidität.
    Z. exp. angew. Psychol., 7, 291-331.
Eysenck, H. J. (1967). The Biological Basis of Personality. Thomas,
    Springfield.
Geer, J. H. (1965). The development of a scale to measure fear.
    Behav. Res. Ther., 3, 45-53.
Janke, W. (1963). Fragebogen zur geistigen Aktivität. Gießen, unpublished
Janke, W., and G. Debus (1978). Eigenschaftswörterliste (EWL).
    Hogrefe, Göttingen.
Janke, W., G. Debus, and N. Longo (1979). Differential psychopharma-
    cology of tranquillizing and sedating drgs. In Th. A. Ban and
    others (Eds.), Modern Problems of Pharmacopsychiatry, Vol. 14.
    Karger, Basel. pp. 13-98.
Janke, W., and R. Schmidt (1967). Konstruktion eines Fragebogens zur
    Feststellung der Gesundheits- und Arzneimitteleinstellung.
    Gießen, unpublished.
Lord, F. M., and M. R. Novick (1968). Statistical Theories of Mental
    Test Scores. Addison-Wesley, Reading/Mass.

ACUTE AND CHRONIC EFFECTS OF ANTIDEPRESSANTS IN NORMAL SUBJECTS CONSIDERING PERSONALITY TRAITS

Günter Debus and Klaus Jürgen Ehrhardt

ABSTRACT

The extent and kind of individual differences in the response to anti-depressant drugs is discussed on the basis of the research in this field.
Two original studies concerning this topic are reported. Study I deals with individual differences in the response to a single drug adminis-tration. Study II deals with responses after repeated drug ingestion.

Study I
The effects of the tricyclic antidepressant drug lofepramine versus a placebo were tested after single drug administration in healthy sub-jects. A sample of 46 male students was divided into two subgroups depending on their scores on depression scales commonly used in clin-ical psychology and psychiatry. A repeated measurement design was used, balancing for sequence. The instruments included self-report measures, performance tests, as well as the registration of physiological varia-bles. The data obtained show that lofepramine increases heart rate, but does not affect performance. In contrast, positive subjective ef-fects previously found in other studies in high-depressive groups could not be replicated.

Study II
A sample of 23 male students, with relatively high scores on a depres-sion scale was selected. Lofepramine or placebo were administered to 12 and 11 subjects respectively, for eight days. The instruments were the same as in the first study. The data show a positive emotional ef-fect for lofepramine in comparison to placebo at the seventh and eighth day of drug administration.
The results agree with the assumption that antidepressant effects could be demonstrated in human normals, when subjects with high depres-sion scores were selected and when drug ingestion was repeated. Several questions are noted, however, which have to be studied before final conclusions can be drawn.

KEYWORDS

Antidepressant drugs; lofepramine; acute effects; chronic effects;
differential drug effects and trait variables; depression scales;
self-report measures; performance tests; physiological variables;
drug response and depression

INTRODUCTION

In the field of Differential Psychopharmacology the drugs primarily
investigated are the sedating and stimulating ones (Janke, Debus and
Longo, 1979). There are almost no studies investigating individual
differences in the response to antidepressant drugs. Two questions
arise when studying individual differences in the response to antidepressant drugs:
(1) How long after drug ingestion should we look for drug responses
and individual differences in these responses? As it is well known,
antidepressants have different effects in patients over time. In the
first two weeks they have more or less sedating properties, there-
after they show their antidepressant effects.
(2) The second question concerns which type of personality characteristic could be regarded as a meaningful variable for explaining inter-
individual drug response differences with antidepressants. There is
no theory which would suggest a certain personality characteristic if
one did not refer to neuroticism or depression because of face validity.

As a rule studies investigating antidepressant drugs in human subjects
try to evaluate general properties of drug action, e.g. effects on
activation and performance, as well as physiological responses seen
in both depressive patients and normal subjects. Most authors do not
look for individual differences. In case of any discussion about individual differences the question is asked whether or not therapy-
typical and therapy-relevant emotional effects of antidepressant drugs
can be shown in normal humans under certain conditions.

Several authors commenting on this question conclude that psychopharmacological studies with normal subjects may be inappropriate for
evaluating antidepressant effects (e.g. Hollister, 1972).

The first criticism made is that such effects are expected to occur
in depressive patients only. A second point is that antidepressant
effects only develop after repeated administrations of the drug, and
thus cannot be shown after a single drug administration, which is the
usual procedure in studies with normals. Results from single administration studies seem to support such a view, since sedation, performance decrement, and autonomic disturbances were the effects most
often observed.

Imipramine (25 mg - 200 mg) has been the most frequently investigated
drug in normals (e.g. Bättig and Fischer, 1964; Blackwell and others,
1972; DiMascio and others, 1964; Grünthal, 1958; Heimann and others,
1968; Herrmann and McDonald, 1979; Hollister, 1964; Ideström and
Cadenius, 1964; Karniol and others, 1976; Lehmann and Hopes, 1977a,
1977b; Pöldinger, 1963; Schmitt and Seifert, 1960; Wittenborn and
others, 1976). Other drugs under investigation have been desipramine
(DiMascio and others, 1964; Herrmann and McDonald, 1979; Hollister,

1964; Pöldinger, 1963), dibenzepine (Broeren and Schmitt, 1964),
maprotiline (Matussek and Aarons, 1974), nomifensine (Wittenborn and
others 1976) and lofepramine (Lehmann and Hopes, 1977).

Sedative effects in normals have consistently been reported by most
authors (e.g. Blackwell and others, 1972; DiMascio and others, 1964;
Karniol and others, 1976; Lehmann and Hopes, 1977a, 1977b; Pöldinger,
1963). Performance was either unchanged (e.g. Bättig and Fischer,
1964; DiMascio and others, 1964 and Ideström and Cadenius, 1964) or
impaired (Heimann and others, 1968; Herrmann and McDonald, 1979;
Lehmann and Hopes, 1977a,1977b; Wittenborn and others, 1976). The
autonomic responses, among others, were heart rate acceleration (e.g.
DiMascio and others, 1964; Ideström and Cadenius, 1964; Lehmann and
Hopes, 1977a, 1977b) and typical anticholinergic effects like dryness
of the mouth (Blackwell and others, 1972). When emotional effects were
observed (e.g. DiMascio and others, 1964; Lehmann and Hopes, 1977a,
1977b, after imipramine 2-3 hours p.a.), they were in the negative
direction, i.e. depressed mood. They probably represent secondary
effects, that is, emotional responses to severe sedation, performance
decrement, or autonomic disturbances. Antidepressant drugs have effects on the EEG after a single administration. They are not specific
to antidepressants, however, since they can also be observed after
administration of anticholinergic drugs without antidepressant action
(Saletu, 1976).

Only a few studies with repeated administrations to randomly selected
normals are reported in the literature. The findings of Degwitz (1964,
1967) are not unequivocal, since a placebo group was not included.
The placebo-controlled study by Zlatnikova and others (1974) fails to
show antidepressant effects. In a study by Matussek and Aarons (1974)
maprotiline showed sedating effects (tiredness). Other studies (e.g.
Clayton and others, 1977; Keeler and others, 1966; Seppälä, 1977) have
only investigated effects upon performance but not upon emotional variables.

So far, the majority of empirical findings does not suggest that there
is a chance of demonstrating some kind of antidepressant effects in
normal humans. Yet, the results of two studies (DiMascio and others,
1968; Lehmann and Hopes, 1977a, 1977b) showed individual differences
in the expected direction. DiMascio and others (1968) selected normal
subjects scoring high or low on a depression scale of the Minnesota
Multiphasic Personality Inventory (MMPI). After a week-long administration of imipramine (150 mg/day) the "high depressive" group
showed a significant reduction in their depression scores compared
to the "low depressive" group. Under placebo conditions there were
no response differences dependent on personality. Yet, there is a lack
of statistical evaluation as no statistically significant drug-placebo
differences are reported, and the interaction effect between drug and
personality has not definitely been tested. A replication of this study
under identical conditions has not been attempted to date. Recently,
Lehmann and Hopes (1977a, 1977b) assigned normal subjects to subgroups
according to their scores on the subscale "Depression" from the Freiburg Personality Inventory (FPI) (Fahrenberg and Selg, 1970), and
tested the effects of two drugs, imipramine (100 mg) and lofepramine
(140 mg). Surprisingly, the authors found that both antidepressants
affected mood positively in "high depressive" subjects. No emotional
effects were observed in "low depressive" subjects. Such positive
emotional effects in the former group were already seen 45 min after

oral application. As time went on, these effects became less pronounced
(lofepramine) or were replaced by negative emotional effects (imipramine).

Our own investigations started from the findings of the two studies
mentioned, in which individual response differences were reported.

STUDY I: SINGLE ADMINISTRATION OF LOFEPRAMINE

Introduction

The purpose of the first study was to assess the replicability of
Lehmann and Hopes' findings. Our experimental design was therefore
quite similar to theirs in most respects. The sample (healthy students)
subjects' classification on the basis of a depression scale (FPI),
application modus (single, oral), as well as doses, testing materials,
and experimental setting were comparable. Digressing from Lehmann and
Hopes we tested only one drug (lofepramine, 140 mg), an imipramine
analogue (Eriksoo and Rohte, 1970). We attempted a broad evaluation
of depression so as to get more information about factors modifying
drug response. The number of subjects was considerably higher in our
study.

Method

Subjects. Fifty-one paid, male student volunteers participated in the
experiment. Five subjects did not complete the experiment for reasons
unrelated to the drug conditions. The age of the remaining 46 subjects
ranged from 19 to 37 years ($\bar{X}$=23.7), the weight ranged from 52 to 84
kgs ($\bar{X}$=72.2). Subjects on medication or with acute or chronic diseases
were excluded on the basis of a health questionnaire (resp. a physical
examination if any doubts remained). At the outset, data concerning
trait variables were obtained for all subjects in order to check if
depressive symptoms were to be found within the normal range.

Design. A 2x2x2 factorial design was used with two levels of the personality factor ("high depressive" vs. "low depressive" subjects),
two levels of the drug factor (lofepramine, 140 mg vs. placebo), and
two levels of drug-placebo sequence (lofepramine-placebo; placebo-
lofepramine). The 46 subjects were divided into two subgroups on the
basis of their score on the FPI depression scale.

TABLE 1   Means and Standard Deviations for Depression Score,
           Age and Weight for Low and High Depressive Sub-
           groups of Study I

Subgroups	Depression FPI score	Age (Years)	Weight (kg)
Low depressive	$\bar{X}$ = 7.2	$\bar{X}$ = 23.7	$\bar{X}$ = 72.7
23 subjects	s = 3.9	s = 4.0	s = 8.0
High depressive	$\bar{X}$ = 18.1	$\bar{X}$ = 23.7	$\bar{X}$ = 71.6
23 subjects	s = 3.2	s = 3.2	s = 8.7

Table 1 shows means and standard deviations for depression scores, age, and weight. Differences between the two subgroups are highly significant for the depression score, but are nonsignificant for age and weight.

All subjects received both drugs in a counterbalanced plan. The drug sequences are shown in Table 2. A double-blind procedure was used for application of the drugs.

TABLE 2   Drug Sequences for Low and High Depressive Subgroups

Subgroups	Sequence of Drugs		Number of Subjects
	Day 1	Day 2	
Low depressive	Lofepramine	Placebo	11
	Placebo	Lofepramine	12
High depressive	Lofepramine	Placebo	12
	Placebo	Lofepramine	11

Instruments

a) Instruments for behavioral assessment:
EWL-ak-Eigenschaftswörterliste aktuell (Janke and Debus, 1978): The adjective check-list contains 161 adjectives (e.g. cheerful, sad, finicky) which the subject can accept or reject as descriptive of his or her momentary state (state EWL). Fifteen aspects of mood are arranged in six scales: activation, disactivation, extraversion/introversion, irritability, general well-being, and depression/anxiety.

Picture rating. Ten emotion-provoking slides (5 inkblots, and 5 expressive paintings by depressive patients) were shown for one minute each. All of them had to be rated along the following dimensions: pleasant-unpleasant, sad-cheerful, anxiety-provoking, exciting-calming, and anger-provoking.

MKSL-ak-Mehrdimensionale körperliche Symptom-Liste-aktuell (Erdmann and Janke, 1975): The momentary intensity of 99 bodily symptoms representing 11 organ systems was rated (state MKSL).

b) Instruments for performance assessment:
Four motor performance tests, two perceptual tests as well as a subjective time guess were taken and stored by an electronic device.

Tremor. A needle had to be held within a hole of 3 mm diameter so that the rim was touched as little as possible (60 sec).

Tapping. Subjects had to tap a plate with a metallic pin, first at a comfortable personal speed, later at maximal speed (15 sec each).

Aiming. Subjects had to tap a plate with a metallic pin so that the pin entered small holes without touching their edges. The number of mistakes was recorded.

Simple reaction time. A button was to be pressed following a light
(12 times in 50 sec with variable interstimulus intervals).

Negative afterimage. A red slide was shown for 20 sec. For the next
3 min the subjects were instructed to fixate the board and press a
button for the duration of the afterimage. Cumulative time was recorded.

Flicker fusion. The alternation frequency of a red flicker (at a dis-
tance of 2.5 m from the subject) was raised and lowered twice between
5-60 flashes per second. A button had to be pressed when the flicker
became continuous and vice versa.

Time guessing. Subjects had to press a button for a subjective duration of 10 sec.

c) Instruments for physiological measures:
Heart rate was obtained for 3 min periods measured by a finger plethys-
mograph connected to a Beckman polygraph. Blood pressure was taken by
the method of Riva-Rocci while subjects were kept sitting.

d) Instruments for personality measures:
In order to assess personality traits concerning depressive symptoms
the following questionnaires were used:

Bf-S - Befindlichkeitsskala (v. Zerssen, 1976): A scale consisting of
28 adjective polarities indicating elevated and depressed mood.

DS - Depressions-Skala (Dietsch and Janke, 1977): A questionnaire of
a preliminary form consisting of 198 statements which are evaluated
according to 12 scales refering to different aspects of depression.

EWL-hab - Eigenschaftswörterliste-habituell (Janke and Debus, 1978):
The adjective check list was employed in a modified version in order
to assess the frequency of mood states during day-to-day life.

FPI - Freiburger Persönlichkeits Inventar (Fahrenberg and Selg, 1970):
A questionnaire consisting of 9 scales based upon 212 statements altogether.

MKSL-hab - Mehrdimensionale körperliche Symptom-Liste-habituell
(Erdmann and Janke, 1975): A list of somatic symptoms which have to
be checked concerning their frequency of occurrence in every day life;
the 99 items are evaluated according to 11 symptomatic aspects.

SDS - Self-Rating Depression Scale (Zung, 1965): A scale consisting
of 20 statements.

Assessment procedure. Subjects were tested in groups of 3-6. Each subject sat in a compartment similar to those used in language labora-
tories. All subjects came for three sessions with a one-week interval between sessions. Each session lasted four hours.

The first session served as an adaptation to the laboratory situation.
The subjects filled in the personality questionnaires and completed
two practice trials on each test. They were instructed to adhere to
their normal day-to-day life, not to undergo sleep deprivation, use

medication or drink more than small amounts of alcohol.

For the experimental sessions subjects came fasting and were given a standard breakfast without caffeine at the institute at 8.30.

A complete test sequence was carried through once before and twice after drug application (45-110 and 120-175 min p.a.; see Table 3). The picture rating was only done twice.

Data analysis. Three-factor analyses of variance were computed. The first factor (independent groups) was the degree of depression measured ("high" or "low"), the second (independent groups) drug sequence, and the third (dependent groups) was the drug factor (lofepramine or placebo).

Correlational and factor-analytical computations were performed on the various depression measures and other personality variables in order to obtain information about the validity of the FPI-depression scale.

TABLE 3   Time-Schedule for the Experimental Sessions

Time	Tests	Duration (min)	Time after Application
8.30	standard breakfast	20	
8.50-9.45	EWL, MKSL (state)	20	
	performance test	20	
	physiological measures	15	
9.45	lofepramine or placebo	5	
9.50-10.00	picture rating	10	
	pause	30	
10.30-11.25	EWL, MKSL (state)	20	
	performance tests	20	45-100 min
	physiological measures	15	
11.25-11.35	picture rating	10	100-110 min
	pause	10	
11.45-12.40	EWL, MKSL (state)	20	
	performance tests	20	120-175 min
	physiological measures	15	

Results

Drug effects on subjects classified on the basis of the FPI-depression
score. No rating scale (EWL-ak, picture rating) showed significant
differences due to the drug factor, neither for the group as a whole
(N=46), nor for the subgroups (N_1=23; N_2=23). The EWL scale "general
well-being" consisting of the subscales "self-confidence" and "elevated
mood" was of major interest, since Lehmann and Hopes had found differential responding to drugs here. This scale differentiates well
($p < .001$) between high and low depressive groups (on the basis of the
FPI), but a drug effect could not be demonstrated within three hours
of recording after drug administration (Fig. 1, see next page).

Performance variables were uninfluenced by the drugs used. The subjective evaluation of somatic symptoms (state MKSL) showed no drug-
dependent changes. Recordings of heart rate, however, revealed an increase in the lofepramine-group towards the end of the session. While
this effect is not yet apparent 90 min after application, heart rate
is by four beats/min higher in the lofepramine-treated group than in
the placebo group at 170 min p.a. ($p < .01$).

Validity of the FPI-depression scale. One purpose of the present study
was to evaluate further the FPI-depression scale used by Lehmann and
Hopes to classify their subjects. It is to be questioned if this scale
actually measures what it is supposed to and whether it shows communalities with scales commonly used in clinical studies for measuring
the degree of depression in patients. We thus employed several other
scales, especially depression scales, to obtain more information about
the validity of the FPI-depression scale. Correlations between scores
on the various depression scales, as well as a factor analysis were
carried out.

Table 4 shows the results from the factor analysis (main component
model, varimax rotation) based upon 44 scales and 46 subjects. As the
table shows, considerable factor loadings (a $>$ .30) were observed with
the FPI-depression scale on four factors: a "somatic" factor, two "depression" factors, as well as a "dominance" factor.

Table 5 contains the highest correlations (r=.50) found between the
FPI depression-scale and the others used in this study.

We can conclude that the FPI-depression scale reflects a broad trait
variable including somatic, general activational, social, and cognitive aspects. It correlates considerably with clinical rating scales
of depression (r=.60; .47).

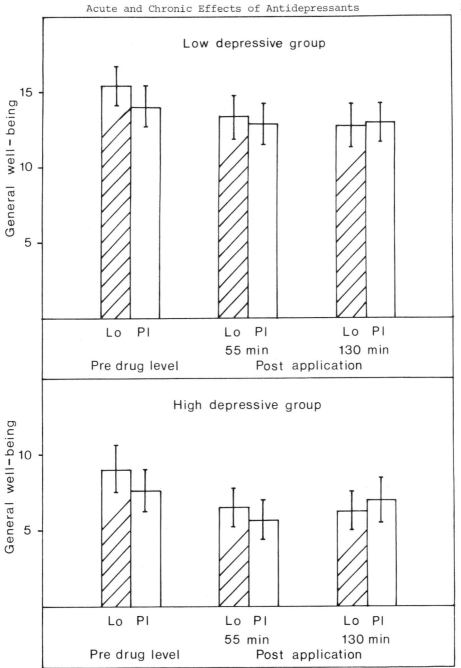

Fig. 1. Mean scores in the scale "general well-being"
         (state EWL) for "low and high depressive" sub-
         jects of the lofepramine group (Lo - hatched
         bars) and the placebo group (Pl - unhatched
         bars); pre drug level, 55 and 130 min p.a.

TABLE 4   Factor-loadings (a) and Communalities (h^2) of Scales in a 6-Factor Solution (N=46). Variables with the Highest Loadings and the FPI Depression Scale have been included.

	Factor Scale		a	h^2
1	muscular symptoms	(MKSL-hab)	.86	.89
	cardiovascular symptoms	(MKSL-hab)	.81	.84
	nervousness	(FPI)	.71	.77
	depression	(FPI)	.40	.83
2	depressed mood	(Bf-S)	.75	.75
	depression	(DS)	.74	.84
	depression	(SDS)	.66	.73
	depression	(FPI)	.45	.83
3	dominance	(FPI)	.76	.70
	aggressiveness	(FPI)	.75	.74
	irritability	(FPI)	.75	.78
	depression	(FPI)	.39	.83
4	sociability	(FPI)	.81	.69
	extra-/introversion	(EWL-hab)	.66	.73
	retardation	(FPI)	-.53	.63
	depression	(FPI)	<.30	.83
5	social rejection	(DS)	.84	.95
	missing understanding	(DS)	.71	.59
	depression	(FPI)	<.30	.83
6	guilty feeling	(DS)	.70	.79
	suicidal-thoughts	(DS)	.51	.49
	depression	(FPI)	.42	.83

TABLE 5   Product-moment Correlations (r > .50) be-
           tween the FPI-Depression Scale and Other
           Scales Applied in the Study (N=46)

Scale		Depression (FPI)
depression/anxiety	(EWL-hab)	.67
guilty feelings	(DS)	.67
depression	(DS)	.66
tension	(DS)	.65
nervousness	(FPI)	.63
loss of social contact	(DS)	.61
depression	(SDS)	.60
desactivation	(EWL-hab)	.59
irritability	(FPI)	.58
cardiovascular symptoms	(MKSL-hab)	.58
anxiety	(DS)	.58
irritability	(EWL-hab)	.58
aggressiveness	(FPI)	.58
sensory hypersensitivity	(MKSL-hab)	.57
retardation	(FPI)	.55
respiratory symptoms	(MKSL-hab)	.53
desactivation	(DS)	.53
suicidal thoughts	(DS)	.53
muscular symptoms	(MKSL-hab)	.52
digestive symptoms	(MKSL-hab)	.52
social rejection	(DS)	.50
low self-esteem	(DS)	.50
relaxation	(FPI)	-.50
⋮		
depressed mood	(Bf-S)	.47

Drug effects in subjects classified on the basis of different scores.
Further evaluations were done in order to control the missing specificity of the FPI-depression scale. Subjects were classified according to the scales loading high on the separated factors (see 6 in
Table 4). Averaged standard scores were used for classification. The
balance of drug sequences was in no instance seriously disturbed. A
three-way analysis of variance was then carried through with these
classifications. The results from this analysis were similar to those
from the first one; a drug trait interaction could not be found for
any of the subjects classifications. F-values in no instance reached
significance.

Discussion

The major result from Lehmann and Hopes' (1977a, 1977b) study was that
a single administration of lofepramine elevated mood in healthy, but
relatively depressed subjects. We were unable to replicate this effect in the present study. What factors could have contributed to such
contradictory results, how are the two experiments different?

Healthy male subjects were used in both experiments and both samples
were divided at the median into a "high" and a "low depression" group
on the basis of FPI scores, which were employed in both studies. There
are no significant differences in age, weight, or depression scores
between the subgroups of both studies. The number of subjects, however, was considerably higher in the present study (46 vs. 24)!

Both studies are well-controlled laboratory experiments. Application
of the medication was double-blind in each case and followed a cross-
over design. Lehmann and Hopes compared the effects of lofepramine
(140 mg) to imipramine and placebo. Thus, all subjects came for three
experimental sessions with drug-free intervals of one week respectively. We used the same dosage of lofepramine in our study, but employed
only a placebo group as control. Subjects came for one training and
merely two experimental sessions.

Both studies employed factorial designs with an identical procedure
concerning the personality factor (depression), but different ones
concerning the drug factor (three-level repeated measurements in the
Lehmann and Hopes' study vs. two levels in the present study). The
possible occurrence of serial effects with repeated measurements has
to be considered. The risk is possibly considerable if a highly potent
drug is used. Such was the case in the Lehmann and Hopes' study. Imipramine had quite strong negative effects on mood, performance, and
autonomic functioning later than one hour after drug ingestion, whereas lofepramine scarcely differed from placebo. In the Lehmann and
Hopes' study the number of subjects for each of the six possible per-
mutations was not balanced for the high and low depressive groups
(personal communication). We see a possible explanation here for their
results not being replicable.

The differing results cannot be due to different instruments for measuring mood, since both studies used the same (state EWL). Time of experiment (morning), inter-session intervals (one week), as well as
procedure in each session (baseline and time of testing) are quite
similar. There are several differences in the experimental setting,
however: Lehmann and Hopes tested the subjects singly, we used groups
of 4-6 subjects. We employed a few other performance variables, but

took no EEG. It seems rather unlikely, though, that such minor differences in the situation should be responsible for the mood changes
observed by Lehmann and Hopes.

One might question if the depression scores of the samples in both
investigations are comparable. The depression scores in the Lehmann
and Hopes' study (low depressive group $\bar{X}$=5.3; s=2.9; high depressive
group $\bar{X}$=15.1; s=3.5) are not significantly different from the ones in
the present experiment, however (Table 1).

Thus, two questions arise in the end: (1) Can we expect antidepressive
drug effects in healthy subjects (within the normal range of depressive deviations)? (2) Can we expect these effects after a single application of the drug?

The first question may be answered in the positive, although, up to
date, there is not enough empirical evidence. By using appropriate
designs which take into account individual characteristics of emotionality (depression) there may be a real chance for showing antidepressant effects in normals.

A positive answer to the second question, however, seems to be in
doubt. The results of the present study do not support such a hypothesis. Studies in other research areas, e.g. pharmacokinetic or biochemical studies, do not favour this hypothesis, either.

          STUDY II: ONE WEEK ADMINISTRATION OF LOFEPRAMINE

Introduction

It was the purpose of the second study to test the effects of lofepramine during a one-week administration. Because of economic reasons
only a group of selected subjects with high depression scores could
be treated. It was predicted that a kind of antidepressant effect
would appear in the group after repeated drug administration.

Methods

Subjects. Twenty-four "subdepressive" but clinically healthy male
students participated in the experiment as paid volunteers. Selections
of subjects out of 72 interested students was done on the basis of a
personality questionnaire (FPI) and a health questionnaire completed
during the notification at the institute. They were accepted if the
FPI depression score exceeded a cut off point; when they were without a history of psychiatric or organic, e.g. hepatic, renal or cardiac, disorder, and did not take any medicaments concurrently. During
the experiment they were instructed to adhere to their normal day-to-
day life, to avoid sleep deprivation and not to drink more than small
amounts of alcohol. One subject did not complete the experiment for
unknown reasons. Table 6 shows means and standard deviations for depression scores, age and weight, which can be compared to the corresponding data of study I in Table 1.

TABLE 6   Means and Standard Deviations for Depression
          Score (FPI), Age and Weight for the High De-
          pression Group of Study II

Group	Depression Score (FPI)	Age (Years)	Weight (kg)
High depressive subjects (N = 23)	$\bar{X}$ = 14.8 s = 6.1	$\bar{X}$ = 22.5 s = 2.7	$\bar{X}$ = 75.6 s = 9.6

Drug condition. On eight days the subjects took 70 mg lofepramine or
placebo in the morning (on day 1 and day 8 in the lab) and 70 mg lofepramine or placebo in the evening (except on day 8). A sham control of
regular drug intake was performed by collecting urine probes at day 1,
4 and 8.

Assessment procedure and instruments. Day 1 and day 8 testing was
done in the lab, in groups of six persons. The procedure was identical for both days and quite similar to that of study I (see Table 3):

Subjects came fasting and received a standard breakfast without caffeine at the institute at 8.30. The first trial served as practice
trial to be acquainted with the performance tests and adapted to the
lab. At 9.30 baseline was taken beginning with the subjective variables and followed by the performance tests. (Day 8 the practice trial
was also done but, due to knowledge, was done more quickly, so that
the beginning of the baseline and all consecutive procedures were
20 min earlier.)

After application of the drug subjects had to fill in personality
questionnaires (FPI, SDS, DS, Bf-S). There was a pause of 20 min
while a urine probe was taken and subjects had time for relaxed reading. The second test trial began exactly two hours after application
with assessment of subjective mood, somatic symptoms and performance.
It was finished 160 min after application.

The tests were the same as in study I. Furthermore two questionnaires
were given. During the seven days between the experimental sessions
in the lab the subjects had to complete a questionnaire about the
sleep every morning and an EWL (modified for the mood during the day)
every evening.

Data analysis. Verum and placebo group were compared at different
trials and different days by simple t-tests and U-tests (Mann-Whitney)

Results

There are no significant drug-placebo differences in the performance
area. The cardiac acceleration effect found for lofepramine in study I
still has not been replicated. In the emotional area, however, there
are significant drug-placebo differences, here concerning the subscales "anxiety" and "depression".

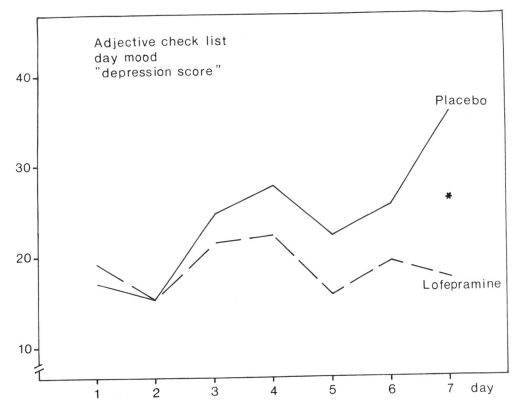

Fig. 2.   Mean depression scores of the adjective check list
           "day mood" for the seven days with placebo resp.
           lofepramine medication; *signifcant drug-placebo
           difference at p ∠ .05.

Figure 2 shows the results of the depression-subscale of the adjective
check list, which was given every evening and which reflects the day
mood. There are no drug-placebo differences on the first day of drug
administration. On the seventh day, however, the depression scores
are lower under lofepramine than under placebo. The same proves true
for the anxiety scale. When the subjects came to the lab on the eighth
day, they again showed different mood ratings under the two conditions.

Figure 3 shows the results of the depression-subscale of the adjective
check list, which was given during the testing session at the lab and
which reflects the actual mood. At the second testing time on the
eighth day, depression is scored higher under placebo than under lofepramine. For this method, however, the anxiety-subscale fails to show
corresponding results.

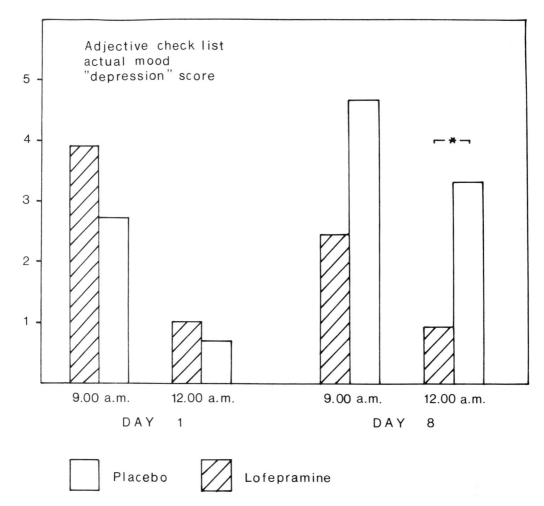

Fig. 3. Mean depression scores of the adjective check list
         "momentary mood" for the first and eighth day with
         placebo resp. lofepramine medication; * significant
         drug-placebo difference at p < .05.

Discussion

The results obtained seem to support the hypothesis that antidepressant effects could be demonstrated in human normals, when subjects
with high depression scores were selected and when drug ingestion was
repeated. The result confirms the findings of DiMascio and others
(1968).

There remain further questions, however:
(1) Despite the drug-placebo difference concerning the depression scores after repeated drug administration there is no clear reduction of the depression scores under lofepramine. Contrary to expectation, the drug-placebo difference becomes significant because of the incrementing depression scores under placebo. It is not difficult to explain this result, although it remains unsatisfying.
(2) Because of the puzzling result just mentioned it is difficult to determine on which day of drug ingestion the antidepressant effects develop. As the drug-placebo difference depends on the course of the scores under placebo it seems conceivable that any manipulation of testing parameters may alter the placebo response and thus the beginning of the development of the "antidepressant" effect.
(3) Since mean time curves admittedly may cover individual differences in time course, one has to consider this point. Yet, in the case given it does not make any sense, because there is no steady improvement under lofepramine.
(4) There is not enough information about the meaning of the personality characteristics studied by means of the questionnaires used.

GENERAL CONCLUSIONS

The investigation of individual differences in response to antidepressant drugs has just begun. A lot of effort will be necessary to clarify the problems connected with the present subject. It seems evident that studies with antidepressant drugs are much more extensive than those with other drugs according to our present knowledge of the necessity of repeated ingestions. Further studies will have to emphasize among other issues the evaluation of the relevant personality characteristics, the specification of the kind of drug responses, and the time aspects of the course of drug responses.

REFERENCES

Bättig, K., and H. Fischer (1964). Die Wirkung von Pharmaka auf psychische Leistungsfähigkeit und Persönlichkeitsfaktoren. Schweiz. Z. Psychol., 23, 26-38.

Blackwell, B., O. Lipkin, J. H. Meyer, R. Kuzma, and W. V. Boulter (1972). Dose responses and relationships between anticholinergic activity and mood with tricyclic antidepressants. Psychopharmacologia, 25, 205-217.

Broeren, W., and W. Schmitt (1964). Differentielle testpsychologische Effekte antidepressiver Pharmaka bei Normalpersonen. Neuropsychopharmacology, 4, 412-415.

Clayton, A. B., P. G. Harvey, and T. A. Betts (1977). The effects of two antidepressants, imipramine and viloxazine, upon driving performance. Psychopharmacology, 55, 9-12.

Degwitz, R. (1964). Zur Wirkungsweise von Psycholeptika anhand langfristiger Selbstversuche. Nervenarzt, 35, 491-496.

Degwitz, R. (1967). Leitfaden der Psychopharmakologie. Wiss. Verlagsanstalt, Stuttgart.

Dietsch, P., and W. Janke (1977). Mehrdimensionaler Depressionsfragebogen. Unpublished paper, Düsseldorf.

DiMascio, A., G. Heninger, and G. L. Klerman (1964). Psychopharmacology of imipramine: a comparative study of their effects in normal males. Psychopharmacologia, 5, 361-371.

DiMascio, A., R. E. Meyer, and L. Stifler (1968 Supp.). Effects of imipramine on individuals varying in level of depression. Am. J. Psychiatry, 124, 55-58.

Erdmann, G., and W. Janke (1975). Mehrdimensionale körperliche Symptomliste. Unpublished paper, Düsseldorf.

Eriksoo, E. O., and O. Rohte (1970). Chemistry and pharmacology of a new potential antidepressant. Arzneim. Forsch., 20, 1561-1569.

Fahrenberg, J., and H. Selg (1970). Das Freiburger Persönlichkeitsinventar FPI. Hogrefe, Göttingen.

Grünthal, E. (1958). Untersuchungen über die psychologische Wirkung des Thymoleptikums Tofranil. Psychiatr. Neurol., 136, 402-408.

Heimann, H., C. F. Reed, and P. N. Witt (1968). Some observations suggesting preservation of skilled motor acts despite drug-included stress. Psychopharmacologia, 13, 287-298.

Herrmann, W. M., and R. J. McDonald (1979). A multidimensional test approach for the description of the CNS activity of drugs in human pharmacology. Pharmacopsychiatr.-Neuropsychopharmacol., 11, 247-265.

Hollister, L. E. (1964). Effect of centrally-active drugs on mobilization of free fatty acids. Arch. Int. Pharmacodyn., 149, 362-365.

Hollister, L. E. (1972). Prediction of therapeutic uses of psychotherapeutic drugs from experiments with normal volunteers. Clin. Pharmacol. Ther., 13, 803-808.

Ideström, C. M. and B. Cadenius (1964). Imipramine-Desmethylimipramine, a pharmacological study on human beings. Psychopharmacologia, 5, 431-439.

Janke, W., and G. Debus (1978). Eigenschaftswörterliste (EWL). Hogrefe, Göttingen.

Janke, W., G. Debus, and N. Longo (1979). Differential psychopharmacology of tranquilizing and sedating drugs. Mod. Probl. Pharmacopsychiatry, 14, 13-98.

Karniol, I. G., J. Dalton, and M. Lader (1976). Comparative psychotropic effects of trazodone, imipramine and diazepam in normal subjects. Curr. Ther. Res., 20, 337-348.

Keeler, M. H., A. J. Prange, and C. B. Reifler (1966). Effects of imipramine and thioridazine on set and attention. Dis. Nerv. Syst., 27, 798-802.

Lehmann, E., and H. Hopes (1977a). Experimentelle Untersuchungen der psychophysiologischen Wirkung eines neuen Antidepressivums (Lofepramine im Vergleich zu Imipramine und Placebo). Arzneim. Forsch., 27, 1100-1104.

Lehmann, E., and H. Hopes (1977b). Differential effects of a single dose of imipramine and lofepramine in healthy subjects varying in their level of depression. Prog. Neuro-Psychopharmacol., 1, 155-164.

Matussek, N., and M. Aarons (1974). Wirkung akuter und chronischer Applikation von Maprotilin und ihre Beziehung zum Plasmaspiegel bei gesunden Versuchspersonen. Arzneim. Forsch., 24, 1107-1111.

Pöldinger, W. (1963). Comparison between imipramine and desimipramine in normal subjects and their action in depressive patients. Psychopharmacologia, 4, 302-307.

Saletu, B. (1976). Psychopharmaka, Gehirntätigkeit und Schlaf. Karger, Basel.

Seppälä, T. (1977). Psychomotor skills during acute and two-week treatment with mianserin (Org GB 94) and amitriptyline, and their combined effects with alcohol. Ann. Clin. Res., 9, 66-72.

Schmitt, W., and H. Seifert (1960). Experimentalpsychologische und klinische Untersuchungen mit dem Iminodibenzylderivat Imipramin. Med. Exp., 3, 52-81.

Wittenborn, J. R., C. F. Flaherty, W. E. McGough, K. A. Bossange,and
   R. J. Nash (1976). A comparison of the effect of imipramine, nomi-
   fensine and placebo on the psychomotor performance of normal males.
   Psychopharmacology, 51, 85-90.
Zerssen v., D. (1976). Die Befindlichkeits-Skala. Beltz, Weinheim.
Zlatnikova, J., U. Consbruch, R. Degwitz, and R. Hampel (1974). Über
   die Wirkung von Amitriptylin in langfristigen Selbstversuchen.
   Arzneim. Forsch., 24, 1103-1106.
Zung, W. W. K. (1965). A self-rating depression scale. Arch. Gen.
   Psychiatry, 12, 63-70.

RELATIONSHIPS BETWEEN PERSONALITY AND PHARMACO-THERAPEUTIC RESPONSES AMONG DEPRESSED PATIENTS

J. R. Wittenborn

ABSTRACT

Some individual differences in response to antidepressant drugs may be a reflection of individual difference in the pretreatment severity of the various symptoms. Among patients having a given level of a particular symptom, however, there are individual differences in remissive changes in that symptom. These differences in the responsiveness of a given symptom to a particular medication pose the central prediction problem in clinical psychopharmacology.

After a preliminary review of methodological considerations, the present report surveys the inquiries that have examined the possibility that pretreatment differences in non-symptomatic respects are associated with treatment-related responses in symptom levels. The evidence for such predictive possibilities is relatively meager, and it appears that the pretreatment metabolic characteristics of the patient may offer as much predictive potential as do pretreatment epidemiologic or characterologic differences.

KEYWORDS

Prediction; global improvement; antidepressant drugs; symptom change; individual differences; MHPG; multivariate, partial correlation.

INTRODUCTION

A useful discussion of the prediction of antidepressant drug effects involves many clarifying distinctions. With few exceptions, the behaviour of depressed patients and of other individuals as well seems to be in constant change which varies from patient to patient in kind, as well as in amount. These changes seem to be multiplely determined and in part reflect changes in the circumstances of the patient's life and of his perception of his circumstances. The changes may reflect the course of pathological processes that may or may not be directly related to his depressive state. The changes may be treatment-induced, and records of change may also reflect differences between or within the observers.

Since the behavioral changes generated by antidepressant medication
may be no different from those generated by a diversity of other influences, the possibility that drug-related changes are confounded
with changes having some other origin can never be disregarded and
must be reckoned with in any effort to gauge or anticipate changes in
response to treatment. Accordingly, it has become customary to
associate a given psychotropic medication with any change that does
not occur in the absence of the medication.

This interpretation of the problem has resulted in a widespread in-
vestigational use of placebo comparisons. These placebo comparisons
must be conducted under the familiar conventions of random assign-
ments of either the drug in question or an indistinguishable placebo.
The subjects should be drawn from a relatively homogeneous population,
and assignment to treatment, care of patients, and assessments of
changes should all be under doubleblind conditions. The research alternative to the use of indistinguishable placebo involves the determination of at least some portion of a dose-response curve. Instead
of using comparisons with placebo where drug-no drug is the independent variable and the dependent variable is some measure of behavioral
change, the independent variable is the amount of medication (other
than zero amount), and the dependent variable remains some measure
of relevant change. Although these paradigms for comparison may be
simply described, the actual preparation for and conduct of such research can be an onerous task requiring sedulous vigilance from start
to finish.

Planning an effective assessment of drug response requires some preliminary knowledge of the drug, such as probable effects and latency
of effect, and some knowledge of the condition under treatment. If
the period of observation is too short, there may have been too little
time for the pertinent behavior changes to have occurred. If the period of observation is too long, spontaneous remissive changes can
have modified the placebo group in the same manner as the drug group
has been therapeutically modified.

There is always the possibility of confounding in the form of concurrent psychotherapeutic influences or other palliative influences
of staff, family, or other patients. The amount and nature of these
influences may vary in consequence of the apparent need of the patient.
For these and other reasons, therapeutic effects of a given drug are
subject to underestimation.

When change in some measurable aspect of a depressive state is accepted as a suitable criteron for antidepressant effect, one must consider how this effect can be expressed in terms of summaries that are
familiar and involve formal quantitative manipulation. These manipulations should include a conventional test of statistical significance
of inter-treatment changes. These tests are often accepted as sufficient
evidence of therapeutic effect despite the fact that the test may bear
no necessary relationship with the magnitude of either the effect or
its practical significance. Since virtually every investigator is
familiar with procedures for testing the statistical significance of
differences between means, the significance of mean differences between
groups provides the principal and often the only terms whereby treatment effects are summarized, compared, and communicated to others.
Sometimes the mean posttreatment assessment for the treatment group
is compared with the respective mean for the placebo group, regardless

of any pretreatment differences between the groups. Sometimes the average of the pretreatment-posttreatment change within a group is used to express treatment effects and is compared with the respective change in the placebo group. Most investigators, however, are aware that a simple difference between pretreatment and posttreatment measures contains the unreliability of the pretreatment measurement, as well as that of the posttreatment measure, and they strive to reduce instrumental error by subtracting from the posttreatment score only that portion of the pretreatment score which is correlated with the posttreatment score. Such corrections based on the regression of the posttreatment score on a pretreatment score correct not only for pretreatment differences between the drug and the placebo groups, but correct for some of the irrelevant variability within the groups. This approach (e.g., analysis of covariance or analysis of residual scores) generates a measure of change that is probably more pertinent and sensitive than a simple pretreatment-posttreatment difference, or worse, an uncorrected posttreatment score. It is apparent, therefore, that the meaning of a test of the significance of a treatment effect can vary with the manner in which treatment effect is quantified.

A mean is commonly used as if it implied that all members of the sample change to an equal degree. Despite this uncritical use, it is generally acknowledged that the amount and speed of improvement varies from patient to patient, that some patients may not have changed during the period of observation, and that others may have worsened. Despite its arithmetic convenience and its advantages for parametric analyses, the mean is not sufficiently informative for clinical purposes, and some other basis for comparison, e.g., the portion who improved to some specified degree, the portion who became asymptomatic, or the portion who worsened, may have more clinical pertinence than the mean and should be included in the quantification of therapeutic effects.

Although the mean may not be the best approach to assessing or even identifying significant clinical changes, something of interest has happened to at least some of the patients if there are significant differences in mean change between the treatment and the placebo group. Because of the intrinsic heterogeneity of all clinical samples, however, it is possible that some patients may be changed in an important way without this change's being reflected in a statistically significant contrast between the means. If, for example, a drug helps some members of a heterogeneous sample and hinders others (e.g., helps young patients, but impairs old patients), there might not be an important change in the mean, but there could be significant change in the sample variance so that the variance of the experimental group would be increased significantly more than the variance of the control group. In a heterogeneous sample, a drug might modify the rank order or the relative standing of the members of the group (e.g., allay the anxiety among those who were initially most severe and generate misgivings among those who were initially free from anxiety). There might be no treatment-group contrast between treatment group means, but the magnitude and possibly the sign of the pretreatment-posttreatment correlation in the treatment group might be different from that found in the placebo group.

All diagnosable psychopathologies are characterized by a somewhat different spectrum of symptomatic manifestations. Nevertheless, very few patients diagnosed as suffering from a particular psychopathology will be found to manifest all the symptoms that are said to be charac-

teristic of that diagnosis, and it may be expected that patients having
a given diagnosis will differ from each other with respect to the symptoms they manifest, as well as with respect to the severity of the
symptoms. The patients may differ also in the order in which the symptom
emerge during the development of the episode and the order in which they
may remit during the course of recovery.

It will be useful for the purposes of the present discussion to distinguish between two points of view: (1) Some students of psychopathology have found it comfortable to assume that the familiar diagnostic
entities represent respectively different diseases, and that although
there is some diversity in the symptomatic respects in which the disease may disturb behaviour, any symptomatic manifestations of the
diagnosed psychopathologies may yield in response to an effective treatment. On this basis, those who hold to the disease point of view consider a rating of overall severity or a rating of global improvement
in response to treatment to provide an assessment, which is not only
sufficient, but also may be preferable to ratings of specific symptomatic manifestations.
(2) There is a second point of view which does not depend upon an
assumption that each diagnosable psychopathology is an expression of
some specific underlying process of mental disease. This simplistic,
direct approach regards the manifest symptoms as an occasion for initiating treatment and accepts the symptoms as a proper basis for selecting a treatment among the available alternatives. The remission
of these symptoms leads to the assumption that the treatment has been
effective.

It is assumed that the interests of the patients are best served by
an approach that considers the amelioration of his symptoms in terms
of medications that are known to be effective for those symptoms.
Where there is a choice of equally effective medications for those
symptoms of a given patient, the preferred medication is the one that
has been most effective in patients having pretreatment nonsymptomatic
characteristics similar to the characteristics of the patient under
treatment. Among such nonsymptomatic pretreatment qualities could be
included age, demographic factors, personality attributes,and the
history of the present or prior episodes, including response to treatment. It is important to distinguish between those pretreatment individual differences that are target symptoms for the treatment and other
pretreatment individual differences that are not expected to change in
the course of treatment.

The pretreatment level of a given symptom is sometimes used as a predictor of posttreatment improvement in that particular symptom, in
some associated symptom, or in some unspecified group of symptoms which
includes the symptom used as a predictor. Correlating pretreatment
"part" scores with posttreatment "whole" scores which comprise the part
score is often disguised by a procedure where the pretreatment level of
a given major symptom is correlated with rating of global improvement.
A high correlation between the pretreatment level of a major symptom
and a posttreatment global improvement score reflects the fact that
individuals whose pretreatment level of a major (i.e., pathognomonic-
ally important) symptom is high may experience a large reduction in
that symptom and as a consequence be awarded a high rating of global
improvement. The opportunity for a relatively large global improvement is obviously diminished when the pretreatment level of a major
symptom is low. A high "predictive" correlation between a given pretreatment symptom and a global improvement rating may be a reflection

of the fact that the symptom in question is remitting in response to
treatment. When the correlation between a pretreatment symptom and improvement is viewed in this manner, questions of procedural economy
and analytical clarity may be raised. The identification of those symptoms that show remissive changes in response to a treatment can best
be approached by a direct method which examines the significance of
the improvement in the respective symptoms and does not confound the
prediction of improvement with the assessment of improvement.

In its simplest form the predictive model involves two variables: y,
a criterion of efficacy (e.g., some measure of a treatment-related
change in some symptom) and x, some variable (e.g., age of the patient)
that is operationally independent of both y and the treatment per se.
If there is a relationship of predictive potential, it can be shown
that y varies as a function of x. As a first approximation, this function is usually regarded as linear in nature, particularly in studies
of human behavior. The summarizing coefficient for the strength of this
relationship can be a correlation coefficient or some other measure of
contingency. The predictive utility of such post hoc relationships,
however, requires cross validation in an independent sample, a step
that is neglected by most investigators although they may involve the
word "prediction" in the title of their reports.

SOME DESIDERATA

The use of pretreatment individual differences for predicting the individual's response to a given pharmacotherapy depends upon a series
of preliminary accomplishments. The necessary preconditions for useful prediction of individual response to a given pharmacotherapy may
be described in a diversity of ways, but the following outline is proposed for the present purposes:

I   Implicit in the predictive effort is the assumption that there is
     a dependable, i.e., reproducible, treatment effect. A verifiable
     therapeutic effect in turn implies that certain conditions have
     been met.
     A.   Any assessment used as one of the criteria of effectiveness
          should be identifiable as at least part of the distress that
          brought the patient to treatment and should have an unambiguous
          meaning. Such freedom from ambiguity requires that the assess-
          ment be conducted in a formal standardized manner and repre-
          sent some definite aspect of the behavioral deviation under
          treatment. For example, a symptom rating of anxiety has a more
          definite meaning than a global rating of severity of illness.
     B.   Obviously, the criterion measure of change must be reliable,
          and any assessment that verifies a therapeutic effect in in-
          dependent samples must, of necessity, possess a de facto re-
          liability, whether or not the reliability had been pre-estab-
          lished by formal trials. The reliability of the criterion is
          critical for predictive purposes because prediction requires
          a substantial correlation between a treatment-associated change
          in a more or less fallible measure of effect with a more or
          less fallible predictor variable. Thus, the intrinsic predictive
          potential can be obscured by the instrumental fallibility (i.e.,
          unreliability) of the pretreatment assessment, of the posttreat-
          ment assessment, and of the predictor variables. Since instru-
          mental error is by definition variable and unrelated with any-

thing including itself, these three sources of unreliability are independent and, therefore, cumulative in their effect on any measure of predictive relationship. Instrumental errors impose an important limitation on verifications of treatment effects and should be minimized.

C.   In order that a therapeutic effect be verified by independent replication, the samples should be drawn from a common population and be equivalent with respect to such qualifying factors as demographic and clinical history. The essential features of the sample should be documented in all research reports.

D.   The research reports should specify the dosage range, the schedule, the mode of administration, and the duration of treatment.

E.   In order for therapeutic effects to be verified, the research reports must describe the context in which the treatment is conducted, and this description should include documentation of confounding influences, whether in the form of concurrent medication, psychotherapy, untoward side effects, or unrelated pathology.

F.   Both the original report of efficacy and the independent confirmation should be based on a double blind placebo control. In the treatment of psychopathologies, particularly those that tend to remit spontaneously, comparisons with a standard drug in the absence of placebo control has no definite meaning unless the drug under investigation is found to be more effective than the standard drug. Studies which show the drug under investigation to be equivalent to the standard drug have little communication value. In a given study, the lack of contrast between the drugs can be explained in many ways and does not require the conclusion that both drugs are effective and equally so.

G.   Since there is a diversity of ways in which data may be summarized, research reports must specify both the manner in which the basic observations are quantified and the manner in which the quantitative expressions for the treatment-associated changes are developed. It is important as well to state explicitly the quantitative nature of the intergroup comparisons and the nature of the tests of significance that have been applied.

II Potential predictors of therapeutic effects can be identified on an ex post facto basis in consequence of surveys. In typical surveys (often called predictive studies), any number of pretreatment factors are examined for their association with one or more criteria of therapeutic effect. Although these candidates for predictive use are often presented to the reader as predictors, it is rare indeed that attempts are made to confirm the potential predictive merit by independent cross-validating inquiry. Regardless of the pertinence that may inhere in their substantive nature, a promising predictor may be expected to have certain qualities:

A.   A promising predictor must possess a content that is readily conceptualized and subject to explicit definition and quantitative determination. This quantification must have a de facto reliability. At the very least this means that the procedures involved in generating the predictor datum are defined in a manner sufficiently explicit to permit them to be "standardized".

B. The pretreatment variables that have been surveyed for predictive potential may be divided into two classes:
1. characteristics that are the object of treatment, i.e.,
symptoms or groups of symptoms under treatment (or groups
of patients characterized by groups of symptoms associated
with the disorder)
2. characteristics that are not the object of treatment, presumably do not change during the course of treatment, and
were characteristic of the patients prior to the episode.
Symptoms, symptom complexes, or groups of patients characterized by symptom complexes are not appropriate predictor variables. The examination of such qualities as potential predictors
is at best a clumsy, indirect, and sometimes misleading evaluation of the therapeutic sensitivity of characteristics that
should be regarded as objects of treatment. For the present
purposes, a true predictor is not a quality that emerges at
the time of the episode and changes as a result of an effective
treatment.

The present approach identifies the predictive task as one of
determining the degree to which patients who have a symptom
that is expected to yield in response to treatment may be separated before treatment in terms of the expected response of
that symptom to the treatment in question. The looked-for
guide to the desired prediction is some pretreatment attribute
or circumstance that is correlated with treatment-induced remissive changes. Such distinguishing pretreatment attributes
are not expected to be modified by the treatment.

C. A pretreatment attribute or circumstance that has been found
to be associated with remissive changes subsequent to a given
treatment may be associated as well with remissive changes
following some other treatment or no treatment at all. This
possibility must be examined as a part of the post hoc exploration for possible predictors. Thus, the association between
the principal predictor and a remissive symptomatic response
in the group receiving active medication must be compared with
the magnitude of that association in the group receiving
placebo.

III After a pretreatment variable has been shown to be correlated with
some remissive change in response to the medication under consideration and is not found to be similarly correlated with a respective change in consequence of placebo, there remains the task
of establishing the predictive utility of this potential predictor.
A. If the correlation between the predictor and the criterion of
change is verifiable in independent trials and is not found
in the placebo group, the predictor is not merely a characteristic of those who show remissive changes regardless of
whether they are treated. As a consequence, a further test of
the utility of the predictive relationship is in order. The
utility of such a predictive relationship lies in its value
as a guide to the choice of the most efficacious treatment
for a given patient. If an alternative therapeutic principle
is available (e.g., a monoamineoxidase inhibitor as contrasted
with a tricyclic substance for antidepressant use), it is
necessary to show that a pretreatment quality (e.g., a paranoid suspiciousness) has a predictive function for a specific
symptom (e.g., anxiety) for MAO inhibitors, but has no com-

parable predictive relationship for changes in anxiety among
patients treated with tricyclic medication.

B. The final proof of predictive practicality requires an application of the predictive relationship in a situation where it
might actually be applied. Such proof would require a trial
where the therapeutic consequence of a procedure which employed the predictive knowledge in assigning the alternative
treatment to patients was compared with the therapeutic consequence of assigning the alternative treatment without benefit
of the predictive knowledge. If the sample of patients in which
predictive knowledge was used responded significantly better
(particularly with respect to the symptom for which the predictor was explicit) than the sample where the predictive knowledge was not used, the predictive knowledge might have sufficient merit to justify its general use in selecting alternative
treatments for individual patients.

C. Having established the predictive practicality of a relationship, there remains the issue of the "cost-benefit" ratio.
The "cost-benefit" concept may be expressed in different ways.
The relationship may be expressed in terms of the convenience
of the therapeutic team, the advantages for the patient, or
the economy of society as a functioning process.

ILLUSTRATIVE STUDIES

The English language reports of antidepressant drug effects comprise
a voluminous and diversified literature, but relatively few studies
provide a systematic examination of relationships between pretreatment
characteristics of the patients and their response to antidepressant
medication.
The reports cited here are representative of the principal approaches
to "predictive" inquiry in the clinical psychopharmacology of depression

Most of the studies did not compare the relationship between pretreatment attribute and therapeutic response in the medicated group with
the respective relationship between pretreatment attribute and therapeutic response in a comparable placebo group. Thus, most of the reports of a potential predictive relationship did not address the
question of whether the relationship was unique to the treatment under
consideration or might be found among patients who received no treatment.

The literature contains several reports of studies which do not provide placebo comparisons, but do describe a relationship between nonsymptomatic pretreatment characteristics of depressed patients and
the overall response to a psychotropic medication. These uncontrolled
reports can generate uncertainty concerning the relationship between
characteristics of patients and response to antidepressant drugs. For
example, in 1962, Kiloh and others found age over 40 to be associated
with a good response to imipramine. In 1963, however, Hordern and
others reported that older patients and post menopausal patients
responded more favorably to amitriptyline than to imipramine, but in
1968, McConaghy and others reported that patients over 40 responded
no better to amitriptyline than did patients under 40. It is probable
that the inclusion of placebo comparison groups would have eliminated
some of the uncertainty generated by these reports. Possibly the inter-
drug differences were minor relative to a contrast with placebo.

Some of the reports of studies without a placebo control have described relationships between specific pretreatment symptoms and improvement in some global melange of unspecified symptoms. If the medication is effective in reducing a major pretreatment symptom, all other things equal, the higher the pretreatment symptom rating the greater the potential diminution in a global score which, in some manner, includes the major symptom and other associated symptoms. Some investigators classified or typed the patients on the basis of groups of pretreatment symptoms and then examined the relationship between the patient's symptom-based class and global response to treatment.

An interesting study following this general model was reported by Prusoff and Paykel (1977). Their depressed patients were classified as either "psychotic" or one of three subtypes of "neurotic" according to their symptoms as represented in a modification of the Hamilton Depression Scale.
These different classes of patients were compared with respect to their treatment-related change (analysis of covariance) in global severity rating. This report confirms earlier reports of a similar inquiry (Paykel, 1972; Paykel and others, 1973) and indicates that the nonpsychotic (i.e., nonendogenous) neurotic patients comprise subtypes that respond differentially to amitriptyline. Specifically, the anxious subgroup did not respond as well as the other neurotic groups or as well as the psychotic group. Since this covariance approach "corrects" the posttreatment global severity rating by considering pretreatment global severity rating, the authors might claim that they had eliminated any confounding between pretreatment symptoms implicit in the symptom based classification and the "corrected" posttreatment general severity. Nevertheless, one cannot be sure that the various determiners (e.g., "anxiety") of the pretreatment classifications had the same respective importance in the pretreatment rating of global severity as they had in the posttreatment rating of global severity. The reader cannot be certain that the covariance analysis freed the relationship between the pretreatment classification and change in global severity from confounding with pretreatment symptoms that determined both the predictor class and the posttreatment general severity rating. In this study, the symptom-based pretreatment classification, anxious depression, may be a predictor only in the sense that it is defined by symptoms less responsive to amitriptyline than symptoms defining other classes of patients.

The structure of the Prusoff and Paykel (1977) report is similar to that of an earlier report by Overall and others (1966). These collaborators grouped depressed patients on the basis of their ratings on the various symptoms comprising the BPRS. They used change in the mean of the 16 BPRS symptoms as a criterion of therapeutic effect and found that patients classified as "anxious" responded better to thioridazine than did patients classified as "retarded". This finding could be interpreted to mean that patients with pretreatment symptoms of anxiety and tension could be expected after treatment with a tranquilizing drug to show improvement in a composite score which included symptoms of anxiety and tension, and patients with pretreatment symptoms of withdrawal, retardation, and blunted affect would not respond to a major tranquilizer. The Overall and coworkers (1966) study was offered as evidence that different drugs have different patterns of symptomatic effect and was not presented as a predictive inquiry.

The typological or classificatory approach to the predictive problem was examined by Wittenborn (1969) in a manner designed to minimize

any confounding between the classification of the patient and pretreatment symptoms that were a target of therapy. A sample of 106
women hospitalized for treatment of depression and assigned to imipramine treatment were classified in the following step-wise manner:

Step 1:   Involutional.
     Select patients for whom the first depressive hospitalization
     occurred after the age of forty-five.
Step 2:   Schizophrenic qualities.
     From the patients remaining after Step 1, select those who
     now have, or in prior hospitalizations were reported to have,
     schizophrenic qualities, whether pseudoneurotic, schizo-
     affective, or other.
Step 3:   Manic-depressive.
     From the patients remaining after Steps 1 and 2, select those
     who have had at least one prior manic episode and one prior
     depressive hospitalization.
Step 4:   Reactive.
     From the patients remaining after Steps 1, 2, and 3, select
     those for whom the current hospitalization is a part of a
     first depressive episode and for whom there are clear indica-
     tions of external causes.
Step 5:   Residual.
     Include the remaining depressed patients, regardless of sym-
     ptoms, as a residual group.

These five classes of patients were compared on the basis of therapeutic response as indicated by a 26-item symptom rating scale (modified
WPRS). The responses of the patients in the involutional, schizophrenic
quality, and manic-depressive classes were all relatively unfavorable
to imipramine, while the responses of the patients in the reactive and
residual classes were favorable. On this basis the five subclasses
were reduced to two , those who tended to respond favorably and those
who tended to respond unfavorably.

In order to assure that the favorable and unfavorable responses to
these classes were drug related and not a difference that would emerge
in response to placebo, data for a comparable sample of 65 placebo patients were secured and compared with a comparable group of 66 imiprami
patients.

For three symptoms indicative of a social and emotional withdrawal
(indifferent to own appearance, does not smile, and spends all time
alone), the patients who were in the favorable class tended to get
better and those in the unfavorable class tended to get worse, regardless of the treatment. Thus, for these three symptoms, the changes
were not drug related.

There was also a group of five symptoms which suggested an hostile,
anti-social state as indicated by restlessness, assaultiveness, irrelevant use of words, avoidance of people, and fear of impending doom
In the imipramine group, particularly, these five symptoms tended to
improve among the patients with a favorable classification, and worsen
among those with an unfavorable classification.

Some investigators have used pretreatment biological characteristics,
particularly the excretion of 3-methoxy-4-hydroxyphenylglycol (MHPG),
in anticipating response to antidepressant medication. In 1972, Maas
and others reported that depressed patients who excreted relatively
small amounts of MHPG prior to treatment were rated as having a better

overall response to tricyclic medication (imipramine or desipramine) than patients whose excretion of MHPG had been relatively high prior to treatment. In 1974, Beckman and Goodwin used 16 unipolar depressed patients to compare the response to imipramine with the response to amitriptyline in terms of the pretreatment excretion of MHPG. They reported that the relationship between global therapeutic response and pretreatment MHPG excretion was negative for imipramine, thereby confirming the prior report of Maas and others (1972), but that the relationship was positive for amitriptyline, i.e. patients whose pretreatment level of MHPG was relatively high responsed better to amitriptyline treatment than those for whom pretreatment level of MHPG was relatively low. The predictive potential of the relationship between pretreatment MHPG excretion and response to antidepressant medication was applied in the selection of an appropriate treatment for depressed patients (Cobbin and others, 1979). An experimental group of depressed patients was assigned either to amitriptyline or to imipramine, nortriptyline, or desipramine on the basis of the relationships described by Beckman and Goodwin (1975). The therapeutic response of this experimental group was compared with the response of similar patients who had been treated with tricyclic drugs in the same treatment setting, but without guidance based on the differential MHPG principle described by Beckman and Goodwin. It was found that the patients in the experimental group for whom alternative tricyclic medication had been selected on the basis of pretreatment MHPG levels improved significantly more than the patients who had been treated without consideration of pretreatment MHPG level in selection of medication.

Although it has been found that there is a decrease in MHPG during the course of tricyclic antidepressant medication, MHPG level is not ordinarily considered to be an objective of antidepressant medication. Since pretreatment level of MHPG can be either positively or negatively correlated with therapeutic outcome depending upon whether the medication assigned is amitriptyline or imipramine, pretreatment MHPG is not considered to be confounded with symptoms of depression.

The relationship between pretreatment MHPG and response to treatment was not examined for a placebo group, but it was established that MHPG has contrasting implications for response to two different tricyclic antidepressants (imipramine and amitriptyline). Low pretreatment MHPG is not predictive of all remissive changes. Various aspects of this relationship have been confirmed by independent investigation (Rosenbaum and others, 1980).

Whether biological predictors of differential therapeutic response are intrinsically more pertinent than the great diversity of phenomenological predictors that have been explored by other investigators is a question that may well be asked, but cannot be answered at this time. It seems, however, that the many different phenomenological investigators, despite their prolific efforts, tend to start somewhere' near the beginning and rarely advance to a position where they are willing or able to confirm relationships reported by themselves or others.

Despite the fact that inquiries have been designed to show interaction between specific nonsymptom pretreatment factors and specific response to alternative treatments, very little evidence of such interaction has been found for antidepressant medication, and numerous studies have failed to find any evidence of interaction. A series of

four reports, which included features of specific nonsymptom predictor
variables and specific, as opposed to global, criterion measures was
provided by Raskin and his collaborators (Raskin and others, 1973;
Raskin, 1974; Raskin and Crook, 1975, 1976). In the 1973 report, Raskin
and others described two studies. One provided comparisons among diazepam, phenelzine, and placebo. The other compared chlorpormazine,
imipramine, and placebo. The eight pretreatment predictor variables
were age, sex, marital status, education, social desirability, number
of prior episodes, amount of prehospitalization medication, and pretreatment severity of illness. Six of these could be considered nonsymptomatic and independent of any treatment effects. This report of
collaborative studies was based on large samples (555 in the diazepam study and 325 in the imipramine study). In this report the criterion of therapeutic effect was severity of depression at three
weeks. In the analyses some of the variables (age, sex, and marital
status) were treated categorically in a search for interactions with
treatment effect. None was found. The other predictors were treated
as continuous variables with separate regression analyses for each
of the treatment groups. There was no significant difference between
the treatments in regression equations. This lack of differentiating
predictive indications characterized both studies described in the
1973 report.

Since the samples were sufficiently large, separate subsamples could
be made on the basis of categorical predictors, and within one of
these subsamples (married men) there were intertreatment group differences in the regression weights for certain variables, particularly
age and education. Among the married men, the good responders to imipramine were over 40 and had good educational backgrounds. In contrast, the good chlorpromazine responders among the married men were
relatively young. These nonsymptomatic pretreatment factors were not
discriminative among married female patients, and they bore no relationship to treatment response in the placebo group. The analysis
of these data was continued in a later report (Raskin, 1974). In this
later analysis, various specific symptomatic aspects of drug response
were examined, and a significant interaction was found. Among young
females, hostility was exacerbated by imipramine.

Response to chlorpromazine and imipramine is differentially influenced
on the basis of sex and race also (Raskin and Crook, 1975). In this
report, based on data from 555 white and 159 black depressed patients
in various collaborating mental hospitals, chlorpromazine, imipramine,
and placebo were compared on the basis of 20 different criterion
measures. Although there were no drug-by-race interactions, there
were significant drug-by-race-by-sex interactions. These were found
for eight of the 20 outcome measures. The responses of white men and
women were similar, but it was clear that for the black men imipramine was most efficacious, particularly for ratings of depression
and social participation, but chlorpromazine was most beneficial for
the black women, particularly for the relief of tension, anxiety,
and insomnia.

Raskin and Crook (1976) applied diagnostic distinctions in their
search for pretreatment characteristics that would interact with drug
response in depressed patients. They generated four classes or types
of patients by intercorrelating and factor analyzing 880 depressed
patients for a sample of 33 variables presumably pertinent to an endogenous-neurotic distinction. Four groups of patients were defined

in this manner. Group 2 was identified as neurotic depressives and group 3 was accepted as endogenous depressives. Although some of these variables were symptomatic in character, most of them were not, and as a consequence the possible confounding between the pretreatment typology and the criteria of therapeutic response was limited and acceptable for the present purposes.

Twenty-one different measures of drug response were applied and showed numerous indications that the drugs were more effective than placebo. Nevertheless, none of the four diagnostic groups interacted with any of the three treatments examined in the first study. Specifically, there was no evidence that chlorpromazine, imipramine, or placebo was better in any respect for one diagnostic group than for other groups. A second sample comparing diazepam, phenelzine and placebo was included in this report. These medications failed also to show evidence of being in some respect superior for one or more of the diagnostic groups. The interaction between drug response and patient type was explored. There were no more significant interactions than would have been expected on the basis of chance alone. Since one of the types they have generated could be identified as endogenous and another as neurotic, this study could not support a commonly held belief that imipramine is a poor choice for neurotic patients and a preferred treatment for endogenous patients. In fact, patients who fell into the neurotic class responded particularly well, regardless of whether they were treated with imipramine or chlorpromazine.

Rickels and others (1970) compared amitriptyline, chlordiazepoxide, and placebo in a sample of 243 mildly depressed outpatients. The predictive variable was a distinction between clinic and private practice patients, and the criteria of change were the several symptomatic components of the Physician Depression Scale (PDS). When treated by amitriptyline, the private practice patients showed somewhat greater improvement than the clinic patients in mood and in psychomotor retardation. This relationship was reversed in the patients receiving placebo, however. In this group, private patients improved less than clinic patients. Later Downing and Rickels (1972) examined the relationship for many pretreatment variables. Some were symptomatic in nature,such as the subscores of the Physician Depression Scale; others were concerned with the patient's medical and social history and certain demographic factors. The treatments were amitriptyline and placebo. There were two significant relationships between treatment outcome and pretreatment factors unrelated with the patient's current symptoms or manner of treatment; specifically, education and social class were related with response to amitriptyline. Other social and demographic factors did not interact with treatment effect.

The present review of illustrative studies provides little indication that nonsymptom pretreatment individual differences have an important relationship with posttreatment status, particularly symptomatic status. In the available studies global or composite ratings were the most frequently used criterion of therapeutic effects. Many investigators tended to limit their inquiry to individual differences in global response as a function of individual differences in pretreatment symptoms (or groups of symptoms) that could be a target of therapeutic effect and could, therefore, be confounded with the criterion of global response.

Although aspects of the patient's medical or social history have been examined as potential predictors of therapeutic effect, there is little evidence concerning the potential predictive value of pretreatment expressions of the patient's personality, particularly the personality qualities that may be indicative of enduring traits as contrasted with expressions of his state at the time that he is presented for treatment.

Accordingly, certain aspects of a complex investigation by Wittenborn, 1966a, 1966b) are reviewed with sufficient detail to illustrate some methodological and substantive features of this approach to the predictive quest. The sample   comprised women in their childbearing years who had been recently hospitalized because of a depressive episode. None of the women was considered to be schizophrenic, addicted or suffering from a desease of the central nervous system. They had been assigned in random order under doubleblind conditions to treatment with placebo, iproniazid, imipramine, or ECT. Dosage was regulated according to the apparent requirements of the patient. The post-treatment assessment, which was a duplicate of the pretreatment assessment battery, was conducted when the patient was ready to leave the hospital or at the end of a maximal treatment period of ten weeks.

For the present purposes, the most interesting criteria of pharmaco-therapeutic response are changes in the symptom rating scale scores (WPRS) (Wittenborn, 1964) for depression, anxiety, and phobia. The most interesting predictor variables include two state measures (the pretreatment WPRS ratings of paranoia and the presence of suicidal behavior (56% of the women had made suicidal gestures)) and two trait measures of the patient's premorbid personality (a) an irresponsible tendency to displace hostility and deny blame, b) a self-critical, dependent disposition). The pretreatment paranoid quality and a record of suicidal gestures may be considered expressive of the patient's personality at the time of the episode. The tendencies to displace and to be self-critical were based on social worker's interviews with family informants. These interviews covered a standard body of information and were directed toward a description of the patient's premorbid history and premorbid personality traits. The composition of the paranoid score for symptom ratings (WPRS), as well as the scores based on the social worker's description of the personality (Wittenborn and others, 1964), was based on separate factor analyses of data from patient samples and has been confirmed by independent replication.

A multivariate discriminant analysis was used to show that the battery of criteria of therapeutic response did distinguish among the several treatments considered, and canonical correlation was used to show that there were significant relationships between the criteria of therapeutic response and the measures of predictive interest, including the several aspects of personality.

Since the various personality characteristics may be expected to be interecorrelated, an attempt was made to examine the role of each personality quality independently of the other personality qualities. Partial correlations were used for this purpose.

TABLE 1   Significant Partial Correlations between Personality
           Qualities and Posttreatment Scores* for Depression

Personality Quality	Placebo n = 50	Iproniazid n = 32	Imipramine n = 50	ECT n = 47
Paranoia (state)		.54	.52	
Suicidal (state)		-.44	-.35	
Displacing (trait)	-.35			
Self-critical (trait)			.53	

* Adjusted for pretreatment differences

Table 1 summarizes the significant partial correlations between remissive changes in the depressed symptom scores and scores for the
four aspects of personality. Correlations having a negative sign indicate that the personality quality is associated with a diminution
of depression.

The partial correlations for the placebo group indicate that the
patients with a displacing, irresponsible personality may show more
spontaneous reduction in depression than those who do not tend to
manifest the displacing disposition.

The partial correlations for the iproniazid group show that patients
who have pretreatment paranoid symptoms may show less remissive
change in depression than people who are free of such symptoms. In
the iproniazid group the patients who had suicidal tendencies showed
greater reduction of depressive symptoms than those who had not mani-
fested suicidal behavior.

The imipramine group was similar to the iproniazid group in the sense
that pretreatment paranoid symptoms were inversely related with reduction in depression and that patients who had been suicidal showed
remissive changes in depression. In addition, however, the correlations for the imipramine group showed that the self-critical, dependent patient tended not to be among those who responded with remissive
changes in depression.

It should be observed that the size and sign of the correlation coefficients are descriptive of the within-treatment group pattern of
association and provide no indication of whether the average change
in the group showed improvement or worsening in depression. A subsequent table will indicate that all treatment groups tended to improve more than the placebo group.

TABLE 2 Significant Partial Correlations between Personality
         Qualities and Posttreatment Scores* for Phobia

Personality Quality	Placebo n = 50	Iproniazid n = 32	Imipramine n = 50	ECT n = 47
Paranoia (state)				.38
Suicidal (state)			.34	
Displacing (trait)			-.39	
Self-critical (trait)			.42	

* Adjusted for pretreatment differences

Table 2 summarizes the relationship between personality and remissive
changes in phobic symptoms. Neither iproniazid nor placebo involved
any of the personality qualities with phobic changes in a significant
manner. In the imipramine group, however, a suicidal state was
associated with relative increases in phobia. This finding is contrary to the association between suicidal state and remissive changes
in depression. The explanation for this seeming paradox may lie in
the particular significance of phobia for suicidal patients. Patients
with a premorbid displacing disposition tended to show remissive
changes in phobia, but the self-critical premorbid disposition was
associated with a worsening of phobias as it has been for depression.
It is interesting to observe that the paranoid patients became more
phobic in response to ECT.

The partial correlations between personality qualities and diminution
in anxiety are summarized for the various treatment groups in Table 3.

TABLE 3 Significant Partial Correlations between Personality
         Qualities and Posttreatment Scores* for Anxiety

Personality Quality	Placebo n = 50	Iproniazid n = 32	Imipramine n = 50	ECT n = 47
Paranoia (state)		.49		
Suicidal (state)				
Displacing (trait)	-.45		-.34	
Self-critical (trait)			.44	

* Adjusted for pretreatment differences

In the placebo group, anxiety is diminished among the patients who are characterized by the displacing quality. In the iproniazid group, it is apparent that the paranoid patients lost less anxiety than the nonparanoid patients. In the imipramine group, the patients with a premorbid tendency to displace showed a diminution in anxiety. Patients with the self-critical dependent personality quality were less likely to show a diminution in anxiety than are those without it. In general, the premorbid self-critical dependent disposition has adverse implications for symptomatic remission among depressed patients treated with imipramine.

It is apparent that remissive changes in certain symptoms of depression vary with personality qualities of the patient, as well as with the manner in which the depressive episode has been treated. This finding suggests that the presence of certain personality qualities may prove to be a useful consideration in selecting the treatment most appropriate for generating the desired symptomatic change. In this connection, it is interesting to compare the relative importance of a given treatment with the various personality qualities. For the present purposes, this question is approached by viewing a given treatment (e.g. iproniazid) versus no treatment (i.e. placebo) as forming a dichotomized variable in a composite sample which comprises both placebo-treated and iproniazid-treated patients. Biserial correlation coefficients may be computed between the dichotomous treatment-no treatment variable and the remissive changes in various symptoms of depression. Partial correlations can be used to express the net relationship between any one variable (e.g. treatment or a personality quality) and remissive changes in one of the symptoms.

The bottom row of Table 4 indicates that when the effect of personality differences is held constant statistically, there is a significant tendency for the patients who received iproniazid to show a greater loss in depression, phobia, and anxiety than the patients who received placebo.

TABLE 4   Significant Correlations between One Variable and
          Adjusted Posttreatment Scores When the Effect of Other
          Variables is Partialled Out

Variables	Composite Sample of Placebo and IPRONIAZID Groups (n=82)		
	Depression	Phobia	Anxiety
Paranoia (state)		.26	.32
Suicidal (state)			
Displacing (trait)		-.24	-.26
Self-critical (trait)			
*IPRONIAZID or Placebo	-.26	-.23	-.28

*Biserial correlations; a negative correlation implies that, relative to placebo, the active treatment is associated with a diminution of the symptom.

As could be anticipated from Tables 1,2, and 3, Table 4 also shows that in this composite sample the patients who had a premorbid displacing disposition tended to show remissive changes in phobia and anxiety. Patients with pretreatment paranoia did not respond as well in these symptomatic respects as patients who were without paranoia. When the magnitude of these various partial correlations is compared, it is apparent that the differences are small and insignificant. It would appear, therefore, that the presence of pretreatment paranoia or of premorbid displacing disposition may be as important a factor in the remission of phobia and anxiety as whether the patient received iproniazid or placebo. Whether a patient receives iproniazid is not the only factor in symptomatic remission, and it may not be the most important. It may be noted in this composite sample, however, that diminution of depressive symptoms per se was not significantly related with personality, but was significantly related with the presence of iproniazid.

The bottom line of Table 5 indicates that when the variance due to personality differences is partialled out, whether the patient received imipramine or not is significantly related with changes in one symptom only-- phobia.

TABLE 5   Significant Correlations between One Variable and
          Adjusted Posttreatment Scores When the Effect of Other
          Variables is Partialled Out

| Variables | Composite Sample of Placebo and IMIPRAMINE Groups (n = 100) | | |
	Depression	Phobia	Anxiety
Paranoia (state)			
Suicidal (state)		.31	.26
Displacing (trait)	-.26	-.28	-.33
Self-critical (trait)	.21	.26	.27
*IMIPRAMINE or Placebo		-.24	

*Biserial correlations; a negative correlation implies that, relative to placebo, the active treatment is associated with a diminution of the symptom.

In this imipramine-placebo composite sample, however, the presence of the premorbid displacing disposition is associated with diminution in all three symptoms under study. The self-critical premorbid disposition, in contrast, has a detracting relationship with remission in all three symptoms. In this composite sample, the suicidal state also has a detracting relationship with remissive changes in phobia and anxiety, a possibility anticipated by Table 2.

Table 6 shows a powerful anxiolytic effect of ECT. Within the limits of these comparisons, ECT had a numerically more conspicuous anxiolytic effect than the pharmacotherapies and appears possibly to be a more important factor in the diminution of anxiety than any of the personality variables, regardless of the treatment group in which their effect was assessed.

Table 6 Significant Correlations between One Variable and Adjusted Posttreatment Scores When the Effect of Other Variables is Partialled Out

Variables	Composite Sample of Placebo and ECT Groups (n = 97)		
	Depression	Phobia	Anxiety
Paranoia (state)		.23	
Suicidal (state)			
Displacing (trait)	-.22		-.31
Self-critical (trait)			
*ECT or Placebo	-.29		-.37

*Biserial correlations; a negative correlation implies that, relative to placebo, the active treatment is associated with a diminution of the symptom.

The interactions between treatment and personality, if confirmed, could have substantial clinical utility. For example, Table 7 illustrates that reduction of anxiety in response to imipramine varies greatly as a function of whether the depressed patients had a high or a low order of the premorbid self-critical quality.

Table 7 Anxiety Scores for Depressed Patients Who Had a High Standing on the Self-critical Trait and Patients Who Had a Low Standing

Self-critical Trait	Mean Anxiety Score					
	Pretreatment		Posttreatment		Adjusted Posttreatment	
	Placebo	Imipramine	Placebo	Imipramine	Placebo	Imipramine
High Above +.5 SD	3.2 (n=13)	4.1 (n=14)	2.2 (n=13)	2.8 *(n=14)	.66 (n=13)	.97 *(n=14)
Low Below +.5 SD	3.2 (n=37)	3.9 (n=36)	2.2 (n=37)	1.1 *(n=36)	.53 (n=37)	-.70 *(n=36)

*p>.05

In general the data show that in these depressed patients the average anxiety level is diminished over the course of treatment, regardless

of whether the patient received placebo or imipramine or of whether the
patient had a high or a low order of the self-critical disposition.
Nevertheless, at posttreatment, the patients who had a high order
(.5 S.D. or above) of the premorbid self-critical disposition and were
treated with imipramine had more anxiety than the placebo patients with
an equally high order of premorbid self-critical disposition. In contras
those patients receiving imipramine and who had a low order (below
.5 S.D.) of the self-critical disposition had much less anxiety than the
respective placebo patients. When differences in pretreatment anxiety
were held constant for the imipramine and placebo groups, the differences were not only confirmed, but the constrast also became more
striking.

The statistical summaries presented in the Wittenborn reports
(Wittenborn, 1966a, 1966b) were designed to show the relative importance
of various personality qualities as factors in symptomatic response
among young depressed females. Since most personality measures are inter
related, an attempt was made to show the importance of each factor independently of the effect of other factors, and partial correlation
coefficients were computed for this purpose. Because of this attempt to
minimize overlapping, the present findings are not directly comparable
with first order correlations or mean differences, such as commonly
used. In view of this difference in approach, it is gratifying to find
some consistency between the present results and those of other investigators, particularly with respect to such qualities as suicidal tendencies and self-critical personality. Paranoia, too, has been reported
as associated with unfavorable therapeutic response. Pollock and others
(1965) reported an unfavorable response to imipramine among patients
with paranoid features, a finding that corresponds with the Wittenborn
data.

The early literature contains many reports that associate suicidal tend
encies with response to pharmacotherapy. Kiloh and others (1962), Robin
and Langley (1964), and Uhlenhuth (1966) have reported that suicidal
behavior was associated with a relatively poor response to imipramine.
Paykel also (1971, 1972) has observed a poor response to tricyclic
drugs among patients with suicidal ideation. In the present reports
suicidal behavior tended to be characteristic of patients whose phobias
showed a relatively poor response to imipramine. In contrast, suicidal
behavior was associated with a reduction in depressive manifestations
among patients treated with imipramine or iproniazid.

At the time that the data presented here were gathered, attempted
suicide was a felony in some parts of the U.S. and could result in
imprisonment unless the patient was sufficiently ill to be hospitalized
It is quite possible, therefore, that patients who made definite suicidal attempts as part of the current episode responded to pharmacotherapy in a way different from that of patients who have suicidal
ideation, but made no suicidal attempt as a part of the current episode
These secondary aspects of suicidal behavior may have played a compli-
cating role in the manner in which suicidal patients responded to
treatment. Therapy which reduced depression could increase phobia and
anxiety among persons who were subject to prosecution because of recent
suicide attempts.

There is surprisingly little recent literature bearing directly on the
relationship between personality qualities and response to antidepressant pharmacotherapy, and much of the literature prior to 1967 has
been reviewed by Janke and Debus (1968), by Raskin (1968), and by

Wittenborn (1968). In a recent study of mixed samples of anxious and depressed patients, Stein, Downing, and Rickels (1978) found that patients who had feelings of personal adequacy tended to show a greater remission of depressive features than patients with low self-esteem, regardless of the nature of the treatment. These findings support a prior report by Downing and Rickels (1967).

It is possible that the sense of personal adequacy that had favorable prognostic implications in the Rickels reports is the positive aspect of the self-critical dependent quality included in the present Tables 1-6. Among patients treated with imipramine, the present tables show that the self-critical dependent quality is associated with relatively high posttreatment symptoms of phobia, depression, and anxiety. Nevertheless, the present relationship between relatively high posttreatment symptoms and the self-critical quality was found among those patients who were treated with imipramine only and not among those who were treated with placebo, iproniazid, or ECT. In this way, the present data differ from the Rickels findings. Had Rickels and his collaborator made special analyses to distinguish the effects of different treatments, they might have found that the feelings of adequacy would have been most highly related with outcome in patients treated with imipramine.

In a recent report, Donnelly and others (1978) introduced the possibility that the relationship between personality manifestations and pharmacotherapeutic responses may be sex-related. In their procedure, depressed patients who responded favorably to lithium therapy and those who did not respond favorably were compared in terms of their pretreatment responses to the various items of the MMPI. The nine most discriminating items were selected for the sample of 18 women, and independently the nine most discriminating items were selected for a sample of 9 men. Responses to the respective sets of discriminating items were combined to give a lithium-response score for the women and a lithium-response score for the men. These scores were subsequently secured for an independent sample of 18 women and 8 men. This scoring procedure formulated on the basis of discriminating trends in the initial sample discriminated without error in the second independent sample.

The authors did not offer an interpretation of the possible psychological significance of the discriminating scores. Upon examination of the items, however, it would appear to this reviewer that among the items that identified the women who were lithium responders a quality of cautious sensitivity could be discerned. Among the items that identified the men who were lithium responders, a kind of acceptant, positively-toned realism seemed to be implicit. To test these or any other psychological conceptualization based on a given set of items, it would be desirable to use the conceptualization to generate new items and see whether these new items have the expected discriminating property in an independent study of drug responders.

A somewhat different approach to the relationship between pretreatment MMPI responses and response to lithium was published by Steinberg (1979). He reported that responders had lower pretreatment depression and psychasthenia MMPI scores than the nonresponders. This can be construed as consistent in implication with the Donnelly and others (1978) report which suggested that the men who were good lithium responders had a positively-toned, realistic outlook.

CONCLUSIONS

Despite numerous and diverse research efforts, there has been virtually
no progress during the last 20 years among those who have sought to
show that the relationship between nonsymptomatic pretreatment characteristics of depressed patients and response to alternative pharmacotherapies differed from pharmacotherapy to pharmacotherapy in a pre-
dictively useful way. Very few of the relationships described in the
various exploratory studies have been confirmed by independent replication, and the predictive utility of these relationships has not been
demonstrated in clinical situations. It is possible that the alternative
antidepressant therapies do not differ from each other in the pattern
of their relationships with pretreatment demographic, historic, and
phenomenological characteristics of patients. It is possible also that
response to treatment is not qualified in any important degree by
pretreatment factors which are not symptomatic and not a part of or confounded with the treatment per se. An alternative to these discouraging
Null Hypotheses is the equally discouraging hypothesis that there is
something wrong with current research.

There are many criticisms that could be offered, but whether they can
provide an explanation for the current stasis is not known. Certainly
the methods of assessment in current use are, for the most part,
imprecise and have a significance which is dependent upon the user and
the context in which they are used. There is also a preference for
"quick and easy" assessment procedures which may reflect the judgment
of the user more than   the objective basis for his judgment. It is
also true that most research samples are heterogeneous and poorly
documented so that the portion of the sample that contributes to or
obscures any particular trend may not be identified, and any attempt
at replication of studies is compromised by the possibilities that the
samples may be incommensurable in some important respect.

The literature describes few efforts to cross validate relationships
of predictive potential. Nevertheless, some studies have provided confirmation of the results of prior inquiries. Unfortunately, the strengt
of relationships established by cross validation is relatively meager,
and further inquiry will be necessary to discover whether refinements
in procedure will reveal trends of practical importance. It must be
admitted as well that some reports appear to be based on poorly designed inquiries or inquiries designed in such a way that more question
may be raised than settled.

When contrasted with the rapid evolution of studies which indicate
relationships between pretreatment MHPG and differential response to
psychotropic substances, the phenomenological approach has been un-
rewarding. Although the MHPG findings appear to be confirmable, the
course of subsequent inquiries may find this approach to be disappointing, also.

REFERENCES

Beckman, H., and F.K. Goodwin (1975). Antidepressant response to
    tricyclics and urinary MHPG in unipolar patients. Archives of
    General Psychiatry, 32, 17-21.
Cobbin, D.M., B. Requin-Blow, L.R. Williams, and W.O. Williams (1979).
    Urinary MHPG levels and tricyclic antidepressant drug selection.
    Archives of General Psychiatry, 36, 1111-1115.

Donnelly, E.F., F.K. Goodwin, I.N. Waldman, and D.L. Murphy (1978). Prediction of antidepressant responses to lithium. American Journal of Psychiatry, 135, 552-556.

Downing, R.W., and K. Rickels (1967). Pre-treatment self estimates and clinical improvement with tranquilizer therapy. Diseases of the Nervous System, 28, 671-674.

Downing, R.W., and K. Rickels (1972). Predictors of amitriptyline response in outpatient depressives. The Journal of Nervous and Mental Disease, 154, 248-263.

Hordern, A., N.F. Holt, C.G. Burt, and W.F. Gordon (1963). Amitriptyline in depressive states. British Journal of Psychiatry, 109, 815-825.

Janke, W., and G. Debus (1968). Experimental studies on antianxiety agents with normal subjects: Methodological considerations and review of the main effects. In D.H. Efron, J.O. Cole, J. Levine, and J.R. Wittenborn (Eds.), Psychopharmacology - A Review of Progress 1957-1967, Public Health Service, U.S. Department of Health, Education and Welfare.

Kiloh, L.G., J.R.B. Ball, and R.F. Garside (1962). Prognostic factors in treatment of depressive states with imipramine. British Medical Journal, 1, (Part 2), 1225-1227.

Maas, J.W., J.A. Fawcett, and H. Dekirmenjian (1972). Catecholamine metabolism, depressive illness, and drug response. Archives of General Psychiatry, 26, 252-262.

McConaghy, N., A.D. Joffee, W.R. Kingston, H.G. Stevenson, I. Atkinson, E. Cole, and L.A. Fennessy (1968). Correlation of clinical features of depressed out-patients with response to amitriptyline and protriptyline. British Journal of Psychiatry, 114, 103-106.

Overall, J.E., L.E. Hollister, M. Johnson, and V. Pennington (1966). Nosology of depression and differential response to drugs. Multidiscipline Research Forum, 195, 162-164.

Paykel, E.S. (1971). Classification of depressed patients: A cluster analysis derived grouping. British Journal of Psychiatry, 118, 275-288.

Paykel, E.S. (1972). Depressive typologies and response to amitriptyline. British Journal of Psychiatry, 120, 147-156.

Paykel, E.S., B.A. Prusoff, G.L. Klerman, D. Haskell, and A. DiMascio (1973). Clinical response to amitriptyline among depressed women. The Journal of Nervous and Mental Disease, 156, 149-165.

Pollack, M., D.F. Klein, A. Willner, A. Blumberg, and M. Fink (1965). Imipramine-induced behavioral disorganization in schizophrenic patients: physiologic and psychologic correlates. In J. Wortis (Ed.), Recent Advances in Biological Psychiatry, Plenum Press, New York. Chap. 7, pp. 53-61.

Prusoff, B.A., and E.S. Paykel (1977). Typological prediction of response to amitriptyline: A replication study. International Pharmacopsychiatry, 12, 153-159.

Raskin, A. (1968). The prediction of antidepressant drug effects: Review and critique. In D.H. Efron, J.O. Cole, J. Levine, and J.R. Wittenborn (Eds.), Psychopharmacology - A Review of Progress 1957-1967, Public Health Service, U.S. Department of Health, Education and Welfare.

Raskin, A. (1974). Age-sex differences in response to antidepressant drugs. The Journal of Nervous and Mental Disease, 159, 120-130.

Raskin, A., and T.H. Crook (1975). Antidepressants in black and white inpatients. Archives of General Psychiatry, 32, 643-649.

Raskin, A., and T.H. Crook (1976). The endogenous-neurotic distinction as a predictor of response to antidepressant drugs. Psychological Medicine, 6, 59-70.

Raskin, A., H. Boothe, J.G. Schulterbrandt, N. Reatig, and D. Odle (1973). A model for drug use with depressed patients. The Journal of Nervous and Mental Disease, 156, 130-142.

Rickels, K., P.E. Gordon, B.W. Jenkins, M. Perloff, T. Sachs, and W. Stepansky (1970). Drug treatment in depressive illness. Diseases of the Nervous System, 31, 40-42.

Robin, A.A., and G.E. Langley (1964). A controlled trial of imipramine. British Journal of Psychiatry, 110, 419-422.

Rosenbaum, A.H., A.F. Schatzberg, T. Maruta, P.J. Orsulak, J.O. Cole, E.L. Grab, and J.J. Schildkraut (1980). MHPG as a predictor of antidepressant response to imipramine and maprotiline. American Journal of Psychiatry, 137, 1090-1092.

Stein, M.K., R.W. Downing, and K. Rickels (1978). Self estimates in anxious and depressed outpatients treated with pharmacotherapy. Psychological Reports, 43, 487-492.

Steinberg, F.A. (1979). The delineation of an MMPI symptom pattern unique to lithium responders. American Journal of Psychiatry, 136, 567-569.

Uhlenhuth, E.H. (1966). Some non-pharmacologic modifiers of the response to imipramine in depressed, psychoneurotic outpatients: a confirmatory study. Unpublished manuscript.

Wittenborn, J.R. (1964). Wittenborn Psychiatric Rating Scales Manual. Rutgers Interdisciplinary Research Center. New Brunswick, New Jersey.

Wittenborn, J.R. (1966a). Assessment of clinical change. In J.O. Cole and J.R. Wittenborn (Eds.), Pharmacotherapy of Depression, Charles C. Thomas, Springfield, Illinois.

Wittenborn, J.R. (1966b). Factors which qualify the response to iproniazid and to imipramine. In J.R. Wittenborn, and P.R.A. May (Eds. Prediction of Response to Pharmacotherapy, Charles C. Thomas, Springfield, Illinois.

Wittenborn, J.R. (1968). Prediction of the individual's response to antidepressant medication. In D.H. Efron, J.O. Cole, J. Levine, and J.R. Wittenborn (Eds.), Psychopharmacology - A Review of Progress 1957-1967, Public Health Service, U.S. Department of Health, Education and Welfare.

Wittenborn, J.R. (1969). Diagnostic classification and response to imipramine. In P.R.A. May and J.R. Wittenborn (Eds.), Psychotropic Drug Response, Charles C. Thomas, Springfield, Illinois.

Wittenborn, J.R., A. Dempster, H. Maurer, and M. Plante (1964). Pretreatment individual differences as potential predictors of response to pharmacology. The Journal of Nervous and Mental Disease. 139, 186-194.

Part IV

DRUG RESPONSE VARIABILITY AND SITUATIONAL FACTORS

WHAT DIFFERENTIATES A DIFFERENTIAL PSYCHOPHARMACOLOGY?

Hans-Peter Krüger

ABSTRACT

The methodological implications of a differential psychopharmacology
are discussed. It is shown that the technique of stratifying subjects
with personality scores depends on one basic assumption: the personality score is not affected by the other experimental factors. Two experiments are reported in which pre- and posttest (after the experiment)
scores were measured. The pre-post-differences showed themselves to be
affected by the medication. It is argued that in psychopharmacological
experimentation an additional step must be included. All non-treatment
factors must be examined for their stability in the course of the
experiment. If they are stable, usual evaluation may take place. If
changes are attributable to the treatment, personality scores must be
regarded as dependent variables. They have to be evaluated together
with the other observables with a multivariate model. Additionally, a
procedure like this yields as "experimental differential psychology"
a self-reliant contribution to the problems of differential psychology.

KEYWORDS

Differential psychopharmacology; differential psychology; drug-personality interaction; methodology of differential psychopharmacology;
personality traits; neuroticism.

I. THE PATTERN OF EXPERIMENTATION IN PSYCHOPHARMACOLOGY

The general pattern of experimenting in psychopharmacology is given by
the expression

$$R = f (D,S)$$

where R = reaction, D = drug and S = situation. The effect in R is
interpreted as a consequence of the factors D and S, given by
independent definition in physical (e.g. db white noise) and chemical
(e.g. 5 mg from a benzo–diazepine) terms. The differential approach
in psychopharmacology (as introduced by Eysenck, in Germany by Lienert
and Janke) is comparable with the evolution from behaviorism to neo-
behaviorism. A "cognitive" element named personality is inserted in

the formular above:

$$R = f (D,S,P)$$

with P = personality. This pattern is also instructive for the way in
which experiments are conducted. Since D,S, and P as factors can be
varied independently, experiments in psychopharmacology are regularly
multifactorial. Our further considerations will emphasize above all the
consequences of this model for the experimental design.

In psychopharmacology a large number of results extended the influence
of the two independent factors personality and situation. First these
factors were thought to be only modifying the drug response, but more
and more a constitutive function was noted.

In a systematic overview, Janke and Debus demonstrated (Debus and Janke,
1978; Janke and others,1979) the essential effects of situation and
personality on drug response. Following these authors, the present
state of an individual is influenced by the drug, by the situation and
by long-term characteristics, more generally by personality. The present
state is modified by these factors, resulting in a primary drug response
covert to the experimenter. This primary response is the equivalent to
the neo-behavioristic internal response, which in interaction with the
possibilities to react in the experimental situation yields the overt,
observable response named here "secondary drug response".

The advantage of such a model is obvious: most of the experimental
results can be ordered. But it is obvious too that the high generality
hides some problems:

- There is no attempt to make understandable the interaction between
  personality and situation.
The personality factor is an experimental tool to control the'psychological situation' of the subjects, ending in a reduction of variance.
The experimenter states the hypothesis that the organismic factor is
a generalized reaction to situations of which the experimental situation is part. The personality factor yields groups of subjects with
comparable reactions (given the validity of the trait for the actual
state). Introduction of a personality variable is in fact a declaration
by the experimenter that the same situation describable in objective
terms is psychologically not the same for all subjects. We have had
an extended discussion in personality theory about the model of person-
situation interaction. The controversy is still going on, recently
with Eysenck & Eysenck's (1980) rejection of the arguments from
Mischel (1968). But without respect to the ending of this discussion
one fact still remains: the results of personality research do not
allow to speak of situation and personality as independent factors. In
the experimental procedure the factors personality and situation may
be varied independently. Extraversion and a noise condition are independent in an experimental and statistical view. But psychologically'
they are highly dependent: a zero correlation between personality and
situation would render personality theory superfluous.

- There is no attempt to make understandable the interaction between
  drug and situation.
Do subjects treated with a tranquillizing drug experience a situation
in the same way as subjects with placebo? Since the work of Lewin it
is accepted that situation is the 'state of the actual field' which

must be defined in psychological terms. Objective descriptions may only
be an approximation to the description of the psychological situation.

-There is also no attempt to make understandable the interaction between
 personality and drug.
Are the reactions to drugs different for subjects with different personality scores without changing the personality? Or: Does the drug change
the long-term characteristic (personality trait) itself or the portion
of short-term characteristics (state) in the personality concept? Anew
these factors are independent: each drug condition may be applied to
each personality condition in stochastic manner. Thus, the conditions
for the internal validity of the experiment sensu Campbell and Stanley,
(1963) is guaranteed. But the problems are essentially the same as in
the case of situational variables.

II. A PRAGMATIC VIEW ON PERSONALITY VARIABLES

As this discussion shows, the role of the personality variables is constitutive and may be discussed in highly theoretical terms. But we also
can look at them from a pragmatic view point. There was a practical
need to introduce such modifying variables because drug effects have
been often too small. It is a usual tool in experimentation to reduce
intra-group variance by stratifying the subjects.

Let us start with a single-situation experiment with drug as the only
treatment factor. $V(T)$ is the effect variance due to the drug, $V(E)$
the error variance. By introducing an organismic factor (Edwards,
1968) like personality, $V(E)$ is split into $V(E) = V(P) + V(PxT) +
V(E^*)$ where $V(P)$ is variance due to personality, $V(PxT)$ is the inter-
action between drug and personality and $V(E^*)$ is the new (smaller)
error variance. If the sum $V(P) + V(PxT)$ is small or, equivalently,
$V(E)$ is of comparable size as $V(E^*)$ there would be no need for organismic factors. A 'differential psychopharmacology' would not have
been created. This research is essentially based on the interaction
term $V(PxT)$ with $V(T)$ small or zero.

If an effect in $V(P)$ is observed without an effect on $V(PxT)$, then the
experimenter has chosen an organismic factor which is correlated with
the dependent variable (observable) or, in another view, we have defined two or more subpopulations. The conditions to detect treatment
effects are better now - some variance in the observable is assigned
to organismic differences independent from drug action.

In single-situation experiments significant effects on $V(P)$ and/or
$V(PxT)$ may be considered as an internal validation of the organismic
factor personality. If an anxiolytic drug is given to a sample of
subjects stratified to anxiety and the dependent variable is 'experienced anxiety' we should expect an effect on the organismic factor,
whether as main or interaction term. If not, the validity of the
organismic trait for the actual state in the experimental situation
is questionnable. A 'hidden effect' of the personality factor has to
be seen in the technique of many experimenters to improve drug effects
only in subpopulations (subjects with high neuroticism, high anxiety
and so on). This technique may be effective in some cases but has a
great disadvantage: the validity of the personality variable is only
based on plausability, but is not proved explicitly in the experimental
situation. If variation of the organismic factor is seen as 'treatment

by the nature', the definition of subpopulations is comparable to drug
studies without reference drugs or without placebo. It is impossible
to explain treatment effects as general or as differential only,
because V(T) and V(PxT) are confounded.

In the second case V(PxT) is significant. If additionally V(P) becomes
significant, the organismic factor has led to a differential experience
of the experimental situation which is modified by the drug (e.g.,
subjects with high anxiety show a greater decrease in experienced anxiety than subjects with low anxiety). On the other side, when V(P) is
not significant, the organismic factor is drug-specific, not situation-
specific. Figure 1 shows the possible results.

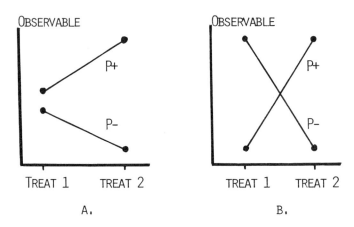

Fig. 1.   Types of interactions between personality
          variables and drug treatment.

In case A (left side of Fig. 1) the personality factor differentiates
between the persons without respect to treatment (main effect). The
personality factor describes the differential experience of the experimental situation. Drug modifies this experience. In case B (right side
of Fig. 1) the experimental situation is the same for the two subpopulations given by the organismic factor (no main effect personality)
which itself shows as situation-indifferent. But reaction to the drug
treatment is clearly dependent on personality.

So, introducing an organismic factor in psychopharmacological experiments we have to decide whether this factor is determining

a. the experience of the situation (a case only interesting in
   differential psychology),
b. the experience of the drug or
c. the reaction to situation a n d drug.

Case B as a double disordinal interaction (see Bredenkamp, 1980) would
be highly desirable. The reaction to drug would be determined by characters of subjects which are independent from situation. Perhaps example
may be found in 'physiological traits' - psychology has not been able
to produce situation-free parameters up to now. Even the purest
'personalist' would not declare that situation should be neglected.

So at the moment one should expect only effects of personality on situation and drug simultaneously. The overview about the effects of the organismic factors 'extraversion' and 'action-orientation' given by Janke and others (1979) reveals in fact that with few exceptions only interactions of our type A are occuring in psychopharmacological research. This indicates that organismic factors change situation as well as drug response.

Interpretation of those interactions is difficult and dependent on the psychophysiological model of the researcher. But before arguing with theoretical terms, a reconsideration of the methodological implications which are underlying the experimental procedure has to take place.

III. THE TECHNIQUE OF STRATIFYING

As mentioned stratifying is a tool to reduce error variance. Usually in statistical textbooks only one desiderat is stated: the stratum variable must be independent from the observable. That is why in experimental practice the stratum variable is measured previous to the experimental action. The independence of the stratum variable is only a question of measurement, not one of the association between stratum variable and observable. If in a teaching experiment comparing two methods of learning, intelligence is introduced as stratum variable, results in performance are highly dependent on this factor (the observable is correlated with the stratum variable). Only error variance is reduced.

But independence in measurement of both variables is only a necessary, but not sufficient condition in designs with stratum variables. The logic of factorial designs (usually evaluated with ANOVA) demands that effects of factors are orthogonal for all cells in two and higher orders. In nonpsychological experiments this demand is usually out of question. Suppose a pharmacologist is interested in the interaction of a certain drug with alcohol. He designs an experiment with two levels of dosages of drug and alcohol. By injecting the drugs in animals he can be sure that at every level of drug every dosage of alcohol is the same. Or: if the observable in this experiment would be 'dosage of alcohol' only a main effect alcohol has to be expected, no other effect is possible. Every main effect of this observable on other factors, every interaction with other factors would render the results uninterpretable, because treatment is no longer guaranteed to be successful.

The desiderat of independence seems trivial in experimenting with treatment factors, though becomes critical in designs with stratifying factors. Eysenck's model of the effects of stimulant action (excitation - introversion) and depressant action (inhibition - extraversion) may be a very dangerous one if you read it in the reverse direction. Then it may be possible that drugs change personality or: personality becomes drug specific. But if the personality factor (thought as independent factor) changes itself during the experimental action, the effects are no longer interpretable. Following these considerations, a precondition for interpretation is the stability of the organismic factor in the course of the experiment. But we have great empirical evidence that personality variables are affected by drugs.

IV. EMPIRICAL EXAMPLES

In an experiment from Kohnen & Krüger (1981) N=72 healthy young subjects
(36 males and females) were divided by random in 3 groups receiving
placebo, 2.5 and 5.0 mg of the benzodiazepine lopirazepam. In the course
of the experiment (2 hours after the oral application of the drug) they
had to solve arithmetic tasks sitting in a circle with 6 members and
being called up by the experimenter one by one. They had to stand up
and to calculate for 1 minute. This call-up situation was shown to be
highly stressing to the subjects (see Kohnen and Lienert, 1980). Days
before the experiment subjects got the FPI (Fahrenberg and others, 1973)
as a personality test which among other scales also measures neuroticism
Scores were thought to stratify subjects. After the experiment (4 hours
after application and 1 hour after the stressing experiences in the
group) subjects got the parallel form of the test. The difference
between the pretest and posttest score of neuroticism (N2 - N1) was
calculated and introduced in the ANOVA as observable with drug treatment as independent factor.

Following our considerations above drug effects in connection with
personality factors can only be interpreted if drug does not change
personality in the course of the experiment. Thus we expected that the
null hypothesis of no difference in the pre-post values is not to be re-
jected.

With F = 3.12 (df 2,69) in the unifactorial ANOVA HO has a probability
smaller than 5%. Changes in neuroticism scores are attributable to drug
levels. This effect is not due to the initial values (the pretest
scores). In the respective ANOVAs we got

a. for the pretest score an F-value of 2.62 (df 2,69),
b. for the posttest score an F = 0.60 (df 2,69).

Both F-values are not significant, a result which supports trait theo-
rists. Also the retest correlations are sufficient: for the placebo
group r(tt) = .25, for 2.5 mg r(tt) = .86 and for 5.0 mg r(tt) = .84
with n = 24 in each group. With exception of the placebo group coefficients are of expected size. Only the calculation of the difference
N2-N1 disturbs the picture. In Fig. 2 A (upper left) the changes N2-N1
are plotted against medication separated for the subjects with high
and low neuroticism pretest score.

The differentiation according to the pretest score (N+,N-) shows that
shift in the neuroticism score is, except to the placebo/N- group,
generally: the posttest scores are the more stable the higher the
dosage. An interpretation may be that highly threatening situations
(as the call up situation is) lead to a repression of anxiety which is
extremely shown by high neurotics in the placebo condition, not by the
subjects with low neuroticism. If the anxiolytic action of the drug is
the liberation of anxiety (as Lader, 1978, suggests) the tranquillizing
agent enables the subjects to 'handle' the situation in its challenging
aspects. The result can be a stabilization of reported neuroticism.

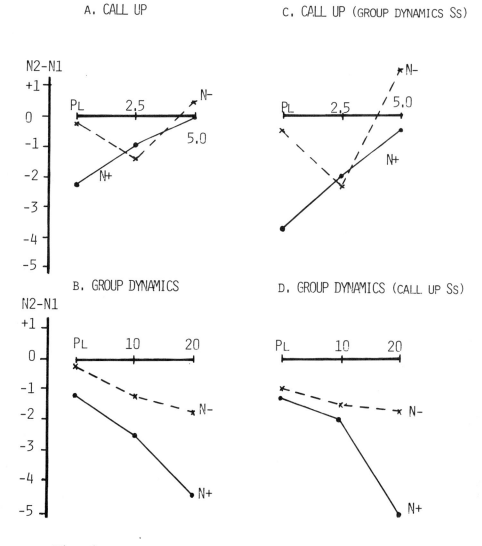

Fig. 2.   Pre-posttest-differences of neuroticism
dependent from medication in two experiments.

This psychopharmacological interpretation is not substantial for our considerations - other models are possible. Essential is the fact that the stratifying factor personality itself changes in the course of the experiment dependent from the treatment factor. In the language of differential psychology this result indicates a greater part of state aspects in the neuroticism score. The methodological implications will be discussed below after we have reported another experiment with comparable results.

In an experimental analog to a group-psychotherapy situation Krüger and Kohnen (1981) realized a wide variety of social situations. The program tried to generate very different situations in groups of 6 persons (3 male, 3 female) as discussions between two or more, but also exercises with touching the others. Phases of medication and self-reflection are also integrated following the lines of the Gestalt-therapy from Perls (1976). In total a more relaxed situation was created with some stressful events (like touching). As tranquillizing agent the benzo-diazepine prazepam in the dosages of 10 and 20 mg was used together with placebo. Four groups of subjects (total N = 24) got previous to the experiment the FPI (yielding the pretest neuroticism score). Four hours after medication and 1 hour after the group dynamics subjects were measured with the parallel scale (posttest score). The results are shown in Fig. 2 B (left below) separated for subjects with high (N+) and low (N-) neuroticism pretest score.

In total the posttest score is lower than the pretest score for all groups. The results are inverse to those reported above: the higher the dosage the lower the posttest score. The retest-coefficients are for the placebo group .55, for the 10 mg group .41 and for the 20 mg group .10 (n = 8). The interpretation of the drug effect would be comparable to those given above. The therapeutic effect of group dynamics is greater in the verum groups which, as in the experiment above, are better able to 'handle' the situation, here in its relaxing aspects.

The effect is with F = 1.89 (df 2,21) not significant (p = 17.5%) in the ANOVA. Essentially for our purposes is another fact. N = 15 subjects of this experiment are the same as in the call up experiment reported above. The two experiments were separated by two months. Now we can ask whether the inverse effects of the two total groups (N = 72 and N = 24) are replicated in the subgroup (N = 15) involved in both experiments. Results are shown in Fig. 2 C (right above) and Fig. 2 D (left below). As may be seen the course of the total group is fully replicated by the subgroup. The same persons show in one situation an increasing, in the other situation a decreasing course of difference scores.

V. DISCUSSION

The retest-correlations showed that a constant character was measured. The changes in scores attributable to the situation and medication indicate that self-description varies if the psychological situation is changed. The psychological situation is influenced by the characters of the situation (threatening call up, more relaxing group dynamics) as well as by the drug. This result gives great hope that psychopharmacology may be used as an 'experimental differential psychology'. But these results also show a great problem for the methodology of a 'differential psychopharmacology'.

The organismic factor neuroticism was thought to be independent in a statistical manner since it was measured before the experiment. Results show that treatment changes this score. The psychological interpretation is simple: neuroticism has to be seen as a combination of a trait and a state variable. The trait-aspect is measured in the high retest-correlation, the state-aspect in the treatment effect. It is another question to think that treatment has changed the trait. Subjects were healthy young people, treatment was a single application - a greater change in the trait cannot be expected. This problem is more one of differential psychology but has no consequence in our discussion of the methodological implications of a stratum variable affected by medication.

Statistically these results indicate that the formal model of ANOVA is violated. Effects of the factors themselves have to be the same for every group in the experimental design. If we have had as observable 'mg tranquillizer in blood' and ANOVA would have shown that the mgs are different for subjects with high and low neuroticism, nobody would interprete the effects on all observables introduced, arguing that medication conditions were different. The same consideration for neuroticism yields difficulties in the interpretation.

What consequences should be drawn? In a substantial sense our results render the concept of neuroticism not questionnable. They emphasize only the necessity for a reconsideration about what portions of this concept are to be seen as trait and state. To what extent is neuroticism a measure of the actual state of the organism? What is rendered questionnable is the method of evaluating experimental designs including stratifying variables by the model of the 'uni-observable' ANOVA (to use a distinction of Lienert & Krauth, 1974) with the stratum variable as factor. If stratum variables can be shown as affected by treatment factors the logic of ANOVA is violated. Interpretation of main and interaction effects is no longer conclusive.

On the other hand, those stratifying variables could be shown as highly effective in psychopharmacology. There are only two ways out of the problematic methodological situation:

1. If stratum variables are affected by treatment they are in fact observables. If dependence of pharmacological effects from those variables is given, a multivariate ('multi-observable') evaluation has to take place. Drug effects are not to be proved with the model of two factors and one observable (factors drug x personality affect observable) but with the model of one factor and two observables (factor drug affects the observables personality x observable). Thus differential psychopharmacology becomes necessarily multivariate.

2. Controlling stratum variables has to be done not by introducing them as factors in the ANOVA but by defining two ore more subpopulations with the stratum. Subjects with high or low neuroticism are no longer viewed as coming from the same population. Doing so, in the ANOVA no common variance can be defined for stratified groups. The way out is to evaluate the drug effects separately for the subpopulations. The two-factorial design recurs to two one-dimensional designs. This procedure is suggested as the most conclusive by Lienert (1981).

Basic requirement for both ways is information about the effect of treatment on the stratum variable. This information can only be gotten with additional experiments. All independent variables in an experiment which not can be randomized (non-treatment factors) have to be

remeasured in the course of the experiment. The first analysis has to
prove whether the difference between pre- and posttest score has an
effect on the treatment-factor or not. Only in the latter case, can
statistical analysis be made as usual.

An effect occuring,   evaluation becomes complicated: the stratum
variable has to be considered as a covariate. It has to be decided
whether (a) the pretest stratum score, (b) the posttest score,
(c) the difference pre-post, or (d) the sum pre + post is the adequate
measure to be introduced in the (now) multivariate evaluation.

A procedure like this has to wait for the end of the experiment before
knowing what has been the independent factors in the experiment. This
is unsatisfying for psychology (and in a strong sense not allowed by
the statistical model). Therefore we want to argue for a multivariate
model which enables the experimenter to plan experiment and evaluation
of data fully in advance. Since it is not clear up to now how great the
portions of situation, of state, of trait are in our personality concepts we should be conservative in evaluating those effects by consider
ing them as observables. This is no disadvantage for differential
psychology: a deeper knowledge about the effect of treatment on personality scores is in fact experimental differential psychology. Thus
differential psychopharmacology with personality as a dependent variabl
yields a self-reliant contribution to differential psychology
(Krüger, 1981).

REFERENCES

Bredenkamp, J. (1980). Theorie and Planung psychologischer Experimente.
    Steinkopff, Darmstadt.
Campbell, D.T., and J.C. Stanley (1963). Experimental and quasi-experi-
    mental designs for research in teaching. In N.L. Gage (Ed.), Hand-
    book of Research in Teaching. Rand McNally, Chicago.
Debus, G., and W. Janke (1978). Psychologische Aspekte der Pharmako-
    therapie. In J.L. Pongratz (Ed.), Handbuch der Psychologie, Vol. 8/
    Klinische Psychologie. Hogrefe, Göttingen.
Edwards, A.L. (1968). Experimental Design in Psychological Research,
    3rd ed. Holt, Rinehart & Winston, New York.
Eysenck, M.W., and H.J. Eysenck (1980). Mischel and the concept of
    personality. Br. J. Psychol., 71, 191-204.
Fahrenberg, J., H. Selg, and R. Hampel (1973). Freiburger Persönlich-
    keitsinventar, 2nd ed. Hogrefe, Göttingen.
Janke, W., G. Debus, and N. Longo (1979). Differential psychopharma-
    cology of tranquillizing and sedating drugs. In T.A. Ban and others
    (Eds.), Modern Problems of Pharmacopsychiatry, Vol. 14. Karger,
    Basel. pp. 13-98.
Kohnen, R., and H.-P. Krüger (1981). What is a tranquillizing drug
    doing in verbal examinations? Paper submitted to Int. Pharmaco-
    psychiatry.
Kohnen, R., and G.A. Lienert (1980). Defining tranquillizers operatio-
    nally by non additive effect in experimental stress situations.
    Psychopharmacology, 68, 291-294.
Krüger, H.-P. (1981). Differentielle Pharmakopsychologie ohne Differen
    tielle Psychologie? In W. Janke (Ed.), Beiträge zur Methodik in der
    differentiellen, diagnostischen und klinischen Psychologie. Fest-
    schrift für G.A. Lienert. Hain, Meisenheim.

Krüger H.-P., and R. Kohnen (1981). Tranquillizer effects in an experimental analog of group-psychotherapy. Paper submitted to Int. Pharmacopsychiatry.

Lader, M.H. (1978). Stress und Angstmechanismus. In P. Kielholz (Ed.), Betablocker und Zentralnervensystem. Huber, Bern. pp. 47-52.

Lienert, G.A. (1981). Vaupee-Variablen im psychologischen Experiment und wie man sie varianzanalytisch kontrolliert. Submitted for publication.

Lienert, G.A., and J. Krauth (1974). Die Konfigurationsfrequenzanalyse: IX. Z. Klin. Psychol. Psychother., 22, 3-17.

Mischel, W. (1968). Personality and Assessment. Wiley, New York.

Perls, S. (1976). Grundlagen der Gestalttherapie. Pfeiffer, München.

AUTONOMIC DRUGS AS TOOLS IN DIFFERENTIAL PSYCHOPHARMACOLOGY

Gisela Erdmann

ABSTRACT

The present paper reports experimental studies on differential emotional responses to adrenergic drugs under different situational conditions.
The results of these studies are used to exemplify the applicability
of autonomic drugs as tools in differential psychopharmacology, namely
(1) as control tools for behavioral response differences due to autonomic side effects of central nervous system drugs, (2) as research
tools for testing theories about autonomic nervous system reactions
as determinants of emotional response differences, and (3) as tools
to develop models for the prediction of situation-dependent emotional
responses to drugs in general.

KEYWORDS

Sympathicomimetic drugs; beta-adrenergic blocking drugs; autonomic
side effects; autonomic system and emotion; situation-dependent drug
responses; drug effects and stress; tranquilizers.

INTRODUCTION

In general, psychopharmacology is only concerned with drugs that are
assumed to directly affect behavior by altering its neurochemical or
neurophysiological basis. Drugs which act mainly on the autonomic
system (or other systems outside the CNS) and which might affect
behavior only indirectly, therefore, are usually not considered.
Nevertheless, there are several reasons why autonomic drugs might be
useful as tools in differential psychopharmacology.

The most obvious reason is that many CNS drugs produce autonomic
side effects. As Janke (this volume) pointed out, such side effects
might act as spurious factors in the determination of behavioral
response differences and therefore cast some doubts on the usual
conclusion that these differences are exclusively or at least
mainly the result of a drug's central action. Drugs which induce autonomic symptoms as their main effects might be useful tools to con-

trol for the response variability due to these kinds of spurious factors.
Before autonomic drugs can be advanced as useful control tools in
differential psychopharmacology it must be shown that drug-induced
autonomic symptoms, indeed, result in behavioral response differences.

In dealing with this question, the present paper will refer to studies
on emotional effects of adrenergic stimulating and blocking drugs in
different emotional situations. Because of the kind of drugs (i.e.
drugs acting on the sympathetic system) and because of the kind of
drug response modifying factors (i.e. situational conditions) considered in these studies, they are of direct relevance only for intraindividual differences in response to drugs with actions on the sympathetic
system, namely stimulants. A further restriction is that only emotional
responses will be considered. Although emotional reactions (e.g. negative feelings) are probably the primary expected effects of drug-induced
autonomic symptoms, this restriction excludes behavioral effects that
might occur secondary to emotional reactions, e.g. changes in performance.

Whether autonomic drugs can result in response differences in terms
of emotional change, is not only relevant for the problem of side
effects, but is important also for theories in differential psychology.
There are several authors who ascribe autonomic nervous system reactions an essential role in the determination of inter- or intraindividual differences in emotional behavior. With regard to interindividual differences, the most prominent author is probably Eysenck.
According to Eysenck (1957, 1966, 1967) the personality dimension of
neuroticism is characterized by differences in the reactivity of the
sympathetic nervous system. Regarding intraindividual differences,
the best-known theory is Schachter's cognitive-physiological theory
of emotions. According to Schachter (1964, 1971, 1975; Schachter and
Singer, 1962) emotions result from the interaction of an unspecific
state of sympathetic arousal and emotion-specific cognitions derived
from the situational context. Since adrenergic drugs can be used to
experimentally vary autonomic nervous system reactions, they are suitable research tools for testing the predictions derived from such
theories (see also Erdmann, 1979; Janke, 1971). (Indeed, because of
their direct actions on the autonomic system and because their use
allows the control of a number of extraneous factors, autonomic drugs
may be considered as the most suitable research tools available in this
area (see also Erdmann, 1982)).

Accordingly, Eysenck (see also Eysenck, this volume) proposed the use
of sympathicomimetic and sympathicolytic agents to test the predictions
derived from the neuroticism-dimension of his theory. As to our knowledge, autonomic drugs were not actually used for this purpose, however. Rather, in his psychopharmacological research, Eysenck was almost exclusively concerned with the personality dimension of "extraversion vs. introversion". Researchers in differential psychopharmacology, who were concerned with neuroticism, did not use adrenergic
drugs, but mostly tranquilizers or other central depressants (for an
overview see Janke, this volume). Schachter, however, tried to support
his theory by experimental studies with adrenergic drugs (Schachter
and Singer, 1962; Schachter and Wheeler, 1962). That this research
stimulated further experiments on the effects of adrenergic drugs
under varied situational conditions is the main reason for considering studies on intraindividual rather than interindividual differences in emotional responses to such drugs in this paper, and for

discussing the results of these studies predominantly in the frame of
Schachter's theory.

Beyond testing the predictions of specific theories, studies on situation-dependent emotional responses to adrenergic drugs might contribute
also to the general understanding of how situational conditions act
in modifying emotional drug responses. In order to provide an explanation for the often observed lack of situational consistency of emotional
drug effects, several authors in differential psychopharmacology
(e.g. Debus and Janke, 1978; Janke, Debus, and Longo, 1979;
Legewie, 1968) refer to Schachter's theory or to an experiment by
Schachter and Singer (1962), on which this theory was mainly based.
Since the drug used in the Schachter-and-Singer-study was adrenaline,
the above authors are assuming that situation-dependent emotional
effects of CNS drugs might follow the same or similar principles
as with adrenergic drugs. If this assumption is valid, studies on
emotional responses to adrenergic drugs under different situational
conditions might be used to develop models for the prediction of situation-dependent emotional drug effects in general.

Whether the predictions derived from studies on situation-dependent
emotional effects to adrenergic drugs might apply also to studies with
CNS drugs will be examined only indirectly in this paper by comparing
the results of the following experiments with those described for
CNS drugs in the literature.

EXPERIMENTAL STUDIES

While it is reasonable to assume that drug-induced adrenergic (or
other bodily) symptoms will be reacted to with negative feelings,
according to Schachter's theory a state of sympathetic arousal will
result in any of a variety of emotions, provided that the appropriate
cognitive cues are available. (According to Schachter it is also
necessary that no other than emotional explanations for the bodily
state are available, i.e. that the subjects cannot attribute the
bodily reactions to the received drug.)

That drug-induced autonomic symptoms will not necessarily result in
negative emotional responses,was the general conclusion from a number
of studies, in which healthy subjects under neutral conditions did
not report any considerable change of emotional feelings after the
administration of sympathicomimetic agents (for summaries see Breggin,
1964; Lader and Tyrer, 1975). As the main evidence for his assumption
of different, i.e. also positive, emotional responses, Schachter cites
the experiment with Singer (1962) on the effects of adrenaline on
emotional reactions (determined by behavior-ratings and self-reports)
of male students under two experimental situations called "euphoria"
and "anger". Although the results of this experiment were in the
direction proposed by Schachter's theory, they were not very convincing:
Neither were there any significant adrenaline-placebo-differences. in
the emotional responses to the "euphoria"-condition; nor were there
significant differences in self-reported emotions between the "anger"
and the "euphoria"-situation under adrenaline. Thus the proposed interaction, according to which a state of sympathetic arousal will result
in different kinds of emotional reactions under different situational
conditions was, actually, not demonstrated. Moreover, the results of
partial (Marshall and Zimbardo, 1979) or modified (Maslach, 1979)

replications of the Schachter-and-Singer-study did not agree even in
the direction of the original findings. In both of these studies,
experimentally induced symptoms of sympathetic arousal led to slight
increases in reports of negative feelings also in the "euphoria"-
situation.

Based on a number of methodological objections against the Schachter-
and-Singer-experiment, Erdmann and Janke (1978) performed a study
which examined if a drug with adrenergic actions can result in both,
negative as well as positive emotional responses (for critiques of
the Schachter-and-Singer-experiment, see also Averill and Opton, 1968;
Birbaumer, 1973; Lazarus, 1967; Leventhal, 1974; Maslach, 1979;
Plutchik and Ax, 1967; Shapiro and Schwartz, 1970; Stein, 1967; Stricker,
1967).[1]

In the experiment by Erdmann and Janke either placebo or 50 mg of the
sympathocomimetic agent ephedrine were orally administered (ephedrine
is also a central stimulant). In order to prevent the subjects from
recognizing bodily reactions as drug-induced, the administration of
drugs was disguised (by false information about the real time of drug-
ingestion). Thirty minutes after the administration of drugs, the subjects of two experimental situations received ficticious feedback,
either positive or negative, about the result of an intelligence-test
administered in a previous session. An emotionally neutral situation
served as control condition. Eight to eleven male students were studied
under the six different conditions.
The adrenergic arousing properties of ephedrine were clearly demonstrable by increases in objective (heart rate, blood pressure) and
subjective (list of bodily symptoms) measures of bodily state. Emotional effects were evaluated by the mood-scale of an adjective
check list. As determined by analysis of covariance with the mood
ratings from baseline as covariates, neither of the main effects was
significant. While the interaction between drug and situational conditions did not reach the convential level of significance ($p < .10$),
the differential interaction between drug treatment and the two experimental situations was significant ($p < .05$).

---

[1] Several of the critiques of the Schachter-and-Singer-study apply
also to the experiments of Marshall and Zimbardo and of Maslach.
One important objection is that in none of these studies were the
effects of the emotional situations controlled by means of an emotionally neutral situation. Indeed, the results of a so-called pre-
experimental inquiry reported by Stricker (1967) indicate that the
"euphoria"-condition used in these studies might result in negative,
rather than positive emotional responses.

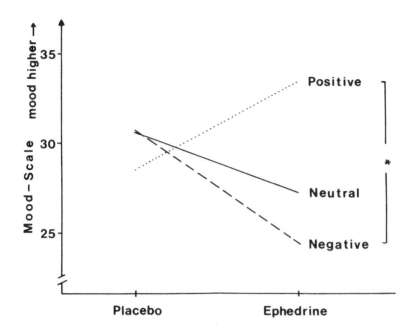

Fig. 1. Adjusted cell means for the mood-scale.
         * ≙ p < .05 for the difference between the cell
         means. (from Erdmann and Janke, 1978)

As Fig. 1 illustrates, a significant difference in reported mood between the two experimental situations was demonstrable only under
ephedrine. This agrees with Schachter's assumption that a state of
sympathetic arousal is necessary for an emotion to occur. The direction of the difference in reported mood between the two experimental
situations corresponded with the intended situational variations.
Thus, as can be predicted from Schachter's theory, a drug with adrenergic actions did, indeed, result in different, i.e. negative or positive, emotional responses, under different situational conditions.

The studies which will be discussed in the following, deal with the
generalizability of Schachter's theory as a model to explain the interaction between adrenergic drugs and situational conditions on the
intensity and quality of emotional responses. The questions are
(1) with regard to the intensity of emotional responses: Provided
    that emotion-relevant situational cues are available, is it
    possible to predict the intensity of the resulting emotional
    response alone from drug-induced changes in the level of adren-
    ergic arousal?
(2) with regard to the quality of emotional responses: Provided
    that the subjects are in a state of (drug-induced) sympathetic
    arousal, is it possible to predict the quality of the resulting
    emotional response alone from the kind of external emotional'
    cues?

Regarding the intensity of emotional responses, results indicating
that drug-induced variations in sympathetic arousal might be less

important than one might expect from Schachter's theory have been
reported by several authors, who under anxiety provoking conditions
could not demonstrate either increases in reported anxiety by sympathicomimetic agents (Erdmann and Janke, 1978; Rogers and Deckner, 1975)
or decreases in reported anxiety by beta-sympathicolytic agents (e.g.
Brewer, 1972; Cleghorn and others, 1970; Eliash and others, 1967;
Gottschalk and others, 1974; Liu and others, 1978; Tyrer and Lader,
1974).

Any definite conclusions as to why the drug conditions did not result
in variations of the intensity of reported anxiety were not feasible
from the results of these experiments, however. The questions raised
by these studies stimulated the following experiment, which aimed at
a more exact examination of the interaction of adrenergic drugs and
situational conditions in the determination of the intensity of
anxiety reactions.

The drug conditions of this study (a more detailed description can be
found in Erdmann, 1982) consisted of the disguised oral administration
of either 20 mg of the beta-adrenergic stimulating agent orciprenaline,
placebo, or 40 mg of the beta-adrenergic blocking agent oxprenolol.
The situational conditions were a neutral control situation and two
experimental situations designed to provoke different degrees of
"anxiety" by means of a public speaking analogue ("moderate" or "high
anxiety", respectively). Subjects of the "moderate anxiety" situation
were told that their speech would be recorded on a video-tape and
evaluated later. Subjects of the "high anxiety" condition were told
that observers in an adjacent room would evaluate their speech simultaneously. Fourteen healthy, male students were studied under each of
the nine conditions of the experiment.

Dependent variables were heart rate, blood pressure, the number of
spontaneous GSR, and standardized self-reports of bodily and emotional
state. During an experimental session, measurements of these variables
were taken twice, before and after the introduction of the experimental
variations (baseline- or treatment-measurements, respectively). The
treatment measurements started 60 min after the administration of oxprenolol, 30 min after the administration of orciprenaline and immediately after the announcement of the speech to the subjects of the
experimental situations.

Analysis of covariance with the corresponding variables from the
baseline period used as covariates yielded significant drug main
effects in cardio-vascular measures (heart rate, systolic and diastolic blood pressure) and significant situational main effects in
all (subjective and objective) measures of bodily arousal, both sets
of main effects corresponding with the intended variations.

For none of these variables did the drug by situation interaction
reach the 5%-level of statistical significance.

Regarding the drug effects, significant differences between orciprenaline and oxprenolol in cardio-vascular measures were also demonstrable
as simple effects under each of the three situational conditions. The
drug-placebo-differences, however, were dependent on the situational
effects under placebo conditions.

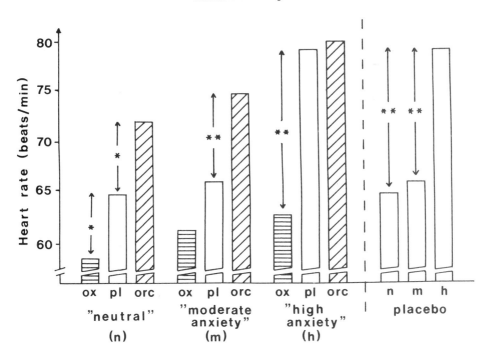

Fig. 2.   Adjusted cell means for heart rate.
           left side: simple effects of drugs under the three
                      situational conditions.
           right side: simple effects of the situational con-
                       ditions under placebo.
           ox = oxprenolol, pl = placebo, orc = orciprenaline.
           n = "neutral", m = "moderate anxiety", and h =
           "high anxiety" situation.
           * ≙ p < .05;   ** ≙ p < .01

As Fig. 2 demonstrates for heart rate (similar results were obtained
for systolic blood pressure), under placebo the "high anxiety" condition as compared to the two other situations led to a significant
increase in heart rate. Oxprenolol blocked this situationally induced
heart rate increase almost completely, resulting in a greater oxprenolol-
placebo-difference in this than in the two other situations (while in
the "neutral" situation the oxprenolol-placebo-difference was significant, under the "moderate anxiety" condition, the oxprenolol-placebo-
difference did not reach the 5%-level of statistical significance
(p < .10)). Orciprenaline increased heart rate under the "neutral" and
under the "moderate anxiety" condition. Under the "high anxiety" condition an increase in heart rate by orciprenaline above the placebo
level was not demonstrated, however.
Effects on reported emotional experience were evaluated by an anxiety-
scale. Analysis of covariance yielded significant main effects of the
situational conditions with significant increases (p < .01) of anxiety-
ratings from the "neutral" to the "moderate" and from the "moderate"
to the "high anxiety" conditions. Neither the drug main effect nor the
interaction between drug and situational treatment were significant.

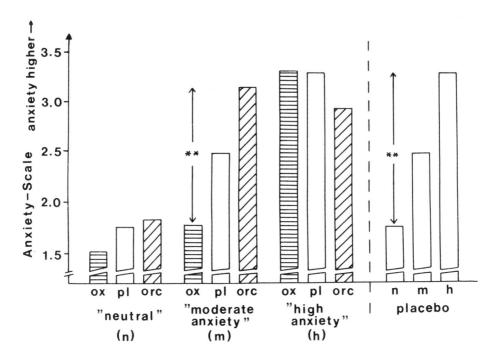

Fig. 3.   Adjusted cell means for the anxiety-scale.
          left side: simple effects of drugs under the three
                     situational conditions.
          right side: simple effects of the situational con-
                     ditions under placebo.
          ox = oxprenolol, pl = placebo, orc = orciprenaline.
          n ="neutral", m = "moderate anxiety", and h =
          "high anxiety" situation.
          ** ≙ p < .01.

Simple effects on anxiety-ratings are illustrated in Fig. 3. As can
be seen, under placebo the anxiety scores increased monotonically over
the three situational conditions. There was a significant difference
only between the "high anxiety" and the "neutral" situation, however.
The drug effects on reported anxiety can be summarized as follows:
(1) There were no drug effects under the "neutral" situation.
This agrees with various studies, where drug-induced sympathetic variations had no emotional effects in a neutral context. These results also
agree with Schachter's theory which states that variations in sympathetic arousal are not a sufficient condition for emotions, but contribute
only to their intensity if emotion-relevant cognitive cues are available
(2) Under the "moderate anxiety" situation, the anxiety scores increased
    monotonically over the three drug conditions. In this situation
    orciprenaline led to significantly higher anxiety scores than ox-
    prenolol.
This agrees with the assumptions derived from Schachter's theory, i.e.
that in the presence of emotion-relevant situational cues the intensity
of an emotional response is predictable from drug-induced changes in
the level of adrenergic arousal.

(3) Under the "high anxiety" provoking situation, there were no differ-
    ences between the three drug conditions.
That orciprenaline did not increase reports of anxiety in this situation was to be expected: In the "high anxiety" provoking situation,
orciprenaline also did not increase physiological measures of adrenergic
arousal. A reduction in measures of adrenergic arousal by oxprenolol was
clearly demonstrable in this situation, however. That this reduction
did not result in a diminuition of reported anxiety does not agree with
the proposal derived from Schachter's theory, that in the presence of
emotion relevant situational cues the intensity of emotional responses
is predictable alone from drug-induced variations in the level of
adrenergic arousal.

Of course, the fact that a blockade of beta-adrenergic reactions did
not result in a corresponding blockade of verbal anxiety does not ex-
clude explanations refering to peripheral physiological factors. Such
an explanation might be that oxprenolol by acting exclusively on the
beta-adrenergic system prevented only a part of the sympathetic reactions induced by the "high anxiety" provoking situation. Another explanation might be that peripheral physiological reactions outside the
sympathetic system, e.g. muscular reactions, were not prevented at all.
The latter explanation, however, is not of relevance for Schachter's
theory, which in its physiological part refers only to the autonomic
system.

More plausible and perhaps even closer to Schachter's thinking might
be an explanation refering to situational characteristics or cognitive
factors, respectively. Such an explanation might be that the "high
anxiety" provoking situation contained such unequivocal emotional cues,
that in evaluating their emotional state or their verbal emotional reactions, respectively, the subjects attended more to the external emotional than to the internal physiological cues. Considering that with
adult healthy subjects emotional responses or their verbal labels are
probably to a high degree conditioned to external stimuli, another explanation might be that the subjects in the "high anxiety" situation -
independent of their bodily state - emitted a well-learned degree of
"verbal anxiety".

With regard to the quality of emotional responses, results indicating
that the situational conditions might be less important than one might
expect from Schachter's theory were obtained in an experiment by Erdmann and von Lindern (1980).

The situational conditions of this study were an emotionally neutral
control situation and an experimental situation designed to induce
"anger" by blaming the subjects for poor performance and lack of cooperation in the experiment. The drug conditions were the same as in
the previously reported study, i.e. consisted of the disguised oral
administration of either 20 mg of the beta-adrenergic stimulating
agent orciprenaline, placebo, or 40 mg of the beta-adrenergic blocking
agent oxprenolol. Fourteen healthy male students were studied under
each of the six conditions of the experiment. During a baseline period
and a treatment period, which started 60 min after the administration
of oxprenolol, 30 min after the administration of orciprenaline, and
immediately after the emotion-induction, measurements of objective
physiological reactions (heart rate, blood pressure, spontaneous GSR)
and standardized self-reports of bodily and emotional state (list of
bodily symptoms, adjective check list) were obtained.

TABLE 1   Summary of the Main-Effects on Cardio-Vascular
           Measures of Adrenergic Arousal

	Oxprenolol	Orciprenaline	"Anger"
Heart rate	- -	+ +	0
Systolic blood pressure	-	+ +	+
Diastolic blood pressure	0	- -	+ +

0 = no change;   +/- = slight increase or decrease;
++/-- = large increase or decrease

Analyses of covariance, in which the corresponding measures of the
baseline period were used as covariates, showed that both situational
and drug conditions, almost completely independent of each other,
affected measures of bodily arousal. As a global summary of the effects
on cardio-vascular variables demonstrates (see Table 1), orciprenaline
and the "anger" situation partly induced increases in different measures
however. Orciprenaline increased heart rate, which was not changed by
the "anger" situation; orciprenaline decreased diastolic blood pressure,
which was increased by the "anger" situation. (The anger situation
also led to an increase in the number of spontaneous GSR, which was
unaffected by both drugs.)

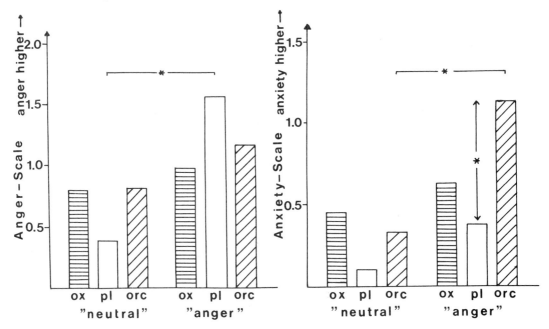

Fig. 4.   Adjusted cell means for the anger-scale (left side) and for
          the anxiety-scale (right side) of the adjective check list.
          ox = oxprenolol, pl = placebo, orc = orciprenaline.
          * ≙ p < .05 for the difference between cell means.
          (from Erdmann and von Lindern, 1980)

Main effects of the "anger" situation on emotional reactions measured by the adjective check list consisted in increases of reported anger and anxiety. In neither case was the main effect of drugs or the drug by situation interaction significant.

As Fig. 4 illustrates, under placebo the anger situation led to a significant increase of anger-ratings, only. The situational main effect on anxiety-ratings resulted predominantly from an increase in the anxiety scores under the orciprenaline condition.

Drug effects on reported emotions can be summarized as follows:

(1) There were no drug effects in the neutral situation.

(2) In the anger situation, there were no drug effects on reported anger.

(3) In the anger situation, orciprenaline as compared to placebo led to an increase in reported anxiety.

With regard to the neutral situation, the results agree with those of the previously reported experiment with the same drug conditions. Likewise, they also agree with Schachter's assumption that differences in the level of adrenergic arousal are not sufficient conditions for the demonstration of emotional response differences. With regard to the "anger" situation, however, the effects of orciprenaline are completely contrary to the expectations derived from Schachter's theory.

The reason why orciprenaline changed the quality rather than the intensity of verbal emotional responses induced by the "anger" situation is not evident from the results of the present experiment.

Regarding the physiological actions of orciprenaline, one explanation might be found in the intensity of adrenergic reactions produced by orciprenaline. One might assume that the pronounced bodily changes after orciprenaline that were unexplainable for the subjects because of the disguised method of drug administration led to feelings of apprehension or anxiety per se. Such feelings might become reinforced or be admitted by the subjects, if any external stimuli are available to which they can be attributed.

Another explanation might be found in the pattern of adrenergic reactions induced by orciprenaline. In fact, the pattern of beta-adrenergic arousal in general and the specific pattern of cardio-vascular reactions produced by the beta-stimulating agent orciprenaline in this study (see Table 1), correspond very well with those autonomic reactions that were described as typical for "anxiety" in studies on physiological response differences between anxiety and anger (Ax, 1953; Funkenstein, King and Drolette, 1954; Schachter, J., 1957; for a summary see also Martin, 1961). On the other hand, the cardio-vascular reactions induced by the "anger" situation in this study, correspond with those reactions that were described as typical for "anger" in the literature. Therefore, one might conclude that under orciprenaline the subjects were placed with an anxiety-like physiological response

pattern into a situation designed to induce "anger" (and actually inducing anger-like reactions under no-drug conditions). Corresponding
to their physiological pattern they reacted with anxiety and not with
anger.
Neither of these explanations excludes the possibility that characteristics of the "anger" situation were not also important for the unexpected increase in anxiety ratings under the orciprenaline-"anger"-
condition. Indeed, it seems plausible to assume that negative comments
on performance can result in anxious-depressive (or "anger-in"-like
responses sensu Funkenstein (1955)), as well. However, since only the
subjects of the orciprenaline condition reacted with "anxiety" to a
considerable degree, an explanation based on situational characteristics
alone is insufficient. Therefore, the result clearly contradicts the
proposal derived from Schachter's theory that the quality of an emotional response is predictable solely from the kind of situation (or
from its emotional effects under placebo conditions, respectively).

With respect to the cognitive part of Schachter's theory, the results
of the present study would require an extension, at least. While
Schachter assumes that emotion-specific cognitions are derived from
the situation and are used to label an unspecific state of sympathetic
arousal, the present results suggest that such cognitions can also be
derived from the state of sympathetic arousal and be used to label a
somewhat ambiguous situation.

                    CONCLUSIONS

The results of the reported experiments clearly demonstrate that emotional effects of adrenergic drugs are to a high degree dependent on
situational conditions.
Situational conditions determine whether such drugs result in emotional effects at all, since both emotion-increasing effects of adrenergic
stimulating drugs as well as emotion-reducing effects of beta-adrenergic blocking drugs were not demonstrable in emotionally neutral situations, but only in situations providing external emotional cues.
The presence of such cues is not a sufficient condition for the demonstration of emotional effects of adrenergic drugs, however. The
results of one of the reported experiments suggest, that such effects
might occur only in situations containing comparably weak emotional
cues.
Situational conditions not only determine whether adrenergic drugs
affect the occurrence or the intensity of emotional responses, but
can also determine the kind of the resulting emotional response. This
was suggested by the results of the experiment reported by Erdmann
and Janke (1978), in which ephedrine resulted in different, i.e. negative or positive, emotional responses under different situations.
That the kind or quality of an emotional response is not only dependent
on the situational condition, however, was evident from the results
of the experiment performed by Erdmann and von Lindern (1980), in
which the beta-stimulating agent orciprenaline led to an increase in
reported anxiety even in a situation which induced anger-like reactions under placebo conditions.

On the basis of these experimental results - at least with respect to
differences in emotional responses due to situational conditions -
the question asked at the beginning of this paper can be definitely
answered: Adrenergic drug effects can, indeed, result in behavioral
response differences.

Regarding the problem of side effects, the present results, of course, do not allow the conclusion that with other drug conditions, the adrenergic drug actions will contribute to situation-dependent emotional effects to the same degree or in the same manner.
The generalizability of the present results might be limited, just because of the disguised method of drug administration. Indeed, experimental results of Schachter and his coworkers (Schachter and Singer, 1962; Nisbett and Schachter, 1966) suggest that emotional effects of sympathetic variations might be less likely to occur if the subjects can recognize these variations as drug-induced. Therefore, one might expect that under the usual conditions of drug administration, the emotional effects of the adrenergic drug actions are weaker than in the experiments reported in this paper.
Another important reason why the present results do not permit any definite conclusions for other drug conditions is that there is no knowledge about how   the central main and autonomic side effects of a particular drug might interact with each other and with the external conditions in determining the final emotional response.

Nevertheless, the fact that the reported experiments clearly demonstrated differential emotional responses to adrenergic drug effects supports the view that such effects have to be considered as one source of variance that should be controlled in studies on the behavioral response variability to CNS drugs.

Regarding theories about autonomic nervous system reactions as determinants of emotional response differences, the fact that the experiments in this paper clearly demonstrated situation-dependent emotional effects of adrenergic drugs principally agrees with Schachter's view that emotions result from the interaction between a state of sympathetic arousal and cognitive factors. With respect to the exact propositions about this interaction, however, the present results are only partly in accordance with Schachter's theory, partly they disagree with it.
In accordance with Schachter's assumptions about the determinants of the intensity of an emotion, it could be demonstrated that - in the presence of situational emotional cues - different degrees of adrenergic arousal can result in corresponding differences in the intensity of reported emotions. However, disagreeing with the prediction derived from Schachter's theory, it could not be demonstrated that the intensity of verbal emotional responses is dependent only on the level of adrenergic arousal.
In accordance with Schachter's assumptions about the determinants of the quality of an emotion, it could be demonstrated that - in the presence of a state of increased sympathetic arousal - different emotional situations can result in corresponding differences in the kind of reported emotions. However, disagreeing with the prediction from Schachter's theory, it could not be demonstrated that the quality of verbal emotional responses is dependent only on the kind of situational emotional cues.

Altogether, the present results provide a sufficient basis for the conclusion that Schachter's theory has only limited value in predicting the interaction between adrenergic reactions and situational conditions in the determination of emotional responses. Given this conclusion, the question to be asked is: What predictions about this interaction can be derived from the present results?
What I would predict, is that - at least with adult healthy subjects - adrenergic reactions can affect emotions or their verbal labels, respectively, in situations containing somewhat ambiguous, but not in

situations containing unambiguous emotional cues. In the presence of
somewhat ambiguous emotional cues, however, adrenergic reactions can
affect not only the intensity but also the quality of the resulting
emotional response.

A very interesting question for the future research in this area might
be, if in the presence of ambiguous emotional cues the quality of the
resulting emotional response depends on the specific pattern of adrenergic arousal, as was suggested in the previous section. Depending on
their differential affinity to alpha- and beta-receptors, adrenergic
drugs induce somewhat different patterns of sympathetic arousal that
correspond well with those patterns that have been described as typical
for either "anger" or "anxiety" by some psychophysiologists (Ax, 1953;
Funkenstein and others, 1954; Schachter, J., 1957). Therefore, such
drugs might be useful tools for experimental tests of the hypothesis
of emotion-specific autonomic response patterns, one of the most con-
troversal hypotheses in the psychophysiology of emotions.

The last question that remains to be asked in this paper is if the
predictions derived from the present studies might apply also to other
drug conditions. Any definite answer to this question has to await
direct comparisons of the emotional effects of adrenergic and
CNS drugs under the same experimental conditions. The possibilities
to examine this question indirectly, by a comparison of the present
results with those reported for CNS drugs under at least
similar conditions, are very limited. The effects of CNS drugs
on experimentally induced emotional states were rather frequently
studied only for drugs that can be expected to reduce emotional
responses (namely tranquilizers and other central depressants), but
not or only very seldom for drugs that might be expected to increase
emotional responses (namely stimulants). Also studies with tranquilizers have used rather selected situational conditions: They refer more
often to unspecific emotional states like noise-induced general emotional tension rather than to specific emotions and - with regard to
specific emotions - they refer almost exclusively to anxiety or
anxiety-like emotions (for reviews see Janke and Debus, 1968; Janke
and others, 1979; Pillard and Fisher, 1978). At least under these
restricted conditions, some obvious similarities in the effects of
CNS drugs with those described for adrenergic drugs in the present
paper can be found, however.

After a comprehensive review of the literature Janke, Debus and Longo
(1979) conclude that with healthy subjects emotion-reducing effects
of CNS depressants are generally not found under non-stress, but
only under stress conditions. This agrees with one of the conclusions
drawn from the present experiments, i.e. that emotional effects of
adrenergic drugs are not demonstrable in emotionally neutral, but
only in situations providing emotional cues.
In their review, Janke and others further concluded that a high degree
of emotionality is no guarantee that emotional stabilization by depressant drugs can be demonstrated. This agrees with another conclusion drawn from the present studies, i.e. that the presence of external
emotional cues is not a sufficient condition for demonstrating emotional effects of adrenergic drugs.
In trying to characterize situational conditions that might affect
the differential efficiency of tranquilizers, Janke and others start
from the observation that these drugs have often been found to reduce
emotional tension induced by noise-stress, but not often found to

reduce emotional responses to anxiety-provoking situations. With regard to anxiety-provoking situations, the often observed lack of
tranquilizer effects agrees with the majority of available studies
that could not demonstrate effects of adrenergic drugs on experimentally induced anxiety. Whether anxiety-reducing effects of tranquilizers
might be more likely to occur in situations containing comparably weak
anxiety cues - as it might be predicted from effects of an adrenergic
blocking drug in an experiment reported here - is unknown. Studies of
the effects of tranquilizers on different degrees of experimentally
induced anxiety are not available in the literature.[2]
On the other hand, there are no studies on the effects of adrenergic
drugs under noise-stress conditions, although such effects might be
expected from the emotional ambiguity of noise-stress. (In that it
lacks any specific emotional contents, noise is an ambiguous stressor,
indeed.) At least similar to the prediction derived from the present
studies, i.e. that adrenergic drugs will affect emotional responses
in situations containing somewhat ambiguous, but not in situations containing unambiguous emotional cues, Janke and others (1979) concluded
that central depressants might be more effective in reducing states
of general emotional tension than specific states of anxiety.

Similarities can also be found in the explanations provided for different emotional effects of CNS and ANS drugs under different situational conditions. With regard to the often observed lack of tranquilizer effects under anxiety-provoking situations, Janke and others
(1979, p.78), for example, state " ... anxiety provoked by situations
such as films or pain-anticipation involves many cognitive factors due
to learning and evaluative processes. These factors, however, may not
be decreased by psychotropic drugs." This explanation is essentially
the same as that provided for the uneffectiveness of a beta-blocking
agent in reducing verbal anxiety under a "high anxiety" provoking situations.
On the other hand, the efficiency of tranquilizers in reducing emotional tension induced by noise-stress might be mediated by a different evaluation of this stressor under drug and placebo conditions, as
it was suggested as an explanation for the efficiency of adrenergic
drugs in affecting emotional responses to emotionally ambiguous situations. According to studies by Krüger (1981; see also Krüger, this
volume) CNS drugs (tranquilizers, central stimulants) significantly
alter the kind of subjective evaluation of noise-stress.

Although there are some similarities in the effects of CNS and ANS
drugs and their interpretation, the present evidence is in no way
sufficient to support the assumption that with both kind of drugs
situation-dependent emotional responses might, indeed, follow similar
principles. Moreover, there are reasons to expect differences.
One reason is that CNS drugs, like tranquilizers, directly act
on structures of the limbic system and the diencephalon, which
might be influenced by autonomic drugs only indirectly. Since these
structures are thought to mediate emotional responses, the emotional

---

[2]In fact, Boucsein (1974) tried to induce different degrees of "anxiety"
by means of two threat of shock conditions in a study with chlordiazepoxide. The two conditions were not differentially effective, however.

effects of these drugs should be stronger and, therefore, less dependent on situational conditions. Another reason is that drugs with central actions will directly interfere with cognitive processes which also might be affected only indirectly by autonomic drugs. Since cognitive factors are thought to mediate the interaction between situational and drug conditions in the determination of the final emotional response, this interactions should be more complicated with CNS drugs.

However, since the neurophysiological actions of psychotropic drugs are at best only poorly understood, some authors regard psychopharmacology less as a subdiscipline of physiological psychology, but as a more general approach in testing the range of variability in behavior (see, for example, Debus and Janke, 1978). For this kind of approach, ANS drugs might be as useful tools as CNS drugs. Considering that (because of their lack of direct psychotropic effects) the range of variability due to situational factors is probably greater with adrenergic drugs, with regard to intraindividual differences they might be the even more useful tools. Considering further that (because of their lack of direct psychotropic effects) their interaction with situational conditions is probably less difficult to explain, they might be also the more useful tools to develop any models for the prediction of such interactions. To what degreee the predictions derived from such models might apply also to more complex conditions, as they are present with CNS drugs, might be considered as a secondary question.

REFERENCES

Averill, J.R., and E. M. Opton (1968). Psychophysiological assessment: Rationale and problems. In P. McReynolds (Ed.), Advances in Psychological Assessment, Vol. I. Science and Behavior Books, Palo Alto, Calif. pp. 265-288.

Ax, A. F. (1953). The physiological differentiation between fear and anger in humans. Psychosom. Med., 15, 433-442.

Birbaumer, N. (1973). Wir denken häufig bevor wir handeln: Angst als kognitive, physiologische und motorische Einheit. In N. Birbaumer (Ed.), Neuropsychologie der Angst. Urban & Schwarzenberg, München. pp. 146-157.

Boucsein, W. (1974). Die Wirkung von Chlordiazepoxyd unter Angstbedingungen im psychophysiologischen Experiment. Arzneim.-Forsch. (Drug Res.), 24, 1112-1114.

Breggin, P. R. (1964). The psychophysiology of anxiety. J. Nerv. Ment. Dis., 139, 558-568.

Brewer, C. (1972). Beneficial effects of beta-adrenergic blockade on examination nerves. Lancet, II, 439.

Cleghorn, J. M., G. Peterfy, E. J. Pinter, and C. J. Pattee (1970). Verbal anxiety and the beta adrenergic receptor: A facilitating mechanism? J. Nerv. Ment. Dis., 151, 266-271.

Debus, G., and W. Janke (1978). Psychologische Aspekte der Psychopharmakotherapie. In L. J. Pongratz (Ed.), Handbuch der Psychologie, Vol. 8/2. Hogrefe, Göttingen. pp. 2161-2227.

Eliasch, H., A. Rosen, and H. M. Scott (1967). Systemic circulatory response to stress of simulated flight and to physical exercise before and after propranolol blockade. Br. Heart J., 29, 671-683.

Erdmann, G. (1979). VNS-Pharmaka als Forschungswerkzeuge in der Emo-
tionspsychologie. In L. H. Eckensberger (Ed.), Bericht über den
31. Kongreß der Deutschen Gesellschaft für Psychologie in Mannheim
1978, Band 2. Hogrefe, Göttingen. pp. 460-462.
Erdmann, G. (1982). Zur Beeinflußbarkeit emotionaler Prozesse durch
vegetative Variationen. (In press)
Erdmann, G., and W. Janke (1978). Interaction between physiological
and cognitive determinants of emotions: Experimental studies on
Schachter's theory of emotions. Biol. Psychol., 6, 61-74.
Erdmann, G., and B. vonLindern (1980). The effects of beta-adrenergic
stimulation and beta-adrenergic blockade on emotional reactions.
Psychophysiology, 17, 332-338.
Eysenck, H. J. (1957). Drugs and personality: I. Theory and methodo-
logy. J. Ment. Sci., 103, 119-131.
Eysenck, H. J. (1966). Neurose, Konstitution und Persönlichkeit.
Z. f. Psychol., 172, 145-181.
Eysenck, H. J. (1967). The Biological Basis of Personality. Thomas,
Springfield.
Eysenck, H. J. (this volume). Psychopharmacology and Personality.
In W. Janke (Ed.), Response Variability to Psychotropic Drugs.
Pergamon Press, Oxford.
Funkenstein, D. H. (1955). The physiology of fear and anger. Sci. Am.,
192, 74-80.
Funkenstein, D. H., S. H. King, and M. E. Drolette (1954). The direc-
tion of anger during a laboratory stress-inducing situation.
Psychosom. Med., 16, 404-413.
Gottschalk, L. A., W. N. Stone, and G. C. Gleser (1974). Peripheral
vs. central mechanisms accounting for antianxiety effects of
propranolol. Psychosom. Med., 36, 47-56.
Janke, W. (1971). Pharmakopsychologie. In W. Arnold, H. J. Eysenck,
and R. Meili (Eds.), Lexikon der Psychologie. Herder, Freiburg.
pp. 763-774.
Janke, W. (this volume). Response variability to psychotropic drugs.
In W. Janke (Ed.), Response Variability to Psychotropic Drugs.
Pergamon Press, Oxford.
Janke, W., and G. Debus (1968). Experimental studies on anti-anxiety
agents with normal subjects: Methodological considerations and
review of the main effects. In D. H. Efron et al. (Eds.), Psycho-
pharmacology. A Review of Progress 1957-1967. U.S. Government
Printing Office, Washington. pp. 205-230.
Janke, W., G. Debus, and N. Longo (1979). Differential psychopharma-
cology of tranquilizing and sedating drugs. In Th. A. Ban et al.
(Eds.), Modern Problems of Pharmacopsychiatry, Vol. 14. Karger,
Basel. pp. 13-98.
Krüger, H.-P. (1981). Differentielle Pharmakopsychologie ohne Diffe-
rentielle Psychologie? In W. Janke (Ed.), Beiträge zur Methodik in
der differentiellen, diagnostischen und klinischen Psychologie.
Festschrift zum 60. Geburtstag von G.A. Lienert. Hain, Meisenheim.
Krüger, H.-P. (this volume). What differentiates a differential
psychopharmacology. In W. Janke (Ed.), Response Variability to
Psychotropic Drugs. Pergamon Press, Oxford.
Lader, M., and P. Tyrer (1975). Vegetative system and emotion. In
L. Levi (Ed.), Emotions - Their Parameters and Measurement.
Raven Press, New York. pp. 123-142.
Lazarus, R. S. (1967). Cognitive and personality factors underlying
threat and coping. In M. H. Appley,and R. Trumbull (Eds.), Psycho-
logical Stress: Issues in Research. Appleton-Century-Crofts,
New York. pp. 151-168.

Legewie, H. (1968). Persönlichkeitstheorie und Psychopharmaka. Hain, Meisenheim.

Leventhal, H. (1974). Emotions: A basic problem for social psychology. In C. Nemeth (Ed.), Social Psychology: Classic and Contemporary Integrations. Rand McNally, Chicago. pp. 1-51.

Liu, K. S., G. Debus, and W. Janke (1978). Untersuchungen zur Wirkung von Oxprenolol auf experimentell induzierte Angst. Arzneim.-Forsch. (Drug Res.), 28, 1305-1306.

Marshall, G. D., and P. G. Zimbardo (1979). Affective consequences of inadequately explained physiological arousal. J. Pers. Soc. Psychol., 37, 970-988.

Martin, B. (1961). The assessment of anxiety by psychophysiological measures. Psychol. Bull., 58, 234-255.

Maslach, C. (1979). Negative emotional biasing of unexplained arousal. J. Pers. Soc. Psychol., 37, 953-969.

Nisbett, R. E., and S. Schachter (1966). Cognitive manipulation of pain. J. Exp. Soc. Psychol., 2, 227-236.

Pillard, R. C., and S. Fisher (1978). Normal humans as models for psychopharmacologic therapy. In M. A. Lipton, A. DiMascio, and K. F. Killam (Eds.), Psychopharmacology. A Generation of Progress. Raven Press, New York. pp. 783-790.

Plutchik, R., and A. F. Ax (1967). A critique of determinants of emotional state by Schachter and Singer (1962). Psychophysiology, 4, 79-82.

Rogers, R. W., and C. W. Deckner (1975). Effects of fear appeals and physiological arousal upon emotion, attitudes, and cigarette smoking. J. Pers. Soc. Psychol., 32, 222-230.

Schachter, J. (1957). Pain, fear, and anger in hypertensives and normotensives. Psychosom. Med., 19, 17-29.

Schachter, S. (1964). The interaction of cognitive and physiological determinants of emotional states. In L. Berkowitz (Ed.), Advances in Experimental Social Psychology. Academic Press, New York. pp. 49-81.

Schachter, S. (1971). Emotion, Obesity, and Crime. Academic Press, New York.

Schachter, S. (1975). Cognition and peripheralist-centralist controversies in motivation and emotion. In M. S. Gazzangia, and C. Blakemore (Eds.), Handbook of Psychobiology. Academic Press, New York. pp. 529-564.

Schachter, S., and J. E. Singer (1962). Cognitive, social, and physiological determinants of emotional state. Psychol. Rev., 69, 379-399.

Schachter, S., and L. Wheeler (1962). Epinephrine, chlorpromazine, and amusement. J. Abnorm. Soc. Psychol., 65, 121-128.

Shapiro, D., and G. E. Schwartz (1970). Psychophysiological contributions to social psychology. Ann. Rev. Psychol., 21, 87-112.

Stein, M. (1967). Some psychophysiological considerations of the relationship between the autonomic nervous system and behavior. In D. C. Glass (Ed.), Neurophysiology and Emotion. Rockefeller University Press, New York. pp. 145-154.

Stricker, G. (1967). A pre-experimental inquiry concerning cognitive determinants of emotional state. J. Gen. Psychol., 76, 73-79.

Tyrer, P. J., and M. H. Lader (1974). Physiological and psychological effects of (+)-propranolol, (±)-propranolol and diazepam in induced anxiety. Br. J. Clin. Pharmacol., 1, 379-385.

NAME INDEX

293

SUBJECT INDEX

Activation and drugs
  basic considerations 33ff, 127ff
  empirical findings 33ff, 127ff,
    185ff

Differential drug effects *see* Drug
    response differences
Differential psychopharmacology
  basic aspects 33ff, 67ff, 97ff,
    127ff, 237ff, 263ff, 273ff
  definition 33ff, 263ff
  in animals 97ff
  in normal subjects 33ff
  in patients 67ff, 237ff

Drug
  absorption 3ff
  abstinence 167ff
  action mechanisms 3ff, 33ff, 97ff
  administration schedule 217ff, 237ff
  distribution 3ff
  effects *see* Drug response differences
  experience 209ff
  interaction 3ff, 67ff
  metabolism 3ff
  postulate *see* Eysenck's drug
    postulate
  response generalizibility 33ff
  response reliability 33ff
  response variability, basic
    considerations 33ff, 67ff, 97ff
      127ff
  self medication 167ff

Drug response differences
  and action - orientation 33ff

and activation 33ff, 127ff, 185ff
and administration schedule 217ff
and age 67ff
and arousal 33ff, 127ff
and attitudes 33ff, 209ff
and constitution 67ff
and disease 67ff
and depression scores 217ff, 237ff
and drug plasma level 3ff, 67ff
and early environmental factors 97ff
and emotional lability 33ff, 127ff
  185ff
and emotional tension 33ff
and environmental factors 33ff, 97ff
  273ff
and extraversion/introversion 33ff,
  127ff, 155ff, 167ff, 185ff, 209ff
and genetic factors 3ff, 67ff, 97ff
and neuroticism 127ff, 155ff, 167ff,
  185ff
and other drugs 3ff, 67ff, 97ff
overview of main factors 3ff, 67ff, 97ff
and peripheral factors 33ff, 273ff
and personality states 33ff, 263ff
and personality traits 127ff, 217ff,
  203ff, 209ff
and physiological state 67ff
and physique 67ff
and predrug level 33ff, 67ff
and pretreatment factors 67ff, 217ff,
  237ff
and race 3ff, 67ff
and sedation threshold 127ff, 155ff
and sex 67ff, 97ff, 185ff
and side effects 33ff, 273ff
and situational factors 33ff, 127ff,
  167ff, 263ff, 273ff
and somatic factors 3ff, 33ff, 67ff,
  97ff